www.harcourt-inter... W9-CES-087

Bringing you products from all Harcourt Health Sciences companies including Baillière Tindall, Churchill Livingstone, Mosby and W.B. Saunders

- ▶ **Browse** for latest information on new books, journals and electronic products

- ▶ **Search** for information on over 20 000 published titles with full product information including tables of contents and sample chapters

- ▶ **Keep up to date** with our extensive publishing programme in your field by registering with eAlert or requesting postal updates

- ▶ **Secure online ordering** with prompt delivery, as well as full contact details to order by phone, fax or post

- ▶ **News** of special features and promotions

If you are based in the following countries, please visit the country-specific site to receive full details of product availability and local ordering information

USA: www.harcourthealth.com

Canada: www.harcourtcanada.com

Australia: www.harcourt.com.au

⚜ Baillière Tindall   ◢ CHURCHILL LIVINGSTONE   Ⓜ Mosby   🅦 W.B. SAUNDERS

Essential Interventional Cardiology

Commissioning Editor: Miranda Bromage/Michael Houston
Project Development Manager: Francesca Lumkin
Project Manager: Hilary Hewitt
Design Director: Jayne Jones

Essential
Interventional
Cardiology

Edited by

Michael S. Norell MD FRCP
Consultant in Cardiology and Coronary Intervention,
Hull and East Yorkshire Hospitals, Hull, UK

E. John Perrins BSc MD FRCP FACC
Consultant in Cardiology and Coronary Intervention,
Yorkshire Heart Centre, Leeds, UK

WB SAUNDERS
An imprint of Harcourt Publishers Limited

© Harcourt Publishers Limited 2001

is a registered trademark of Harcourt Publishers Limited

The right of Michael S. Norell and E. John Perrins to be identified as the authors of this work have been asserted by them in accordance with the Copyright, Designs and Patents Act, 1988.

First published 2001

ISBN 0 7020 2480 5

Cataloguing in Publication Data:
Catalogue records for this book are available from the British Library and the US Library of Congress.

Note
Medical knowledge is constantly changing. As new information becomes available, changes in treatment, procedures, equipment and the use of drugs become necessary. The editors, authors, contributors and the publishers have taken care to ensure that the information given in this text is accurate and up to date. However, readers are strongly advised to confirm that the information, especially with regard to drug usage, complies with the latest legislation and standards of practice.

Existing UK nomenclature is changing to the system of Recommended International Nonproprietary Names (rINNs). Until the UK names are no longer in use, these more familiar names are used in this book in preference to rINNs, details of which may be obtained from the British National Formulary.

Printed in China

Contents

Contributors

Raphael Balcon, MD, FRCP
London Chest Hospital, London, UK

John L Caplin BSc(Hons), MD, FRCP
Consultant Cardiology and Honorary Senior Lecturer in Cardiology
Hull Royal Infirmary, Hull, UK

Michael Cusack BSc (Hons), MB ChB, MRCP (UK)
Specialist Registrar in Cardiology
Cardiothoracic Unit St Thomas' Hospital London, UK

Keith D Dawkins BSc, MD, FRCP, FACC
Consultant Cardiologist Southampton General Hospital
Southampton, UK

Adam J de Belder BSc, MRCP, MD
Consultant Cardiologist, Department of Cardiology, Royal Sussex County Hospital, Brighton, UK

Mark de Belder MA, MD, FRCP
Consultant Cardiologist, South Cleveland Hospital, Middlesbrough, UK

Simon C Eccleshall MB, ChB, MRCP
International Fellow, Amsterdam Department of Interventional Cardiology, OLVG Hospital, Amsterdam, The Netherlands

Duncan F Ettles MB ChB (Hons), MRCP, FRCR, MD
Consultant Cardiovascular and Interventional Radiologist Honorary Senior Lecturer, Department of Radiology, Hull Royal Infirmary, Hull, UK

Anthony Gershlick BSc, MBBS, FRCP
Consultant Cardiologist/Honorary Senior Lecturer, Department of Academic Cardiology, Glenfield Hospital, Leicester, UK

Ever D Grech MBBS, MRCP (UK), MD, FACC
Consultant Cardiologist, Health Sciences Centre, Winnipeg, Canada

Jim Hall MA, MD, FRCP
Consultant Cardiologist, Cardiothoracic Unit, South Cleveland Hospital, Middlesbrough, UK

Roger JC Hall BA, MD, FRCP, FESC
Professor of Clinical Cardiology, Hammersmith Hospital, London, UK

Angela Hoye, MRCP
Specialist Registrar, Hull Royal Infirmary, Hull, UK

James M McLenachan MD, FRCP
Consultant Cardiologist, Leeds General Infirmary, Leeds, UK

Bernhard Meier MD, FACC, FESC
Professor and Chairman, Swiss Cardiovascular Center Bern, University Hospital, Bern, Switzerland

Anthony Nicholson MSc, FRCR
Consultant Cardiovascular and Interventional Radiologist, and President, British Society of Interventional Radiologists, Department of Radiology, Hull Royal Infirmary, Hull, UK

James Nolan MB ChB, MRCP, MD
Consultant Cardiologist, Cardiothoracic Centre, North Staffordshire Hospital, Stoke-on-Trent, UK

Michael S. Norell MD, FRCP
Consultant Cardiologist,
Hull Royal Infirmary,
Hull, UK

E. John Perrins MD, BSc, FRCP, FACC
Consultant Cardiologist,
Department of
Cardiology,
Leeds General Infirmary,
Leeds, UK

Raphael A Perry FRCP, DM, FACC, BMedSci
Consultant Cardiologist,
Cardiothoracic Centre
Liverpool,
Liverpool, UK

Bernard D Prendergast DM, MRCP
Senior Registrar in
Cardiology,
Department of
Cardiology,
Western General
Hospital,
Edinburgh, UK

David R Ramsdale BSc, MB, ChB, FRCP, MD
Consultant Cardiologist
and Director of Cardiac
Catheterisation,
Cardiothoracic Centre
Liverpool,
Liverpool, UK

Simon Redwood MD, MRCP
Senior Lecturer/
Consultant Interventional
Cardiologist,

Cardiothoracic Unit,
St Thomas' Hospital,
London, UK

David H. Roberts MD, FRCP, FACC, FESC, FICA
Consultant Cardiologist,
Victoria Hospital NHS
Trust,
Blackpool, UK

Eric Rosenthal MD, FRCP
Consultant Paediatric
Cardiologist,
Guy's Hospital,
London, UK

Peter Schofield MD, FRCP, FACC, FESC
Consultant Cardiologist,
Papworth Hospital,
Cambridge, UK

Man Fai Shui MD, FRCP
Consultant Cardiologist,
Walsgrave Hospital,
Coventry, UK

Ulrich Sigwart MD, FRCP
Consultant Cardiologist
and Director,
Department of Invasive
Cardiology,
Royal Brompton
Hospital,
London, UK

David Smith BSc, MBBS, FRCP
Consultant Cardiologist,
Cardiology Department,

Royal Devon & Exeter
Hospital (Wonford),
Exeter, UK

Rod Stables MA, DM, MRCP
Consultant Cardiologist,
Cardiothoracic Centre
Liverpool,
Liverpool, UK

Ian R Starkey BSc, MB ChB, FRCP
Consultant Cardiologist,
Western General
Hospital,
Edinburgh, UK

Martyn R Thomas
Consultant Cardiologist,
Department of
Cardiology,
King's College Hospital,
London, UK

Neal G Uren MD, MRCP
Consultant Cardiologist,
Department of
Cardiology,
Royal Infirmary,
Edinburgh, UK

Mark Walters MB ChB, MRCP
Consultant Cardiologist,
Diana Princess of Wales
Hospital,
Grimsby, UK

Foreword

Cardiac intervention without surgery revolutionised the management of cardiac patients, particularly those with coronary artery disease, as much as cardiac surgery did in its time. This book covers all aspects of the subject including the history and development of the various techniques and provides the reader with important insights into both the potential and limitations of the techniques now being used. It also helps readers to understand the courage and tenacity of the pioneers who introduced what was then a very controversial method of treatment. The modern era of cardiology dates from the time Mason Sones first performed coronary arteriography in the late 1950s. This was followed by the first successful coronary surgery using the vein bypass technique in the second half of the 1960s. The adaptation for the coronary circulation of the peripheral balloon angioplasty technique of Dotter, by Andreas Grüntzig was the next landmark. The equipment available to those of us involved in percutaneous transcoronary angioplasty (PTCA as it soon became known) in its early days was very limiting, greatly restricting the application of the technique. This and the soon recognised problem of relatively early restenosis and recurrence of symptoms were the two major challenges from the outset. The problem of restenosis led to a great deal of research, much of it of a very fundamental nature with implications far beyond the horizons of percutaneous intervention. The main directions have been in the area of cell proliferation and platelet activity and thrombosis and their control, and these are covered in Chapters 4 and 5.

Continuing experience and the evolution of the equipment as described in Chapter 1 led to a great expansion of the indications and use of PTCA, but there were still some coronary lesions that could not be treated using balloons. This led to much innovative research in an effort to devise ways of dealing with, for example, complete occlusions and calcified and diffuse lesions. Those techniques developed that proved to be effective and useful and which survived this era to be in use today are described in Section Two.

The development and use of coronary stents, once again 'borrowed' from another branch of vascular disease treatment, was the next major step that greatly improved both the acute phase of treatment and the subsequent recurrence of symptoms. Stents were first designed for the aorta and were miniaturised for use in the coronary circulation, first being implanted by Ulrich Sigwart in Lausanne. Their use is described in Chapter 6.

As a result of all of these changes, the number of PTCAs currently performed exceeds the number of coronary bypass operations almost everywhere they are carried out.

Although percutaneous techniques to deal with congenital lesions predates PTCA with the introduction of balloon atrial septostomy pioneered by Rashkind, there was parri passu with and to a certain extent stimulated by angioplasty, a major development of new techniques to deal with a variety of congenital lesions. They also now encompass valve disease both congenital and acquired. These developments are covered in Section Three.

The availability of all of these techniques has meant a revolution in patient management and the need to redefine indications for the various interventions available. It has been achieved with co-operation with our surgical colleagues whose support has made the whole development possible, especially during the early period.

There have been a number of spin-offs regarding the approach to the circulation and the prevention of complications, and these are described in Section Five.

This book has brought together all the important aspects of percutaneous intervention in a practical and readable fashion. It also looks to the future and attempts to predict what is coming next, often a very unreliable activity. Younger readers will discover how successful that has been.

Raphael Balcon

Preface

We are pleased to have produced this book which describes the current practice of percutaneous cardiac intervention.

This is not a manual of how to perform coronary angioplasty; there is no substitute for scrubbing up and working at close quarters with the patient and the interventional team of nurses, technicians and radiographers together with an experienced angioplasty operator. This book is designed to provide a foundation of core knowledge upon which increasing practical experience can be built.

Percutaneous coronary intervention continues to be a rapidly advancing and highly technological speciality. Any publication that attempts to describe such a field may court danger in being out of date even as the presses are rolling! Nevertheless the basic principles that underlie the practice of coronary angioplasty and the numerous devices and adjunctive techniques it has generated, remain important despite the passage of time. The many contributors to this book are all experienced interventionists and recognised authorities in their particular area of expertise. Like most of us, the work they enjoy most is practising coronary intervention. Inviting them to contribute to this book can only have increased their pressure of work and the many demands for their time. We much appreciate their enthusiasm for this project and are grateful for their help. The British Cardiovascular Intervention Society has been pivotal in the development of this book; many of the authors are past or present council members, and others will hopefully be future ones.

Michael S. Norell and E. John Perrins
September 2000

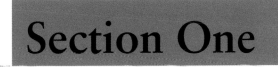

Section One

Fundamental Techniques

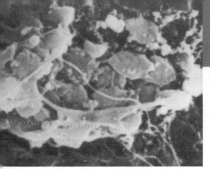

1

History, development and current activity

MICHAEL S. NORELL

KEY POINTS

■ Following the first percutaneous coronary angioplasty in 1977, growth in the procedure has been exponential.

■ It is estimated that in 2000, approximately one million angioplasty procedures will be undertaken worldwide.

■ In the USA the number of percutaneous transluminal coronary angioplasties (PTCAs) performed annually exceeds that of coronary artery bypass graft (CABG) procedures.

■ Despite major technological advances in equipment, and the increasing applicability of PTCA to a variety of patient subsets, the basic principles of the technique remain unchanged.

■ UK rates for PTCA remain below those in the USA and western Europe as a result of restricted resources and limited access to cardiological investigation.

HISTORICAL PERSPECTIVE

Cardiac catheterisation and coronary angiography

More than two decades have passed since Andreas Grüntzig (Fig. 1.1) first attempted the percutaneous relief of a coronary stenosis. This single event, representing the culmination of many years of experimentation, has now passed into legend. Percutaneous coronary revascularisation has emerged as a routine cardiac procedure, but the trials and tribulations of workers in the field of invasive cardiology, whose efforts led stepwise to that day in September 1977, are nevertheless worthy of review.

The era of invasive cardiac investigation and intervention began with the pioneering efforts of Forssman in 1929. The latter half of the previous century had seen Claude Bernard and later, Chaveau and Marey, develop

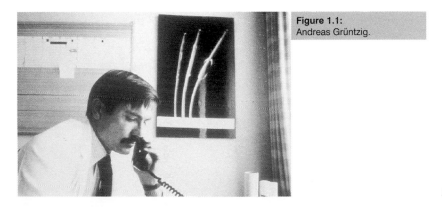

Figure 1.1:
Andreas Grüntzig.

3

the concept of 'cardiac catheterisation' in animal subjects employing intra-arterial or intravenous intubation in horses or dogs, but it was Forssman who demonstrated its feasibility and safety in humans. Taking advantage of his friendship with a nurse, Gerda Ditzen, he was able to cut down on his own cephalic vein and advance a rubber urethral catheter to his right atrium, documenting its progress with X-ray fluoroscopy. Right heart catheterisation was further developed with the work of Cournand and Ranges (1941). while investigation of the left heart proceeded via parasternal, subxiphoid, apical, suprasternal, transbronchial, papravertebral and transseptal approaches until Zimmerman reported the results of retrograde left heart catheterisation in 1949.

Other developments also allowed cardiac catheterisation to progress to a stage recognisable in the present day. In 1953 Seldinger introduced his technique of entering arteries percutaneously. Serious peri-procedural cardiac arrhythmias could be addressed with closed chest cardiac compression (1960) and the introduction of direct current (DC) defibrillation by Lown in 1962. X-ray documentation had been limited to single plate exposures until the image intensifier coupled to film exposure at rapid frame rates resulted in the emergence of true cineangiography. Cardiac events could thereby be visualised in 'real time' incorporating less contrast volume and less radiation exposure to both patient and operator.

By the mid 1950s, visualisation of the coronary circulation had been achieved only by flush injection into the aortic root. A number of modifications to this technique were in use, including power injection into the sinus of Valsalva. It was during one such procedure in 1958, that an National Institute of Health (NIH) catheter inadvertently migrated into the right coronary artery and the subsequent injection of contrast opacified the vessel without the patient experiencing ill effects; Mason Sones had thereby demonstrated that selective coronary arteriography was possible. During the next few years, the first 1000 coronary angiograms were performed with only two deaths and a 2% incidence of ventricular fibrillation. Pre-formed polyethylene catheters were introduced in 1962 and were further modified by Judkins heralding the modern era of comprehensive percutaneous cardiac investigation.

Coronary angioplasty

Initial non-surgical attempts to address arterial obstruction focused on the peripheral circulation. Charles Dotter, together with Judkins in 1964, first reported a successful approach in leg arteries using co-axial sheaths to allow sequential dilatations. In an initial series of nine patients with severe perpheral ischaemia, six improved and four amputations were avoided. However, it was recognised that a better mechanical method of dilatation was required which exerted radial, rather than longitudinal force, on the vessel wall. A latex balloon was initially tried, but it was then appreciated that a non-elastic dilator was preferable. In 1974 Andreas Grüntzig

developed a sausage-shaped polyvinyl chloride (PVC) balloon, mounted at the end of a catheter, which could be inflated to a predetermined diameter to exert a radial force of 3 to 5 atmospheres. This was initially used in the iliac and femoropopliteal system with satisfactory results, and was then extended to address disease in renal, basilar, coeliac and subclavian arteries.

Miniaturisation of this balloon system allowed it to be considered for coronary stenoses. Initial experiments in relieving mechanically produced strictures in canine coronaries, were reported in 1976. In May 1977, after careful planning, Grüntzig together with Richard Myler, decided to attempt balloon dilatation in a patient undergoing bypass surgery in San Francisco. During the operation, a balloon tipped catheter was passed retrogradely up the left anterior descending artery (LAD) from a distal arteriotomy. Following balloon expansion no debris was produced downstream, and reinvestigation after surgery showed that vessel dilatation had been successful. A further 15 peri-operative cases were undertaken in San Francisco and Zurich before true percutaneous transluminal coronary angioplasty (PTCA) was attempted in the human subject.

Gruntzig's description of the first PTCA, performed in Zurich on the 16th September 1977, was later quoted in an article by Hurst:

After working 7 years to develop peripheral arterial dilatation, using animal experiments, post-mortem examinations and intraoperative dilatations, we were ready to use the technique for coronary artery dilatation in man ... It happened in September 1977 that we did coronary angiography on a 37-year-old insurance salesman with severe and exercise induced angina pectoris. The coronary angiography revealed single vessel disease with a proximal stenosis in the left anterior descending artery located immediately before the take-off of a large diagonal branch ... The guiding catheter was placed in the left coronary orifice and the dilatation catheter was inserted ... a roller pump (was in place to start coronary perfusion) through the main lumen of the dilatation catheter (if this became necessary). The stenosis was severe but the catheter slipped through it without resistance. (The balloon was inflated). To the surprise of all of us, no ST elevation, ventricular fibrillation or even extrasystole occurred and the patient had no chest pain. At this moment, I decided not to start the coronary perfusion with the roller pump. After the first balloon deflation, the distal coronary pressure rose nicely. Encouraged by this positive response, I inflated the balloon a second time to relieve the residual gradient ... Everyone was surprised about the ease of the procedure and I started to realise that my dreams had come true.

This first case was reported in a letter to *The Lancet* in 1978. In it, Grüntzig prophetically stated:

This technique, if it proves successful in long-term follow-up studies, may widen the indications for coronary angiography and provide another treatment for patients with angina pectoris.

A report of the first 50 cases was published in the *New England Journal of Medicine* in 1979, indicating success in 32 patients. Stenosis severity fell from 84% to 34%, with a reduction in the translesional pressure gradient from 58 to 19 mmHg. Seven patients required emergency coronary artery bypass graft (CABG); there was a 5% incidence of myocardial infarction, but no procedural deaths. In a book prepared before his untimely death in 1985, Grüntzig wrote:

Whatever becomes of the method I have left one mark on medicine. Forssman demonstrated that man could place a catheter into his heart successfully. Mason Sones studied the coronary arteries selectively by angiography without significant mortality. I have shown that man can work therapeutically within the coronary arteries themselves in the face of an alert, comfortable patient.

In September 1977, coronary revascularisation had entered a new era of rapidly advancing technology. The subsequent 20 years have seen the subspecialty of interventional cardiology become one of the most exciting and rewarding fields in modern medicine.

TECHNOLOGICAL DEVELOPMENTS

The procedure of coronary angioplasty, although modified over the last 20 years by enhanced technology, still conforms to the original descriptions of the technique (Figs 1.2 and 1.3). Under radiographic control and local anaesthesia, the coronary arterial ostium is engaged with a guiding catheter and the target lesion traversed with an atraumatic guidewire. A balloon tipped catheter is then advanced over the guidewire until it reaches the site of atheromatous obstruction, at which point the balloon is inflated with diluted contrast medium. The size of balloon, inflation pressure and the number and duration of inflations, varies according to the lesion characteristics. When the angiographic appearances suggest adequate lesion dilatation, all the equipment is removed and the patient is returned to the ward.

The original Grüntzig balloon material was PVC and of low compliance. It would rupture rather than exceed its designed maximal outer diameter. The catheter shaft incorporated a double lumen which allowed the balloon to be expanded and voided, and for pressure to be monitored at the catheter tip. Other than for a short fixed guidewire, steerability was not possible. Balloon material limited inflation pressures to 5 atmospheres, the catheter shaft diameter was almost 5 French (F) (1.7 mm) and crossing profiles were high. The subsequent 15 years witnessed a rapid growth in technology resulting in marked improvements in guiding catheters and guidewires, as well as in balloon design.

Guiding catheters

Although coronary angioplasty represented an extension of diagnostic angiography, the construction of guiding catheters needed modification as

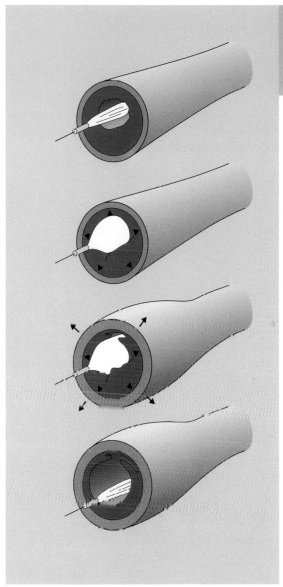

Figure 1.2:
Diagrammatic transverse cross section of coronary dilatation. Note the development of intimal fissuring as a result of balloon barotrauma.

these would need to support the passage of high profile and inflexible balloon catheters through tortuous vessels and across high-grade obstructions, rather than simply allow contrast injection. Initial examples had large outer diameters with poor memory and torque control. In the early 1980s, bonded, multilayer guiding catheters were developed comprising an inner surface of Teflon (to decrease friction), a middle layer of woven mesh (for torque control) and an outer layer of polyurethane (to maintain form). The variety of preformed shapes available for diagnostic

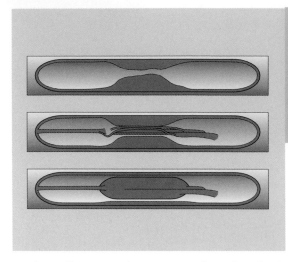

Figure 1.3:
Diagrammatic representation of the principles of balloon coronary angioplasty. The deflated balloon catheter is positioned across a coronary stenosis and inflated (middle). It is then deflated leaving the atheromatous lesion compressed and the stenosis relieved (bottom).

work (Judkins, Amplatz), were reflected in the design of guides for interventional use, with many additional configurations to deal with atypical anatomy (e.g. Voda, Multipurpose, El Gamal, Hockey Stick).

Soft-tipped guides meant a reduced likelihood of catheter induced trauma to the coronary ostium, while thinner walls allowed increased internal lumens to incorporate other non-balloon devices. Nine or 10 F (3 or 3.3 mm diameter) guides were routinely used in the early 1980s, but with advancing technology, notably in reducing the profiles of balloons and other devices, guiding catheter diameters came down in size. While in the early 1990s 8 F (2.7 mm) guides were commonplace, 7 and 6 F (2.3 or 2.0 mm) catheters are now increasingly employed. This results in less femoral arterial trauma and more rapid patient ambulation after the procedure, as well as allowing PTCA to be undertaken from alternative sites of vascular access, particularly the radial artery.

Guidewires

A short wire was fixed to the distal tip of the balloon catheter in 1979, but a major advance was made in 1982 when Simpson developed a long moveable and independent guidewire that was inserted through the central lumen. This allowed better tip control and steerability enabling access to distal coronary lesions. The initial 0.018 wires were later to be reduced in diameter and incorporate a variety of lubricious coatings to reduce friction and enhance passage through severe stenoses. Another modification was the introduction of a low profile balloon able to be moved only over a limited segment of reduced diameter wire (Hartzler 'Micro').

Guidewire control could be restricted by its passage through the balloon catheter lumen and contrast injection was also limited. Furthermore, the exchange of balloons was problematical involving wire extension to avoid having to rewire the target lesion. This was overcome by Kaltenbach's introduction of the long (300 cm) wire technique in 1984. Currently used wires measure 0.014 inches in diameter. The radiopaque distal few centimetres varies in flexbility, as does the shaft, providing increased support when addressing tortuous anatomy with relatively inflexible devices.

Balloon catheters

The balloon catheter itself has sustained a number of major modifications since its original design in 1977. A large variety of balloon lengths and expanded diameters became available, increasing the scope of possible lesions. Balloon material was also developed which could withstand far higher pressures (currently in excess of 20 atmospheres) and yet expand in a predictable fashion. Operators could choose from balloon materials with a range of compliance characteristics to suit particular lesion types. As balloon and shaft design improved, so did trackability and steerability, and as the crossing profile of the balloon reduced it became axiomatic that if a wire could cross the stenosis then so would the balloon catheter.

Balloon preparation was often problematical as the material did not collapse easily with aspiration and thus de-airing was frequently incomplete. Until the development of superior materials, this was overcome with a specific air venting tube which was integral in the Simpson–Roberts balloon catheter system.

The original fixed wire design re-emerged in the mid 1980s with the 'balloon on a wire' concept. This was particularly valuable for distal lesions, or cases when preservation of wire position or balloon exchange was considered not to be a priority. Erbel and Stack produced continuous perfusion balloons that allowed the anterograde flow of blood beyond the inflated balloon and could thereby limit ischaemia during long balloon inflations.

A milestone in balloon catheter development occurred in the 1986 with the introduction of the 'monorail' system by Bonzel. By only requiring a relatively short segment of guidewire to run through the distal catheter tip and shaft, lesions could be independently wired before selection of the balloon catheter, and balloon exchange was simplified. 'Over the wire' systems remained in limited use as they provided easier wire exchange (when occasionally required) and the ability to measure distal pressure. However, the emergence of superior fluoroscopy and digital X-ray systems with online quantitative coronary angiography (QCA), meant that operators could assess the results of angioplasty visually without having to rely on abolition of the translesional pressure gradient. Thus, in Europe, monorail systems represent the majority of activity while in the USA such 'rapid exchange' devices are more restricted by regulatory issues.

As the technique of PTCA necessarily incorporates the temporary occlusion of an epicardial coronary artery, it is not surprising that much research activity capitalised on this model of controlled myocardial ischaemia. A multitude of publications have emerged in the literature as a result of harnessing this therapeutic modility and thereby studying the effects of transient coronary occlusion in man. Examination of these effects has involved action potential changes, coronary sinus blood sampling, electrocardiographic and haemodynamic alteration, and analysis of ventricular contraction during balloon inflation employing echocardiography or contrast left ventriculography.

Such research has clarified the sequence of abnormalities occurring in left ventricular myocardium rendered ischaemic as a result of transient coronary occlusion. Initially diastolic dysfunction (abnormal relaxation and reduced compliance), is followed by systolic contractile changes indicated by hypokinesis, akinesis or dyskinesis of myocardial segments subtended by the treated artery. Electrocardiogram (ECG) abnormalities then develop, manifest as ST segment changes in leads overlying the ischaemic territories. Cardiac chest pain is a final and unpredictable occurrence in this cascade of ischaemic events all of which totally resolve in the reverse sequence when ischaemia is relieved. These ischaemic effects may be mitigated by collateral flow to the index artery, and there is now much interest surrounding the role of preconditioning in this setting.

These, and other technological advances steadily increased the scope of PTCA allowing a larger variety of lesions to be treated more successfully and with greater safety. Angioplasty had grown from a pioneering and unpredictable experiment to become a routine therapy for patients with coronary disease. A further breakthrough was to occur in 1987 which, in significance, was second only to Grüntzig's pioneering efforts; this was the first implantation in man of an intracoronary stent (see Chapter 6).

WORLDWIDE ACTIVITY

Initial enthusiasm for PTCA resulted in an understandable rush to learn the technique. This prompted leaders in the field to convene a workshop in June 1979, in Bethesda, USA, under the auspices of the National Heart, Lung, and Blood Institute (NHLBI). Here it was decided to limit the availability of PTCA to centres with clearly defined and agreed protocols. Even the commercial provider of the equipment agreed to abide by these guidelines such that operators could not obtain balloon catheters without having undergone approved instruction in the technique. Results of procedures were pooled in a unified and systematic fashion so that many of the first insights into PTCA and its outcomes derived from this NHLBI registry.

Between 1977 and 1982 data on 3079 patients were entered into the registry from 106 institutions. Of these patients, 77% were male with a mean age of 54 years, two-thirds having Canadian Heart Class III or IV symptoms. Almost three-quarters had single vessel disease, the left anterior descending artery being the most commonly addressed. Left main stem disease was attempted in 1% and bypass graft dilatation performed in 4%.

At this early stage several drawbacks were apparent when PTCA was compared with coronary artery surgery. First, the initial and long-term results were unpredicatable and the definition of a successful procedure was uncertain; a 20% reduction in stenosis severity was achieved in 67% of the original registry. Secondly, the risks of PTCA were not clearly superior to surgery (myocardial infarction: 5.5%, emergency CABG: 6.6%, death: 0.9%) acknowledging that the majority had single vessel disease. Thirdly, it became apparent that a relatively small volume of procedures was being undertaken by an increasingly large number of operators thus potentially diluting an initially small experience. Finally, technical factors like vessel angulation or tortuosity, distal disease and lesion calcification, eccentricity or chronic occlusion, were anticipated to limit PTCA to perhaps 10 or 15% of patients considered for surgical revascularisation.

The technical advances in PTCA described in this chapter resulted in greater applicability of the procedure and thereby an exponential increase in activity. Emory University in Atlanta, where Grüntzig had undertaken much of his later work, was in the vanguard of interventional research. Their experience, reported in 1985, indicated a learning curve for the technique and improving results associated with increasing experience and the new emerging technology. For example, the circumflex artery became more accessible with steerable systems rising from 7% to 16% of all procedures and enjoying similar success rates as with the other main arteries. Their experience in 3500 consecutive cases set a standard to which other interventional units could aspire with success in 89%, myocardial infarction in 2.6%, emergency CABG in 2.7% and death in 0.1% of patients.

The growth in activity has been seen worldwide, with the USA particularly generating large volumes. It is interesting to note that ten years after the first report of coronary artery bypass grafting in 1968, 100 000 operations had been performed in the USA. However this figure had been overtaken by the number of PTCA procedures (106 000) undertaken within only 7 years of its first reported series in 1978. Recent data suggest that CABG rates in the USA may now be on the decline as PTCA activity continues to increase.

In 1995, there were an estimated 350 000 PTCA cases performed in the USA, with almost half a million undertaken worldwide. In Europe, activity has been similarly increasing from approximately 250 000 in 1995, to almost 300 000 in 1997. Individual European countries differ in interventional activity and thus in the PTCA rates per million of the population. Growth in activity in the UK, although substantial, nevertheless lags behind that of other European countries like France, Germany and Belgium. This discrepency in the UK compared with other western European nations is primarily a funding issue within the National   **11**

Health Service. A lack of resources limits the number of patients coming forward for angiographic investigation, and thereby the number available for revascularisation with CABG as well as PTCA.

In the UK, data on PTCA activity is collected by the British Cardiovascular Intervention Society on an annual basis. Input from participating centres has been voluntary, but nevertheless the volumes recorded have always been in concordance with those suggested by industry sources when equipment sales have been examined. Thus in 1991, 52 centres in the UK undertook 9933 PTCA procedures representing 174 cases per million population. The annual growth in activity has varied between approximately 12% and 19%, the average since 1991 being 15% per year. In 1997, a total of 58 centres reported 22 902 procedures, giving a rate per million of 395.

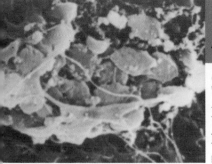

2

Selection of patients for percutaneous intervention

ROD STABLES

KEY POINTS

■ Case selection is an essential element in the practice of percutaneous coronary intervention (PCI) and has a direct and immediate bearing on outcome.

■ The enthusiasm for PCI must be tempered with the realisation that:
- Clinical gains are real but modest.
- Performance is associated with morbidity and mortality.
- Alternative therapeutic strategies exist.

■ The process involves the interaction of a number of factors:
- The training and experience of the interventionist.
- Access to equipment and facilities.
- The availability of surgical or other support.
- The characteristics of the patient.
- The nature of the clinical presentation.
- The details of the epicardial coronary anatomy to be addressed.

■ Assessment of appropriateness can be complex and involves a consideration of symptoms and functional testing.

INTRODUCTION

In the practice of percutaneous coronary intervention (PCI) the aim is to deliver maximum clinical gain at appropriate levels of risk. Case selection is an essential element in this process and is one of the few factors in the control of the cardiologist that has a direct and immediate bearing on outcome. The development of the skill (or art!) of case selection should be a central component of training but is often neglected, with increasing emphasis on procedural issues.

Careful review will identify cases that would be best managed by alternative treatments but can also provide important information to guide the conduct of a proposed intervention. The need for specialised equipment or adjunctive medication can be identified and provision assured. Appropriate scheduling of catheter laboratory, ward and other clinical areas can be performed. Unusual or high-risk cases may demand the collaboration of other interventionists or surgical and anaesthetic colleagues. Furthermore, the process of informed consent is improved if patients can be appraised of a case specific assessment of likely gains and potential risks.

GENERAL CONSIDERATIONS

Most interventionists will accept that PCI has established limitations. The enthusiasm to recommend this form of therapy should be tempered in the light of this reality.

13

Clinical gains are real but modest

No study has been able to demonstrate that management with PCI confers prognostic advantage. In the management of stable angina, randomised controlled trials against medical therapy have shown that an interventional strategy does result in better resolution of symptoms but the gains are modest and attenuate over medium term follow-up.[1–3] The role of early angiography and revascularisation in the acute coronary syndromes is still the subject of debate but it seems likely that an invasive strategy will benefit only a selected proportion of patients. As in the management of acute myocardial infarction, prompt access to facilities and appropriately trained staff may be required at a specific point in the natural history if benefits are to be realised.

Performance is associated with morbidity and mortality

All trials comparing PCI with medical therapy have shown an increased rate of major adverse cardiac events in the intervention group, mostly related to complications at the time of revascularisation.[2,3] All interventionists will be familiar with the potential for other forms of procedure-related morbidity. Although these events may not be reported as formal outcome measures in the trial literature, they have important implications for the patient's perception of outcome and for the consumption of health-care resources.

Alternative therapeutic options exist and are effective

Advances in medical therapy options for symptom management, support of impaired left ventricular function and secondary prevention (particularly lipid lowering[4]) have revolutionised the so-called conservative approach. A major, multicentre trial (COURAGE) has been initiated in the United States and Canada to reassess the value of PCI over continued modern medical therapy.

In the management of more advanced disease, coronary artery bypass grafting (CABG) remains an effective and widely applicable treatment option. A meta-analysis of the first generation trials comparing percutaneous transluminal coronary angioplasty (PTCA) and CABG has been published.[5] Rihal and Yusuf[6] extended these observations to include the Bypass Angioplasty Revascularisation Investigation (BARI) trial producing a combined sample size of 5200 patients. The overall mortality rate was 7.8% and 6.6% in the PTCA and CABG groups respectively (odds ratio 1.20, 95% CI 0.97–1.48). This represents a trend to increased mortality in the PTCA group that approaches conventional levels of statistical significance. The PTCA strategy was also limited by a greater need for repeat revascularisation procedures (34% PTCA vs 3.3% CABG in the first year of follow-up), and less effective relief of angina symptoms.

Preliminary results from the Arterial Revascularisation Therapy Study (ARTS) trial reveal that the advent of coronary stenting has eroded some of the advantage enjoyed by the surgical strategy but there remains a marked difference in the need for additional, unplanned revascularisation by 1 year of follow-up (CABG 3.5% vs PTCA 17%).

CASE SELECTION – ASSESSING APPROPRIATENESS

The process of case selection is complex and multifactorial. Many aspects are difficult to characterise and hence describe. The appropriateness of any given procedure will be influenced by the skills and experience of the interventionist, the availability of other therapeutic options and the attitude of the patient to the potential for benefit and risk. The management of specific clinical syndromes will evolve over time and be influenced by the development of (and access to) new techniques, equipment and adjunctive medications.

These difficulties are perhaps best exemplified by retrospective studies designed to rate the appropriateness of interventional procedures. Most have used the opinions of 'Expert Panels' using a methodology designed by the RAND Corporation and the University of California.[7–10] Raw data from these panels consists of tables of thousands of situation-specific rankings that can be difficult to apply to routine clinical practice. Furthermore the data becomes obsolete over time, can be influenced by the composition of the panel[11,12] and do not necessarily translate from one nation to another.[13]

Other investigators have adopted a more simplified approach. The University of Maryland Revascularisation Appropriateness Scoring System (RAS) combines information on symptoms, clinical presentation, coronary anatomy, non-invasive tests of functional significance, left ventricular function and co-morbidity to derive a simple index of suitability (Fig. 2.1).[14] A German group has developed a computer program to predict the outcome of coronary interventions. Initial weightings for predictive factors were derived from retrospective data and tested on new prospective cases.[15] The potential for artificial intelligence computer systems to 'learn' from cases as they are added to the registry means that this type of tool may be able to remain current with practice evolution, though routine clinical application is still several years away.

The leading professional societies issue guidelines for the practice of coronary intervention and for the management of common clinical presentations. A joint publication from the American College of Cardiology (ACC) and the American Heart Association (AHA) established Class 1, 2 and 3 approved indications for PCI based on simple clinical scenarios.[16] These are now somewhat dated and are to be updated in early 2000 and will be available from the ACC website (*http://www.acc.org*).

CASE SELECTION – A PRACTICAL APPROACH

A structured approach to case selection or risk stratification might consider three elements:

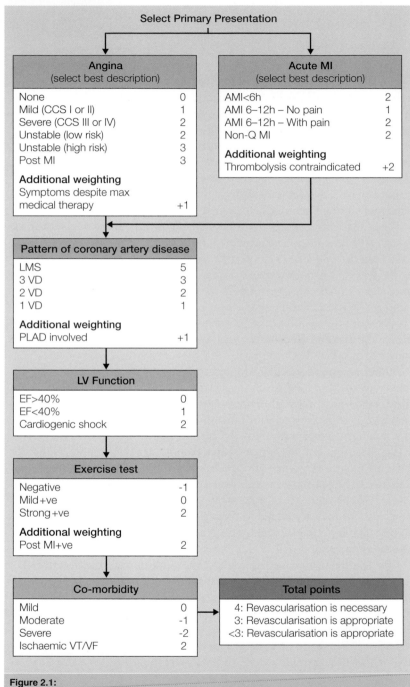

Figure 2.1:
Calculation of the University of Maryland Revascularisation Appropriateness Scoring (RAS). (Adapted from Ziskind et al.[14] AMI, acute myocardial infarction; CCS, Canadian Cardiovascular Society; EF, ejection fraction; LMS, left main stem; LV, left ventricle; MI, myocardial infarction; PLAD, proximal left anterior descending; VD, vessel disease; VT/VF, ventricular tachycardia/fibrillation.)

■ Factors related to the nature of the clinical presentation.

■ Factors related to the clinical characteristics of the patient.

■ Factors related to the proposed target lesion(s).

The established clinical indications for PCI are subject to continued expansion and refinement. Its role in the management of many presentations (for example – acute myocardial infarction, acute coronary syndromes, cardiogenic shock, multivessel disease and small vessel disease) are still the subject of continuing evaluation. A detailed review of this area is beyond the scope of this text and the role of PCI in a number of key clinical presentations is explored in other chapters.

Assessment of the status and clinical characteristics of the patient can be considered in the following terms.

General cardiac status

The state of the circulation has an immediate and significant impact on the performance of any PCI procedure. Cardiogenic shock precipitated by acute ischaemia represents a clear but very high-risk indication. Less florid left ventricular failure is another negative prognostic factor and may compromise the ability of the patient to lie supine on the examination table. The need for elective ventilation or circulatory support (for example intra-aortic balloon pumping) is a marker of adverse outcome. Post-procedural reduced perfusion or hypotension can precipitate subacute vessel closure. In this respect a vaso-vagal response or disturbance of cardiac rhythm with brady or tachycardia can have important implications.

Details of the coronary anatomy

The operator must contemplate the likely impact of transient balloon occlusion or an abrupt closure event at each proposed target lesion. This analysis demands a thorough review of current angiographic findings, including bypass graft conduits, if present. Flow limiting lesions or occlusive disease in non-target vessels increase procedural risk. Procedures to a 'last remaining conduit' represent one extreme in this continuum. In certain clinical situations (for example thrombus laden lesions, saphenous vein graft disease or rotational atherectomy) the sequelae of embolisation of material to the distal vascular bed should be considered.

The left main stem (or right ostium) and proximal portions of the principal vessels may be subjected to mechanical trauma by the guide catheter and other equipment. Plaque or other atherosclerotic disease in these territories increases the risk of vessel dissection or abrupt closure.

Suitability for CABG

Angiographic review should also involve a consideration of the options for surgical therapy, either as an elective alternative to PCI or in a bailout setting. There is merit in involving surgical colleagues in this process. Suitability for CABG will be influenced by co-morbid factors beyond the coronary vasculature, particularly respiratory, renal and hepatic function. Lack of a surgical 'rescue' option increase the risk of any proposed procedure but may of course represent an appropriate procedure for patients in need of revascularisation.

Peripheral and great vessels

Adequate stability of the guiding catheter is an essential pre-requisite for successful PCI. Atherosclerotic or other disease of the peripheral vessels may deny access for the catheter of choice and for additional equipment, for example an intra-aortic balloon pump (IABP). Unfolding or excessive tortuosity of the aorta can further compromise guide catheter positioning.

Procedural morbidity will be increased in cases with widespread vascular disease. The risk of catheter-related embolic release to the head and neck or peripheral vessels is real. Complications at the vascular access site can result in embolisation, occlusion or bleeding. Co-existing hypertension, obesity or systemic anticoagulation can confound these problems.

Renal function

Chronic renal failure (CRF) is an established risk factor for coronary artery disease. Nevertheless emerging data suggests that the results of PCI at any individual lesion may be less favourable in patients with established CRF.[17] For patients with any degree of renal impairment the nephrotoxicity of radiographic contrast can precipitate acute renal failure. Even with precautionary measures such as fluid administration or elective filtration, the scope and duration of any PCI procedure will be limited by the need to minimise exposure to contrast agent.

Diabetes mellitus

Diabetes mellitus (DM) is often a marker of more widespread and diffuse coronary artery disease. This pattern of disease is difficult to manage with PCI and CABG may provide a better revascularisation strategy. In the BARI trial, comparing multivessel PTCA with conventional CABG, the advantages of the surgical approach were most marked in patients with DM.[18]

The reasons for this are not fully established and may extend beyond the simple presence of more extensive disease. At individual lesions, the restenosis rate seems to be higher in diabetic patients. Recent studies suggest that use of a GPIIb/IIIa receptor blocking antiplatelet agent (abciximab) seems to confer particular advantage in diabetic patients.[19] This may suggest that other mechanisms, some platelet mediated, may be

involved.

REFERENCES

1. Hueb W, Bellotti G, Almeida de Oliveira S *et al.* The medicine, angioplasty or surgery study (MASS): a prospective randomised trial of medical therapy, balloon angioplasty or bypass surgery for single proximal left anterior descending artery stenoses. J Am Coll Cardiol 1995;25:1600–1605.

2. Parisi AF, Folland ED, Hartigan P, on behalf of the Veterans Affairs ACME Investigators. A comparison of angioplasty with medical therapy in the treatment of single-vessel coronary artery disease. N Engl J Med 1992;326:10–16.

3. RITA-2 trial participants. Coronary angioplasty versus medical therapy for angina: the second Randomised Intervention Treatment of Angina (RITA-2). Lancet 1997;350:461–8.

4. Pitt B, Waters D, Brown WV *et al.* Aggressive lipid-lowering compared with angioplasty in stable coronary artery disease. N Engl J Med 1999;341:70–76.

5. Pocock SJ, Henderson RA, Rickards AF *et al.* Meta-analysis of randomised trials comparing coronary angioplasty with bypass surgery. Lancet 1995;346:1184–9.

6. Rihal CS, Yusuf S. Chronic coronary artery disease: drugs, angioplasty or surgery. BMJ 1996;312:265–6.

7. Hilborne LH, Leape LL, Bernstein SJ *et al.* The appropriateness of use of percutaneous transluminal coronary angioplasty in New York State. JAMA 1993;269:761–5.

8. Hilborne LH, Leape LL, Kahan JP, Park RE, Kamberg CJ, Brook RH. Percutaneous transluminal coronary angioplasty: a literature review and ratings of appropriateness and necessity. Santa Monica, CA, USA: The RAND Corporation. JRA-01, 1991.

9. Meijler AP, Rigter H, Bernstein SJ *et al.* The appropriateness of intention to treat decisions for invasive therapy in coronary artery disease in the Netherlands. Heart 1997;77:219–24.

10. Bernstein SJ, Brorsson B, Abert T *et al.* Appropriateness of referral of coronary angiography patients in Sweden. Heart 1999;81:470–77.

11. Shekelle PG, Kahan JP, Bernstein SJ, Leape LL, Kamberg CJ, Park RE. The reproducibility of a method to identify the overuse and underuse of medical procedures [see comments]. N Engl J Med 1998;338:1888–95.

12. Ayanian JZ, Landrum MB, Normal SL, Guadagnoli E, McNeil BJ. Rating the appropriateness of coronary angiography – do practicing physicians agree with an expert panel and with each other? [see comments]. N Engl J Med 1988;338:1896–1904.

13. Brook RH, Kosecoff JB, Park RE, Chassin MR, Winslow CM, Hampton JR. Diagnosis and treatment of coronary disease: comparison of doctor's attitudes in the USA and the UK. Lancet 1988;1:750–53.

14. Ziskind AA, Lauer MA, Bishop G, Vogel RA. Assessing the appropriateness of coronary revascularisation: The Universtiy of Maryland Revascularization

Appropriateness Score (RAS) and its comparison to RAND expert panel ratings and ACC/AHA guidelines with regard to assigned appropriateness rating and ability to predict outcome. Clin Cardiol 1999;22:67–76.

15. Budde T, Haude M, Hopp HW *et al*. A prognostic computer model to individually predict post-procedural complications in interventional cardiology: the INTERVENT Project [see comments]. Eur Heart J 1999;20:354–63.

16. Ryan TJ, Bauman WB, Kennedy JW *et al*. Guidelines for percutaneous transluminal coronary angioplasty. A report of the American Heart Association/American College of Cardiology Task Force on Assessment of Diagnostic and Therapeutic Cardiovascular Procedures (Committee on Percutaneous Transluminal Coronary Angioplasty). Circulation 1993;88:2987–3007.

17. Schoebel FC, Gradaus F, Ivens K *et al*. Restenosis after elective coronary balloon angioplasty in patients with end stage renal disease: a case–control study using quantitative coronary angiography. Heart 1997;78:337–42.

18. BARI Investigators. Comparison of coronary bypass surgery with angioplasty in patients with multivessel disease. N Engl J Med 1996;335:217–25.

19. Lincoff AM, Califf RM, Moliterno DJ *et al*. Complementary clinical benefits of coronary-artery stenting and blockade of platelet glycoprotein IIb/IIIa receptors. Evaluation of platelet IIb/IIIa inhibition in stenting investigators. N Engl J Med 1999;341:319–27.

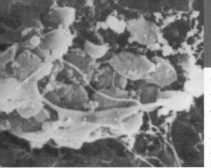

3

Patient investigation, work up and preparation

IAN R. STARKEY

KEY POINTS

Prior to performing PCI, ensure that the following have been considered:

■ **P**reliminary investigations

■ **T**herapeutic alterations

■ **C**onsent

■ **A**nticipation (and possible prevention) of problems.

INTRODUCTION

In 1998, almost 25 000 percutaneous coronary intervention (PCI) procedures were performed in 61 centres in the UK (British Cardiovascular Intervention Society [BCIS] annual survey – unpublished data). It is important to remember that such procedures, while 'routine' for some operators and exciting for others, may be frightening, painful and dangerous for the patients on whom they are performed, even though statistically the success rate is high. Before such a procedure begins, much can be done to diminish the patient's fear and pain, minimise the danger and increase further the likelihood of procedural and clinical success. The essential components of this preparation are:

P Preliminary investigations
T Therapeutics
C Consent
A Anticipation (of possible complications).

There is inevitably some overlap between these elements, all of which require consideration in *all* patients. The emergency nature of some procedures (e.g. primary percutaneous transluminal coronary angioplasty [PTCA] for a patient with an acute myocardial infarction) may curtail the time available for preparation of the patient, but should *never* result in omission of the basic essentials.

PRELIMINARY INVESTIGATIONS

These are needed to allow three questions to be answered:

1. Is percutaneous coronary intervention (PCI) appropriate for this patient?

With few exceptions, PCI should only be considered in a patient with symptoms of coronary artery disease, objective evidence of myocardial

21

ischaemia/infarction and an anatomically suitable lesion(s), as demonstrated by coronary angiography. As a preliminary to such a procedure, therefore, the interventional cardiologist should review the patient's history and the results of any non-invasive and invasive investigations. While all this information should be available in advance of a procedure performed electively, patients with acute coronary syndromes (ACS: unstable angina or acute myocardial infarction) often have combined diagnostic (i.e. coronary angiography) and therapeutic (i.e. PCI) procedures performed. In this situation, it is especially important for the interventional cardiologist to retain a capacity for objective judgement, so that, for instance, a patient who might best be treated surgically does not receive suboptimal treatment simply because it is 'convenient' for him/her to do so.

2. If PCI is appropriate, is he/she fit for the procedure?

Before arrival in the cardiac catheterisation laboratory, *every* patient should have a clinical history documented and a physical examination performed (Fig. 3.1). These should be supplemented by some basic investigations, although the number of these will be kept to a minimum in emergency situations (Table 3.1).

It is of particular importance to discover conditions that might increase the technical difficulty or risk of an invasive cardiac procedure. Some such factors can be corrected but awareness of others may lead to changes in peri-procedural drug therapy (see Therapeutics below), the information provided to the patient (see Consent below) or an ability to predict, and hopefully prevent, possible complications (see Anticipation below).

3. Can anything be done to improve his/her fitness?

This is mostly discussed in the ensuing sections of this chapter. The discovery of some intercurrent medical conditions might appropriately result in the postponement of an elective procedure. Examples would include severe anaemia, active or suspected infection, uncontrolled hypertension and possible/definite pregnancy. On rare occasions, the discovery of a serious intercurrent medical problem (e.g. advanced malignancy) might lead to cancellation of a planned PCI procedure.

TABLE 3.1 – INVESTIGATIONS PRIOR TO PCI
ALL PATIENTS
Full blood count
Blood urea, creatinine and electrolytes
12-lead ECG
Blood group and save
SOME PATIENTS
INR (patients on warfarin)
Chest X-ray (if clinically indicated)
Others (respiratory function tests, plasma glucose, etc. according to clinical indication)

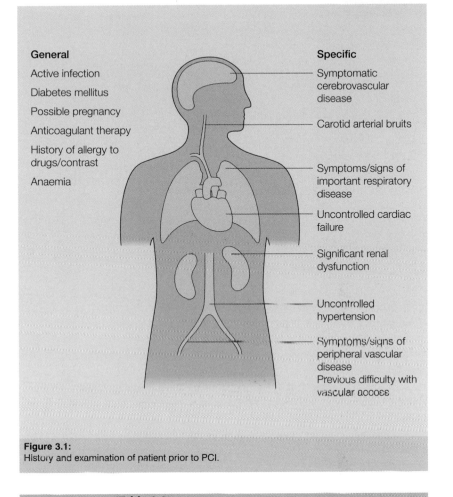

General

Active infection

Diabetes mellitus

Possible pregnancy

Anticoagulant therapy

History of allergy to drugs/contrast

Anaemia

Specific

Symptomatic cerebrovascular disease

Carotid arterial bruits

Symptoms/signs of important respiratory disease

Uncontrolled cardiac failure

Significant renal dysfunction

Uncontrolled hypertension

Symptoms/signs of peripheral vascular disease
Previous difficulty with vascular access

Figure 3.1:
History and examination of patient prior to PCI.

THERAPEUTICS (Table 3.2)

Antianginal drugs

Most patients with symptomatic coronary artery disease are taking regular antianginal medication, which can be continued until, and indeed, after the interventional procedure. Treatment with a long-acting nitrate ± a calcium-channel blocker may actually be of benefit in the prevention of coronary artery spasm during/after the procedure. Although there is no convincing evidence that cholesterol-lowering therapy (e.g. statin drugs) specifically affects the short-term outcome of coronary interventional procedures, such treatment is an important part of the management of patients with coronary artery disease and should, likewise, be continued.

Oral antiplatelet therapy

Most patients with coronary artery disease are taking aspirin, which inhibits the platelet cyclo-oxygenase pathway, thus reducing the formation

23

TABLE 3.2 – DRUG THERAPY PRIOR TO PCI	
DRUG CLASS	ACTION REQUIRED
Oral anti-anginal drugs	Continue
Cholesterol-lowering therapy	Continue
Oral anti-platelet therapy	Ensure that aspirin has been taken
	Consider addition of ticlopidine or clopidogrel
Warfarin	Discontinue if possible (usually not)
	Measure INR and correct excessive anticoagulation
	Take appropriate measures to avoid haemorrhage
	at vascular access site
IV Heparin	Continue
	Measure ACT and consider reduced bolus dose
SC Low molecular-weight heparin	Administer last injection >12 hours prior to PCI
	(if possible)
Platelet GP IIb/IIIa receptor	Continue
antagonists	Use a reduced, weight-adjusted heparin regime
Pre-medication	If necessary, use diazepam 5–20 mg orally
Antidiabetic medication	See text
Other drug therapy	Continue unchanged

of thromboxane A_2, prostaglandin E_2 and prostacyclin. In the unusual circumstance of a patient not taking regular aspirin presenting for PCI, this drug (300 mg) should be given, preferably at least 2 hours before the start of the procedure. Aspirin (75–300 mg daily) should be continued long term thereafter.

In patients undergoing coronary stent implantation, long-term aspirin therapy is usually supplemented by a course (2–4 weeks) of ticlopidine or, more recently, clopidogrel, both of which inhibit adenosine diphosphate (ADP)-induced platelet aggregation.[1] On theoretical grounds, some interventional cardiologists give an initial dose of ticlopidine (250–500 mg) or clopidogrel (75–300 mg) *before* the start of a procedure in which stenting is likely, although there is no convincing published evidence that this approach is superior to commencing such antiplatelet therapy immediately after stent implantation.

Anticoagulant therapy

Some patients may be anticoagulated with warfarin, usually for reasons other than the presence of coronary artery disease (e.g. prosthetic heart valve, atrial fibrillation, venous thrombo-embolic disease). It may be impossible or undesirable to discontinue such treatment, but it is imperative that its effect is measured (by international normalised ratio [INR]), preferably before the start of the procedure and certainly prior to the removal of the arterial access sheath. Excessive anticoagulation should be corrected, but even therapeutic anticoagulation increases the risk of haemorrhage, especially at the vascular access site – anticipation of such a problem should lead to the use of appropriate prophylactic measures (see below).

Most patients with acute coronary syndromes are treated with heparin. Intravenous unfractionated heparin can be continued until the patient's arrival in the catheterisation laboratory. Measurement of the activated clotting time (ACT) will then allow the administration of an appropriate bolus of intravenous heparin, which may not actually be substantially different from that given to a patient not pre-treated with heparin.[2] If a twice-daily regime of subcutaneous low molecular-weight heparin is being used, the last injection should be given at least 12 hours before any planned coronary interventional procedure.[3] At the start of the procedure, an intravenous bolus of unfractionated heparin can then be given in the usual way. In 'emergency' procedures, performed less than 12 hours after the last dose of low molecular-weight heparin, one should consider using a reduced dose of IV heparin (<70 U/kg).

Platelet glycoprotein IIb/IIIa receptor antagonists

The results of randomised placebo-controlled clinical trials of several agents of this type demonstrate a clear benefit in patients with acute coronary syndromes, those undergoing percutaneous coronary interventional treatment or both. A detailed discussion of the use of such drug treatment is outwith the scope of this chapter – suffice it to say that it is clear that PCI can be performed safely after/during administration of such agents provided that a reduced, weight-adjusted heparin regime is used, in order to reduce the risk of major bleeding.[4]

Pre-medication

Despite explanation and reassurance, many patients remain anxious about undergoing PCI. If anxiety is overt and/or the patient expresses a desire for a sedative, a benzodiazepine such as diazepam 5–20 mg orally may be given 1–1½ hours before the start of the procedure. Benzodiazepines are also effectively absorbed when administered sublingually, but this method conveys no great advantage as the onset of action is unlikely to be any more rapid. Some patients undergoing PCI will have had many previous invasive procedures, so that femoral arterial access may be difficult and painful. Prior administration of an opiate drug (pethidine or morphine), combined with generous quantities of local anaesthetic (lignocaine) will be much appreciated by such patients.

Diabetes mellitus[5]

Since patients are usually fasted for several hours before PCI procedures, special precautions may be required to prevent hypoglycaemia in patients with diabetes mellitus. If possible, an elective procedure in a diabetic should be scheduled at the beginning of the list, to avoid the patient having to fast for an unpredictable and excessive length of time.

Treatment with sulphonylureas should be omitted on the morning of the day of the procedure. The administration of significant quantities of glucose-containing IV fluids should be avoided if possible. Insulin treatment is unlikely to be required. Drug treatment can be restarted at the time of the patient's first meal after the procedure.

Although lactic acidosis associated with treatment with metformin occurs only rarely, it is more common in diabetics with impaired renal function. There have been a number of reports of cases of metformin-associated lactic acidosis in patients with acute renal failure precipitated by iodinated contrast material, as is used during diagnostic and therapeutic cardiac procedures. This has led to the manufacturer's current recommendation that metformin should be discontinued at the time of, or prior to, any such procedure and withheld for 48 hours after the procedure. Treatment should be re-instituted only after renal function has been re-evaluated and found to be normal. In all but emergency cases, renal function should be checked in all patients taking metformin *before* the procedure. As metformin is contraindicated in the presence of abnormal renal function, such patients should have their drug therapy reviewed, although PCI can be performed provided that special precautions are taken[6,7] (see Anticipation below).

Patients controlled with insulin should receive no subcutaneous insulin on the day of the procedure. An IV infusion of GKI (e.g. 500 ml 10% glucose with 10 mmol potassium chloride and 15 U insulin at 100 ml/hour) should be commenced before the procedure and continued until a normal diet and subcutaneous insulin can be restarted safely. The blood glucose level should be checked at least every 2 hours using one of the commercially available bedside test strips. Depending on the result, the amount of insulin may require adjustment (if plasma glucose >11 mmol/l, increase insulin to 20 U; if <6.5 mmol/l, decrease to 10 U).

Other drug therapy

In general terms, there is no need for other drug therapy to be discontinued or changed. Even long-term steroid therapy is unlikely to need enhancement, although the need for this should be reviewed in the event of a major complication, especially significant myocardial infarction (MI) and/or emergency coronary artery bypass graft surgery (CABG).

CONSENT[8]

In an emergency, if consent cannot be obtained, medical treatment may be provided to anyone who needs it, provided that the treatment is limited to what is immediately necessary to save life or avoid significant deterioration in the patient's health. With this exception, an interventional cardiological procedure should not be performed without the patient giving his/her informed consent. This implies a two-stage process, involving the provision of information to the patient, who then decides voluntarily whether or not to consent to undergo the proposed procedure.

The information which a patient wants or ought to know, before deciding whether to consent to an interventional cardiological procedure, should include:

- Details of the diagnosis and prognosis, including the likely prognosis if the proposed treatment is not carried out.
- Other options for treatment of his/her condition, including the option not to treat.
- The purpose of the proposed procedure; details of exactly what is involved (including the likely duration of the procedure and the hospital stay).
- Details of what he/she might experience during or after the procedure (e.g. 'will it hurt?'), including a discussion of the risks and the probability of success.
- Advice about whether any part of the proposed procedure is experimental.
- The name of the doctor who will have overall responsibility for the treatment.
- Whether doctors in training will be involved.
- A reminder that a patient can change his/her mind about a decision at any time and has a right to seek a second opinion.

It is important to ensure that this information is provided in such a way that the patient has sufficient time to consider it carefully and ask questions before giving consent. In practical terms, it may well be the case that information is given in stages, sometimes by different people working in different institutions. For instance, a patient may be given information about his/her cardiac condition (and a possible need for an invasive procedure) after coronary angiography performed by a physician/cardiologist working in a District General Hospital (DGH). Staff at the Regional Cardiac Centre might then provide further information about the proposed procedure, both before and at the time of the patient's admission for that procedure. It is important that any information given is both consistent and accurate. Medical staff performing interventional procedures should provide their audited results to colleagues in their referring DGHs.[9] It is also important that the facts provided are relevant to the patient's particular clinical situation. For example, it would be misleading to cite an *average* risk of death during coronary angioplasty as <1% when talking to a patient (or his/her relatives) about performing coronary angioplasty as treatment for cardiogenic shock following acute myocardial infarction – in this fortunately rare clinical situation, the likelihood of survival is considerably less than 99%!

Provided that the patient agrees, especially in high-risk clinical situations, it may well be appropriate to provide information about the proposed procedure to the next of kin (and/or other relatives/friends). In the worst case scenario, it will not be the patient who will be asking what went wrong and why!

Ideally the doctor undertaking the procedure should discuss it with the patient and obtain consent, but if this is not practicable, the task can be delegated to another person, provided that he/she is suitably trained and qualified and has sufficient knowledge of the proposed procedure and its risks.

Although in an emergency a patient can indicate their informed consent orally, it is good clinical practice to make a routine of obtaining

written consent for a cardiac interventional procedure. Following
appropriate discussion, the patient should be asked to give consent for the
treatment of any complications which may arise (e.g. emergency CABG).
It is also important to ascertain whether there any procedures to which the
patient would object and which, therefore, should *not* be performed: the
consent form should be worded appropriately. Most institutions have
special consent forms for Jehovah's witnesses, whose religious beliefs
preclude the transfusion of blood or blood products.

ANTICIPATION

Before and during of a cardiac laboratory procedure, it is imperative for
the interventional cardiologist to maintain an air of calm and cheerful
optimism, as uncertainty will quickly be detected by other members of
staff and the patient, with potentially unfortunate consequences. In reality
it is important to be thinking 'one step ahead' as anticipation of possible
problems is a vital step towards preventing them or at least dealing with
them swiftly and efficiently if/when they occur. While almost anything *can*
happen to any patient, some are especially vulnerable to particular
problems, and appropriate prophylactic measures should be undertaken.

All patients

The 'easy procedure' can only be defined in retrospect and one should
never assume that an apparently straightforward procedure will
necessarily be so. An interventional procedure should only be undertaken
by, or under the direct supervision of, a trained operator, with ancillary
staff (nurses, technicians and radiographers) who experience a sufficient
number of cases in their centre to ensure personal and institutional
competence. It is also vital that the procedure is carried out in a fully
equipped cardiac catheter laboratory, with an adequate range of
equipment and drugs available at all times. This must include *full* facilities
for cardiopulmonary resuscitation, including an intra-aortic balloon
pump. There can be no place for a 'quick angioplasty' performed by an
inexperienced operator in an ill-equipped location.[9]

Most patients

Although emergency CABG is now required in less than 1% of all
reported PTCA procedures performed in the UK, the possibility of surgical
intervention should be anticipated in all but a very small subgroup of
patients in whom a decision is made before the procedure that emergency
CABG would be inappropriate. In practical terms this means that
coronary interventional procedures should be carried out on patients who
have given informed consent for CABG if it should be deemed necessary
and have donated a blood sample for blood grouping ± formal cross-
matching. In other than emergency situations, patients should undergo a
3-hour liquid fast and a 6-hour solid fast before the procedure. The
arrangements for surgical cover for such procedures will vary according to

local conditions, but the generally accepted national guideline is that it must be possible to establish cardiopulmonary bypass within 90 minutes of the referral being made to the cardiac surgical service.[9]

Some patients

It can be anticipated that patients with significant impairment of left ventricular (LV) systolic function may experience considerable haemodynamic deterioration during a cardiac interventional procedure, especially if this is prolonged or complex. If such a procedure is to be performed, systemic circulatory support, most often with intra-aortic balloon pump (IABP) counterpulsation should be used or at least on standby.

Although no patient is immune from the development of 'contrast nephropathy', patients with pre-existing renal dysfunction are especially vulnerable. In such patients, measures which may help to prevent the development of this condition[6] include:

- Minimising the volume of contrast medium used.
- Avoiding concomitant use of other nephrotoxic drugs (especially non-steroidal anti-inflammatory drugs).
- Ensuring adequate hydration (this usually implies the administration of IV fluid to a fasting patient).
- The use of low-osmolar non-ionic contrast media, especially iodixanol (Visipaque®).

A history of 'allergy' to contrast media is often unconfirmed on checking. Serious reactions are unusual following arterial administration, but should be anticipated in patients with a confirmed history of anaphylactic reactions during previous procedures. Pre-treatment with prednisolone 40–60 mg daily, preferably for 3–4 days, may be helpful. In an emergency, hydrocortisone 200 mg IV immediately before the procedure, repeated 4-hourly, is a reasonable alternative. Although chlorpheniramine is often given in addition, there is no convincing evidence that it is of value.

Finally, as has already been stated, patients taking oral anticoagulant therapy are at increased risk of haemorrhage, especially from the vascular access site. A number of measures may lessen this risk, including the use of small-calibre sheaths, conservative heparin dosing and selective or routine use of arterial closure devices and/or pneumatic compression systems.

REFERENCES

1. Brookes CIO, Sigwart U. Taming platelets in coronary stenting: ticlopidine out, clopidogrel in? *Heart* 1999;82:651–53.

2. Blumenthal RS, Wolff MR, Resar JR *et al*. Preprocedural anticoagulation does not reduce angioplasty heparin requirements. *Am Heart J* 1993;125:1221–5.

3. FRISC II Investigators. Invasive compared with non-invasive treatment in unstable coronary-artery disease: FRISC II prospective randomised multicentre study. *Lancet* 1999;354:708–715.

4. Topol EJ, Byzova TV, Plow EF. Platelet GPIIb–IIIa blockers. *Lancet* 1999;353:227–31.

5. Gill GV, Albert KGMM. The care of the diabetic patient during surgery. In: Alberti KGMM, Zimmet P, DeFronzo RA *et al.* (eds) *International textbook of diabetes mellitus*, 2nd edn. Chichester: John Wiley, 1997, pp. 1243–53.

6. Ansell G. Complications of intravascular iodinated contrast media. In: Ansell G, Bettman MA, Kaufman JA *et al.* (eds) *Complications in diagnostic imaging and interventional radiology*, 3rd edn. Cambridge, MA: Blackwell Science, 1996, pp. 245–300.

7. Heupler FA. Guidelines for performing angiography in patients taking metformin. *Cathet Cardiovasc Diag* 1998;43:121–3.

8. General Medical Council. Seeking patients' consent: the ethical considerations. London: General Medical Council, 1998.

9. Joint working group on coronary angioplasty of the British Cardiac Society and British Cardiovascular Intervention Society. Coronary angioplasty: guidelines for good practice and training. *Heart* 2000;83:224–35.

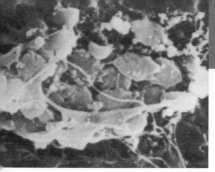

4

Pathology of balloon dilatation and restenosis

DAVID H. ROBERTS

KEY POINTS

- Changes in coronary arteries of patients undergoing PCTA are divided into those observed early (acute) and those observed late (chronic).

- Acute changes as a result of balloon injury are caused by plaque fracture, plaque compression or balloon stretching.

- Balloon injury to atherosclerotic plaque produces various angiographic appearances.

- Chronic changes are a result of healing at the angioplasty site which may change luminal size, leading to restenosis.

- Restenosis occurs in nearly all coronary lesions following intervention.

- IVUS has shown that the amount of residual plaque tissue after coronary intervention is an important predictor of restenosis.

Morphological and histological changes in coronary arteries of patients undergoing percutaneous transluminal dilatation may be divided into two categories.

1. those observed early (acute) (<30 days) after the procedure and
2. those observed late (chronic) (>30 days).

EARLY (ACUTE) CHANGES (Fig. 4.1)

Mechanisms(s) of balloon injury

The majority of atherosclerotic plaques in human coronary arteries are composed of dense fibrocollagenous tissues with varying amounts of calcific deposits and small amounts of intracellular/extracellular lipid ('hard plaques'). The major mechanism of balloon dilatation in such lesions is plaque fracture with intimal cracks or tears extending from the endothelium for variable depths. Fracturing improves vessel patency by creating additional channels for coronary blood flow. Variable degrees of penetration into the vessel media occur (often through the internal elastic lamina) and can produce dissection. This can result in vessel closure.

Plaque compression does not play a major role in balloon dilatation unless the atherosclerotic plaque is composed almost entirely of lipid-laden foam cells without dense collagen and calcific deposits i.e. 'soft plaques'.

Balloon stretching of a plaque-free wall segment can also occur resulting in an initial increase in lumen diameter and cross-sectional area, but gradual relaxation of the overstretched elastic segment reduces the

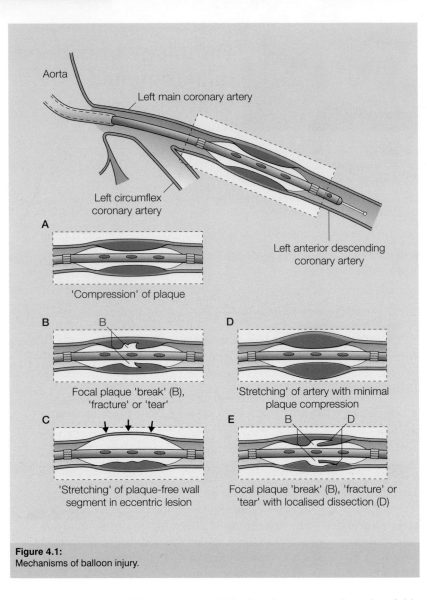

Figure 4.1:
Mechanisms of balloon injury.

lumen back to its predilatation state while the plaque expands and unfolds into the lumen. In addition the normal coronary vessel wall is capable of dynamically reacting to dilatation through various humoral or neurogenic stimuli, producing spasm in the disease-free segments. Such spasm can lead to abrupt closure or severe luminal narrowing (usually responding to intracoronary injection of a nitrate or calcium antagonist).

Angiographic patterns of balloon injury

The morphological patterns from balloon injury to atherosclerotic plaque produce various angiographic appearances. These range from 'no change' following balloon inflation (in densely calcified lesions for example) through to smooth-walled 'stent-like' appearances in soft plaque lesions. Other angiographic appearances can occur:

■ Intraluminal 'haziness' (due to intimal irregularity ± adherent thrombus).

■ Intimal flaps or dissections. Dissections may be localised or extensive with intramural contrast material extending anterograde or retrograde from the dilatation site.

■ Extravasation of contrast material following adventitial disruption, producing coronary staining or even leakage into the pericardium (perforation).

■ Coronary spasm in 'disease-free' vessel wall, as already described.

LATE (CHRONIC) CHANGES

Healing and repair changes at the angioplasty site remodel the atherosclerotic plaque. The healing process may increase or decrease luminal size, the latter leading to restenosis.

Coronary restenosis

Restenosis has been described as the 'Achilles' heel' of the interventional cardiologist, affecting patient morbidity and resulting in additional health-care expenditure. It occurs to a variable extent in virtually all coronary lesions following intervention, usually within 3–6 months. It is usually reported by angiographic criteria or on recurrent symptoms although the correlation between these two is often poor.

Angiographic restenosis

Although a continuous variable with a Gaussian distribution, many angiographic definitions view restenosis as a dichotomous event, i.e. either present or absent. The most common such definition is a stenosis diameter (DS) >50% at follow-up. Several others exist (Table 4.1), which if used,

TABLE 4.1 – ANGIOGRAPHIC DEFINITIONS OF RESTENOSIS

EMORY
Diameter stenosis ≥ 50% at follow-up.
NHLBI I
An increase in diameter stenosis >30% at follow-up (compared to immediately after intervention).
NHLBI II
Residual stenosis <50% after PTCA increasing to diameter stenosis ≥ 70% at follow-up.
NHLBI III
An increase in diameter stenosis at follow-up to within 10% of the diameter stenosis before PTCA.
NHLBI IV
A >50% loss of the initial gain achieved after PTCA.
THORAXCENTER IIA
>0.72 mm lumen loss at follow-up.
From the New Manual of Interventional Cardiology, 1996.

NHLBI: National Heart, Lung and Blood Institute.

can result in inconsistencies in reported data. A restenosis rate of 30% at 3 months, following balloon angioplasty (PTCA) is a convenient figure to give to patients.

Expressing DS% or minimal lumen diameter (MLD) as a cummulative distribution curve (Fig. 4.2) give a better visual estimate of changes in lumen diameter and allows more effective comparisons between different interventions in clinical trials.

It is also important to quantify the relationship between MLD prior to intervention, immediately afterwards and during follow up, in terms of acute gain and late loss (Fig. 4.3). Acute gain is defined as the difference in lumen diameter before and immediately after intervention with late loss defined as the difference in lumen diameter after intervention and at

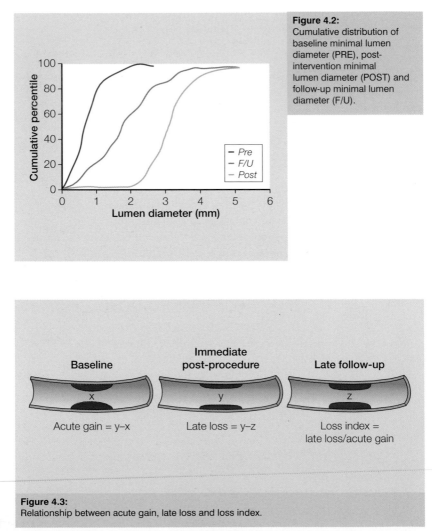

Figure 4.2:
Cumulative distribution of baseline minimal lumen diameter (PRE), post-intervention minimal lumen diameter (POST) and follow-up minimal lumen diameter (F/U).

Figure 4.3:
Relationship between acute gain, late loss and loss index.

follow-up (usually 6 months later). Several studies have shown that for every 1 mm of acute gain in lumen diameter, 50% (i.e. 0.5 mm) is lost over 3–6 months. The loss index is a numerical description of this relationship, defined as late loss divided by acute gain; a typical loss index is 0.5.

Clinical restenosis

Recurrent angina within 3–6 months following PTCA is the usual manifestation of restenosis while myocardial infarction and sudden death are fortunately rare. Published trials often refer to target lesion revascularisation (TLR) as a clinical endpoint for restenosis. This is defined as the need for repeat revascularisation of the original lesion based on recurrent symptoms and a positive exercise test.

Pathophysiology of restenosis

Restenosis is a response to vascular injury through several mechanisms including histopathological changes which lead to neointimal hyperplasia. Early hopes that alternative technologies to PTCA (rotational atherectomy, for example) would leave a smoother residual lumen and cause less injury are unfounded. The neointimal response and restenosis rates are at least as high as with PTCA.

The lesions of restenosis differs distinctly from the original atherosclerotic disease both in time, course of development as well as histopathological appearance. In contrast to atheromatous lesions, restenotic segments consist of cells and interstitial material resembling normal connective tissue with smooth muscle involvement. Data from porcine coronary artery injury has shown that the initial haemostatic changes (platelet activation and deposition with thrombus formation) progress to cellular infiltration of monocytes (becoming macrophages) and lymphocytes from the lumen side of the injured artery. In the final healing phase (day 8 onwards following coronary intervention), these cells proliferate towards the injured media, resorbing residual thrombus with replacement by neointimal cells. Smooth muscle cell migration and proliferation also occurs at this time. These cells produce extracellular matrix, which is the main component of the restenotic process (Figs 4.4–4.6).

There are other components to the restenotic process. Elastic recoil is the difference in vessel diameter during balloon expansion and subsequent deflation. As already described most recoil occurs within 30 minutes of PTCA although a 20% lumen loss occurs in the following 24–48 hours. Further reductions in vessel diameter can occur up to 3 months following PTCA due to shrinkage of the vessel wall from scar contraction within the vessel layers. This is called negative remodelling and has been demonstrated on serial intravascular ultrasound (IVUS) studies. Elastic recoil can result in significant decreases in cross-sectional area, which is associated with a high incidence of restenosis.

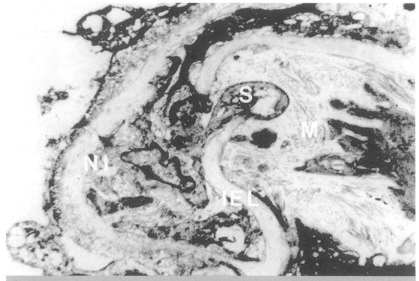

Figure 4.4:
Progress of smooth muscle cell (S) from media (M) to new intima (NI) through the damaged internal elastic lamina (IEL) in a balloon injured artery. Once in the new intima the smooth muscle cell proliferates leading to restenosis. (Courtesy of Dr A.H. Gershlick).

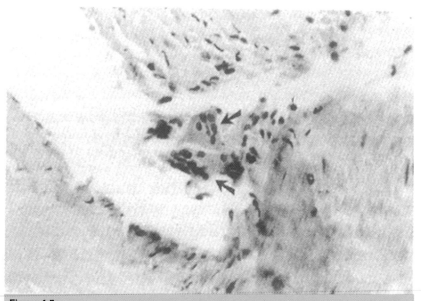

Figure 4.5:
Changes after stent implantation demonstrating the inflammatory nature of stent implantation, with multinucleate giant cells. (Courtesy of Dr A.H. Gershlick.)

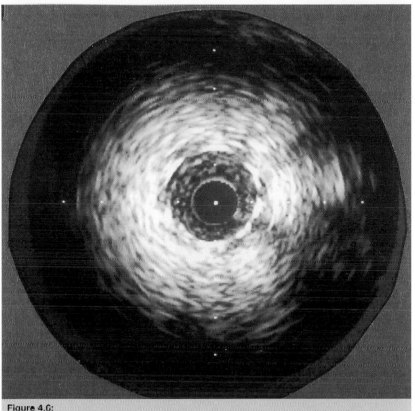

Figure 4.6:
IVUS image showing intimal hyperplasia (low echogenic material) inside fully expanded stent lumen.

Predictors of restenosis

IVUS studies have also shown that the amount of residual plaque tissue after coronary intervention is an important predictor of restenosis. Studies using directional coronary atherectomy have shown that if sufficient plaque tissue can be removed to give a lumen size similar to that of a well expanded stent, a significant reduction in restenosis rate occurs.

There are several angiographic variables associated with increased risk of restenosis (Table 4.2). Clinical variables associated with increased risk

TABLE 4.2 – ANGIOGRAPHIC VARIABLES ASSOCIATED WITH INCREASED RISK OF RESTENOSIS FOLLOWING PTCA

- Long diffuse lesions
- Lesions in saphenous vein grafts
- Ostial stenosis
- Chronic total occlusions
- Small calibre vessels
- Bifurcation lesions
- Proximal left anterior descending lesions

of restenosis are recent onset angina, unstable angina, diabetes mellitus and patients receiving chronic renal dialysis. Recent randomised trials have suggested that the platelet glycoprotein IIb/IIIa receptor inhibitor, abciximab reduces restenosis (possibly by plaque stabilisation) and should be considered in these higher risk groups.

A stent reduces or prevents elastic recoil so that a larger lumen is initially obtained. Two landmark randomised trials, Benestent (Belgium, Netherlands Stent Trial) and Stress (Stent Restenosis Study) have shown significantly reduced restenosis rates with elective single-stent deployment versus PTCA in de novo lesions of native coronary arteries, i.e. an inverse relationship exists between post-procedural lumen diameter and restenosis. After stenting, intimal hyperplasia is actually greater than following PTCA, but the larger initial lumen outways late loss at 6 months, resulting in less restenosis.

Instent restenosis

As the scaffolding properties of a fully expanded stent prevent elastic recoil and shrinkage from negative remodelling, the bulk of instent restenosis consists of an inflammatory process leading to smooth muscle cell proliferation and the production of extra cellular matrix (neointimal tissue), (Fig. 4.4) which is best demonstrated in clinical practice by IVUS (Fig. 4.6).

Several pathological factors influence the degree of instent restenosis. The depth of vascular wall damage and radial strain produced by the stent are influential and over-expansion of the stent may produce a greater neointimal response. Variations in stent design (nitinol versus stainless steel; coil versus slotted tube) confer little benefit but stent coatings (e.g. phosphoryl choline or carbon) may have a role in modifying the restenotic process.

In every-day clinical practice, factors which increase the risk of instent restenosis include:

- Underexpansion of the stent in relation to the reference diameter of the vessel treated (an MLD <3.0 mm).
- Stenting in small diameter vessels (therefore more common in females).
- Placement of long stents or multiple stents.
- Diabetes mellitus.

While randomised trials have shown stenting is preferable to PTCA for treatment in saphenous vein grafts, restenotic lesions and total occlusion it should also be remembered the rate of instent restenosis is higher in these patient groups than in the stented group of the Benestent and Stress trials.

The Washington Hospital Medical Centre has used IVUS plus angiography to characterise the site and type of instent restenosis. They define the site of instent restenosis as focal (<1.0 cm), intrastent, proliferative (beyond stent margins) or total occlusion. The site of instent restenosis is an important factor in deciding the best treatment for this condition.

Current strategies for the treatment of instent restenosis include PTCA (including Cutting Balloon, Chapter 13), repeat stent deployment, debulking techniques, e.g. rotablator, to remove the formed tissue (which are described in Chapters 6 and 10) and techniques to prevent the initial smooth muscle cell response, e.g. radiation (brachytherapy in Chapter 16).

FURTHER READING

1. Freed M, Grimes C, Safian RD. The new manual of interventional cardiology. Birmingham, Michigan: Physicians' Press, 1996.

2. Holmes Jr DR, Vliestra RE, Smith HC et al. Restenosis after percutaneous transluminal coronary angioplasty (PTCA): A report from the PTCA Registry of the National Heart, Lung and Blood Institute. Am J Cardiol 1984;53 (Suppl.):77C–81C.

3. van Beusekom HM, van der Giessen WJ, van Suylen R et al. Histology after stenting of human saphenous vein bypass grafts; observations from surgically excised grafts 3–320 days after stent implantation. J Am Coll Cardiol 1993;21:45–54.

4. Garratt K, Edwards W, Kaufmann U et al. Differential histophathology of primary atherosclerotic and restenotic lesions in coronary arteries and saphenous vein bypass grafts: analysis of tissue obtained from 73 patients by directional atherectomy. J Am Coll Cardiol 1991;17:442–8.

5. Gershlick AH, Baron J. Dealing with instent restenosis. Heart 1998;79:319–23.

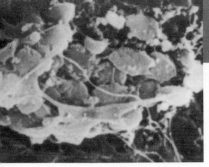

5

Anti-thrombotic pharmacology and angioplasty

ANTHONY GERSHLICK

Platelet-initiated thrombus plays a central role in the pathogenesis of coronary artery disease, especially in the acute coronary syndromes (unstable angina, non-Q wave myocardial infarction and acute MI). Evidence from animal studies, examination of post-mortem material, angioscopic investigations, laboratory markers of platelet activation and the efficacy of antiplatelet drugs have all indicated that platelets are central to thrombotic events, and that they may also play an important role in restenosis through the release of potent vasoactive, prothrombotic, inflammatory and mitogenic factors.

The sequence of events following vessel wall damage

Normal haemostasis is designed to prevent fatal bleeding. When the integrity of the blood vessel wall becomes disrupted mechanisms are initiated to reduce blood loss. The normal vessel wall is lined by non-thrombogenic endothelium, which covers and protects the flowing blood from sub-endothelial pro-thrombogenic collagen and myofibrils. The endothelium is rendered non-thrombogenic by the presence of releasable platelet inhibitors such as prostacyclin and nitric oxide from within the endothelial cells. In atheromatous vessels the balance is tipped towards the prothrombotic state, partly because the lesion induces alterations in local flow with changes in shear rate and because of release of platelet agonists such as adenosine diphosphate (ADP) from red blood cells. The endothelium covering the atheroma is also structurally abnormal being more 'crazy-paving' in shape than cliptoid and the function of the cells has been shown to be abnormal with platelets and white cells adhering to the surface as well as there being craters present (Fig. 5.1). Lower levels of non-thrombogenic mediators such as tPA have also been shown to be present in plaque. The plaque is vulnerable at its shoulders where the cap meets the main body of the lesion. The role of metalloproteinase enzymes and the function of the smooth muscle cells at the cap junction as a cause of potential plaque weakness and disruption is currently the focus of a number of research programmes. Once disrupted the plaque may be more thrombogenic than normal vessel wall. Complex plaque contains cholesterol crystals, fibroblasts, areas of calcification and degenerated red blood cells as well as collagen and thrombin, all of which promote platelet deposition and thrombus formation. The role of platelet-rich thrombus in the generation of the acute coronary syndromes is well recognised. Taking **41** all of the above into account it is perhaps not surprising that angioplasty-induced plaque disruption is a very prothrombotic procedure and without the use of anti-thrombotic agents coronary occlusion would render angioplasty unacceptable. Stents have been shown to activate platelets (Fig. 5.2)[1] and their surface to become covered by a monolayer within 30 seconds (Fig. 5.3). Occlusion rates of up to 20% that were reported in

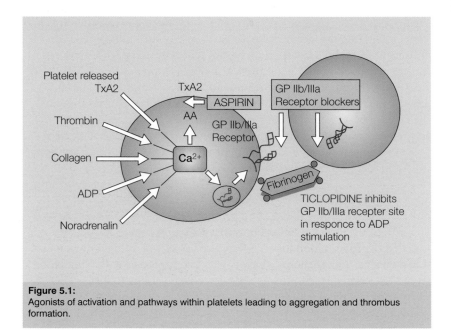

Figure 5.1:
Agonists of activation and pathways within platelets leading to aggregation and thrombus formation.

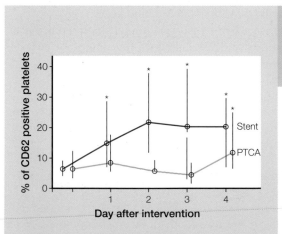

Figure 5.2:
Platelets are activated to a greater degree after stenting than after balloon angioplasty (from Schomig[7] © New England Journal of Medicine).

the early days of stenting meant that there needed to be improvements in non-thrombotic strategies.

Platelet physiology

Exposure of a damaged endothelial cell surface (such as a ruptured atherosclerotic plaque) causes platelets to adhere and to recruit further platelets and haemostatic factors to form a thrombotic plug via a finely balanced sequence of events (Fig. 5.4). Under conditions of relatively high shear (as is present in normal flowing blood) platelets bind to von Willebrand factor (VWF) via the glycoprotein (GP)Iba receptor on their surface. Exposure to vessel collagen and to thrombin (generated locally by

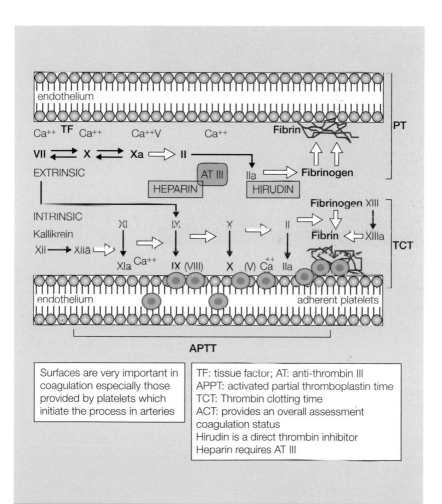

Surfaces are very important in coagulation especially those provided by platelets which initiate the process in arteries	TF: tissue factor; AT: anti-thrombin III APPT: activated partial thromboplastin time TCT: Thrombin clotting time ACT: provides an overall assessment coagulation status Hirudin is a direct thrombin inhibitor Heparin requires AT III

Figure 5.3:
The development of thrombus within an artery.

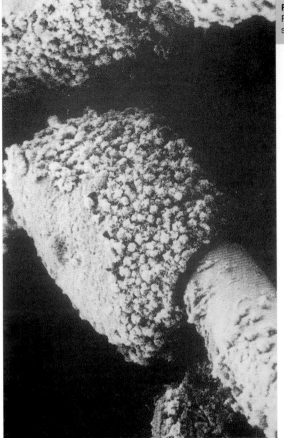

Figure 5.4:
Platelets adhere to stent struts within 30 seconds.

interaction of exposed tissue factor with plasma clotting factors), causes activation of the platelets which leads to a conformational change in the GPIIb–IIIa receptor complex, allowing it to bind fibrinogen and recruit further platelets to the growing thrombus. Platelet activation can be augmented by the additive effects of epinephrine, and enhanced by ADP and thromboxane A_2 released from activated platelets. As the thrombus develops and blood flow declines, the adhesion of platelets to the vessel wall may be enhanced by interactions between additional platelet membrane glycoprotein complexes; GPIa–IIa with vessel wall collagen, GPIIb–IIIa with fibrinogen or VWF, GP1c'IIa (VLA5) with fibronectin and laminin, and the avb3 complex with vitronectin. Platelet activation is accompanied by release of a range of potent vasoactive, pro- and anti-thrombotic factors that contribute to the growing thrombotic plug. In addition adherent platelets activated by a combination of collagen and thrombin undergo changes in the orientation of the plasma membrane causing anionic phospholipids (predominantly phosphatidyl serine) to flip to the outer phospholipid bilayer, producing a negatively charged surface for the formation of the tenase and prothrombinase complexes (clotting factors IXa–VIIIa and Xa–Va respectively). This leads to a local increase in thrombin generation, enhancing the formation of the fibrin clot. Finally, exposure of P-selectin and activated GPIIb–IIIa on the platelet surface allows platelets to bind to leucocytes, recruiting granulocytes and monocytes into the growing thrombus.

Thrombus formation

Damage to the vessel wall initiates thrombus formation. While platelets play a major role, other processes such as release of tissue factor from the vessel wall are important by initiating the extrinsic pathway of coagulation. The final common pathway is well described and the end result of thrombin formation and fibrin depostion is to produce a mesh of platelets, white cells, red blood cells and fibrin which in the presence of luminal narrowing (be this residual plaque or disrupted intima) results in vessel occlusion. The established pathways and the points of potential therapeutic targeting are shown in Fig. 5.4. At the most basic level the control of pro-coagulation during percutaneous coronary intervention (PCI) is dependent on administration of heparin. Monitoring of heparin through determination of the activated partial thromboplastin time (APTT) may be sufficient, but if other agents such as glycoprotein IIb/IIIa receptor blockers are used activated clotting time (ACT) provides a better overall assessment.

Failure to establish laminar flow may be an important in promoting thrombus formation. Thus well deployed stents with good apposition to the vessel wall are less likely to be the nidus for thrombus formation.

Targeting platelet mediated pathways

The thrombotic process following vessel wall damage is initiated by platelet deposition, and activation and subsequent involvment of platelets in coagulation pathways. This makes the platelet an important target for therapeutic strategies. There are a plethora of platelet agonist-mediated signalling pathways as well as adhesive reactions which offer a wide range of potential targets for antiplatelet therapy (Fig. 5.5).

ANTIPLATELET AGENTS

Aspirin

Aspirin is a potent inhibitor of platelet cyclo-oxgenase, an enzyme that converts arachidonic acid to thromboxane A_2, a potent platelet agonist. The effects of aspirin are seen most markedly when platelets are stimulated with weaker agonists such as ADP, or when TxA_2 is generated as a consequence of platelet–platelet aggregation. More powerful agonists such as thrombin and collagen both of which are exposed following balloon damage to the vessel wall, although potent stimulators of the arachidonic acid pathway, do not require thromboxane A_2 generation to

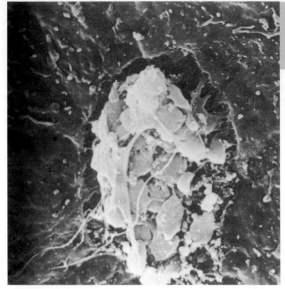

Figure 5.5:
Platelet-rich thrombus, fibrin and white cells adherent to region of de-endothelialised artery.

exert their full agonist effect. Aspirin has been available for over a hundred years and is, for most patients, the agent of choice for first-line therapy, but is not powerful enough an inhibitor on its own. It is well tolerated with few side effects.

During the 1980s there was great debate concerning the 'correct' dose of aspirin since at high doses it inhibits the cyclo-oxygenase in vascular endothelial cells, leading to a reduction in the release of the anti-aggregatory factor, prostacyclin (PGI_2), from the vessel wall. Doses of around 100 mg were found, by Wallentin[2] and others, to inhibit production of TxA_2 in platelets whilst preserving prostacyclin generation by the endothelium. Most patients now receive between 75 and 150 mg aspirin per day, depending on whether they have chronic stable angina or whether it is being given after acute infarction. There are, however, little data to support the correct dose for PCI. Since much of the data on dose comes from non-interventional studies and as balloon angioplasty is such a powerful stimulant to thrombus formation, there is a case to be made for the minimum dose of 300 mg being given with the pre-medication and during follow-up.

Non-aspirin antiplatelet agents
Although aspirin has been shown in large retrospective analysis[3] to be effective in reducing thrombotic events in a wide group of patients, on an individual patient basis it is only partially effective. This is firstly because aspirin affects only one of the various pathways of platelet activation and so it may not be effective in all cases, particularly where the thrombotic stimulus is potent (e.g. through angioplasty generation of collagen and thrombin) which can activate the platelet bypassing the arachidonic acid

pathway. Added to this, in a subset of patients the phenomenon of aspirin insensitivity/aspirin resistance is increasingly recognised. These factors have led to a search for alternative antiplatelet agents.

Ticlopidine/Clopidogrel

Both ticlopidine which has been known for some time, and its more potent chemical analogue clopidogrel, act specifically on ADP-mediated platelet activation. These drugs are thienopyridine derivatives that are metabolised in the liver, but the nature and action of their active metabolites remains unclear. Clopidogrel has approximately six times the potency of ticlopidine and lacks many of its adverse effects on the bone marrow and the GI system. Metabolites of these drugs appear in the circulation 3 hours after treatment and although is has been reported that 3 days are required for the antiplatelet effect to be seen, this has not been borne out in clinical practice. Their specificity for ADP-induced platelet activation means they are potentially of greatest benefit in conditions where shear-stress is a primary factor in causing platelet activation, which may account for the beneficial effects of the drugs in preventing acute occlusion in association with stenting. High shear-stress can activate platelets directly by a mechanism that has an absolute requirement for ADP. In addition, high shear-stress can cause release of ADP from damaged red cells.

A number of clinical studies have assessed the value of ticlopidine, predominantly in the setting of thrombo-embolic stroke and post-angioplasty coronary stenting. The stroke studies suggested benefit with ticlopidine over aspirin[4,5] but side effects such as diarrhoea (15%), skin rash (5–10%) and neutropenia were more common. In a study assessing ticlopidine in unstable angina published in 1990, ticlopidine reduced the combined end-point of vascular death and non-fatal myocardial infarct by 46%.[6] It is however important to note that the control group did not receive aspirin.

Based on these studies ticlopidine was felt to be a potential alternative antiplatelet agent in those patients unable to tolerate aspirin. Its use was limited by a perceived lack of large benefit over aspirin and the higher risk of side effects especially the risk of neutropenia. The complications of stent thrombosis however reawakened interest in this drug. Shortly after stent deployment was introduced, stent thrombosis was reported in up to 20% of patients. By virtue of its nature, acute coronary stent occlusion is associated with a high incidence of major adverse cardiac events (50% myocardial infarction). It became routine therefore to treat all patients with high dose heparin, warfarin and aspirin. Rates of stent thrombosis did not actually fall merely that patients were required to stay in hospital for up to 6 days to cover the period of potential stent thrombosis and to allow the anticoagulation regimen to be adjusted. Additionally femoral artery complications were high. Routine anticoagulation was clearly not the way forward.

Ticlopidine and stenting
A number of developments in stenting altered clinical practise. Stents became more conformable and this change, together with the realisation that there was a need to achieve a good angiographic result, reduced the likelihood of a dead space existing between the stent and the vessel wall. At the same time ticlopidine was tested in the setting of stent deployment. Schomig and others showed, in the ISAR trial, that the incidence of stent thrombosis was 1.6% in those patients treated with ticlopidine compared with 5.4% in those randomised to formal anticoagulation.[7] Other investigators notably Colombo's group have shown that the combination of ticlopidine plus aspirin results in stent thrombosis rates of less than 2% compared with rates of up to 4% with aspirin alone.[8] Thus current recommendations were that patients who undergo coronary stenting should receive ticlopidine and aspirin. Although the stent thrombosis rate is now low for routine stenting it has been shown to be higher in certain patient subgroups such as those with small vessels or in those being stented against the background of acute coronary syndromes. The major adverse cardiac event rate in the STARS trial in the subgroup with small vessels was 28%. From the four trials of ticlopidine and stenting it is also clear that the stent thrombosis rate reflects the patient population risk with higher rates reported from those studies where the patients were less routine.[9]

Side effects from ticlopidine, such as neutropenia (severe < 0.45 × 109/L in 0.9% patients) and thrombocytopenia, meant that haematologic assessment was required for the duration of the course (2 weeks in low-risk patients and 4 weeks in higher risk patients). Haematologic side effects reverse with discontinuation of the drug. Rash (5–10%) and diarrhoea (15%) are other common side effects and are also reversible on discontinuation of the drug.

Clopidogrel was been developed to replace ticlopidine since side effects are less common. This agent has approximately six times the potency of ticlopidine and lacks many of its adverse effects on the bone marrow and the GI system. In the CAPRIE Study[10] 19 000 patients with atherosclerotic cardiovascular disease (ischaemic stroke, myocardial infarction) or peripheral vascular disease,) were randomised to receive either clopidogrel (75 mg) or aspirin. The incidence of significant neutropenia was similar in both groups while those receiving active treatment with clopidogrel had a small but significant reduction in combined end-point (ischaemic stroke, death or myocardial infarct) over the 3-year follow-up – 5.32% for clopidogrel and 5.83% with aspirin.

Recently a European trial has been completed that compared the safety of clopidogrel in 1000 patients receiving coronary stents (the CLASSICS trial). Patients were randomised to one of three groups – standard maintenance, clopidogrel vs loading dose and maintenance clopidogrel vs ticlopidine – all with aspirin. The results have now been published. The incidence of side effects was 9.1% in the triclopidine group, 4.6% in the combined clopidogrel group and 2.9% in the group treated with the pure loading dose of 300 mg ($p < 0.005$). The reduction in side effects was driven by a reduction in cardiological events. However, since side effects such as gastrointestinal discomfort or risks can lead to discontinuation of the drug, which in turn can lead to stent thrombosis, these findings were important.[11] Current recommendations are that to impact on stent thrombosis, 300 mg of clopidogrel are given on return to the ward following 'successful' stenting and 75 mg is administered daily thereafter for 1 month. Aspirin given as a pre-medication should be continued indefinitely. Any stents deemed not to be successfully deployed (edge tear, thrombus) are regarded at risk of thrombotic occlusion and patients tend to be treated with cath lab intravenous glycoprotein IIb/IIIa receptor blocker.

GPIIb–IIIa antagonists

Regardless of the mechanism of activation, the final common pathway for platelet aggregation is the cross-linking of platelets through fibrinogen, bound to GPIIb–IIIa receptor. Early animal studies with monoclonal antibodies (Mabs) to GPIIb–IIIa demonstrated the potent antiplatelet effects accruing from blocking the binding of fibrinogen to activated GPIIb/IIIa receptor. This has lead to a number of fibrinogen receptor antagonists in various stages of clinical application.

Abciximab (c7E3 or ReoPro), is a 'humanised' Fab fragment of a mouse Mab in which the hypervariable, antigen-specific regions of the original 7E3 mouse Mab have been genetically engineered into a human immunoglobulin Fab domain (to reduce immunogenicity and Fc-mediated effects *in vivo*). It is a potent, selective inhibitor of platelet aggregation, but in addition, its preferential specificity for the GPIIIa component of the receptor (the b3 chain of this integrin complex) gives it the potential advantage that it may also block the binding of the vitronectin receptor (avb3), thus inhibiting the binding of platelets to vitronectin in the subendothelium. Several clinical trials of ReoPro have been conducted.

The EPIC study[12] compared ReoPro bolus plus ReoPro infusion with ReoPro bolus plus placebo infusion and with placebo bolus plus placebo infusion in high-risk patients (determined by the presence of acute coronary syndrome and lesion complexity) undergoing angioplasty. The incidence of composite end-point (death, myocardial infarction, or need for unplanned intervention) at 1 month was 8.3%, 11.5% and 12.8% in the three treatment groups. The difference between ReoPro bolus and infusion and placebo bolus and infusion was significant ($p = 0.008$). Most benefit was due to the reduction in subsequent rate of enzyme-determined acute MI. Of the 2099 patients in the trial, 489 were categorised as having refractory unstable angina. In these, the difference in outcome was even more impressive with a rate of composite end point between ReoPro bolus and infusion and placebo bolus and infusion being 4.8% and 12.8% ($p = 0.012$). Again the benefit was in the incidence of enzyme-determined MI (1.8% vs 9.0%; $p = 0.0004$). Long-term follow-up up to 3 years supports continued benefit. The incidence of death, MI and need for revascularisation was 41.1% in the ReoPro group vs 47.2% in the placebo group ($p = 0.009$). The need for revascularisation was the only component of the composite end-point where the difference reached significance (34.8% vs 40.1% [$p = 0.02$]).

In the EPIC trial the combination of uncontrolled heparin plus the ReoPro resulted in an excess of bleeding in the treated group (14% vs 7%).

The EPILOG trial[13] was therefore undertaken to compare standard heparin regimen with weight adjusted heparin. A total of 4800 patients were planned but the trial was terminated at 2792 patients. At 30 days the composite end-point was reached in 11.7% of the placebo group but only in 5.2% of those receiving ReoPro in combination with weight adjusted heparin ($p < 0.001$). There was no significant difference in incidence of major bleeding between groups. These findings have influenced clinical practice, so that patients tend to be given weight adjusted heparin peri-procedurally, especially if the use of ReoPro is likely and are given no further heparin afterwards if ReoPro is administered. Sheath removal while the ReoPro is still running, has reduced bleeding complications, providing the ACT is <150 seconds.

The CAPTURE trial[14] also evaluated the effects of ReoPro on the outcome in patients with unstable angina who went on to angioplasty (18–24 hours ReoPro prior to revascularisation followed by 1 hour ReoPro post-intervention). This study was terminated early with a significant benefit in composite 30-day end-point (11.3% ReoPro vs 15.9% placebo; $p < 0.012$). One interesting and important part of the CAPTURE study was that pre-angioplasty MI (enzyme-determined) was significantly less in the treated group (0.6% vs 2.1% $p = 0.029$). However, by 6 months there was no difference between the groups.

The success of the studies of ReoPro in unstable coronary syndromes has led to this agent being tested in a number of other clinical circumstances. In addition a restrospective analysis of the EPILOG and CAPTURE data suggested that those patients who received stents did better if they had been randomised to the ReoPro group. This observation led to a prospective randomised trial which compared stent alone with stent plus ReoPro with angioplasty plus ReoPro (the EPISTENT Study).

EPISTENT: This trial[15] assessed the effect of ReoPro in the setting of routine stenting in the three groups – stent plus routine medication (control group); stent plus ReoPro; and ReoPro but no stent (ReoPro plus angioplasty group). The composite end-point (death, enzyme-determined

MI and revascularisation) was reached in 10.8%; 5.3% and 6.9% of patients respectively. The difference between stent alone and stent plus ReoPro was significant (p = 0.001), as was the difference between stent alone and angioplasty plus ReoPro (p = 0.007). This suggests that using ReoPro gives an outcome better than using a stent. It needs to be reiterated that the difference between the groups in this study, as in the previous trials, was in the incidence of enzyme determined MI (9.6% vs 4.5% (p = 0.001) vs 5.3% (p = 0.001) vs stent). The incidence of death or urgent revascularisation was not initially different between the groups. There is major debate currently as to the importance of these enzyme changes, with some believing they are merely enzyme leaks and others suggesting that they represent potent predictors of short and longer-term prognosis.

Later outcome data have recently been published[16] and suggests that later (1 year) mortality is influenced by ReoPro (8 deaths [1%] in the treated patients and 19 deaths in the placebo group [p = 0.037]. The real question is whether these differences correlate with enzyme levels at the time of procedure. Target lesion revascularisation was only reduced significantly in a diabetic subgroup of patients.

In the diabetic subgroup the composite endpoint (6-month death, myocardial infarction or target lesion revascularisation) was reached in 25.7% of stent-placebo patients (n = 173), 23.4% of balloon-ReoPro (n = 162) but in only 13.0% of stent-ReoPro patients (n = 156, p = 0.005) Death and MR rates alone were also significantly reduced; 12.7%, 7.8% and 6.2% respectively (p = 0.029).[17]

Such findings have led to ReoPro being administered in various patient groups. The EPIC and EPISTENT data suggest that all patients regarded as high risk coming to percutaneous coronary intervention (unplanned cases or those with acute coronary syndromes – non-Q wave infarcts, primary angioplasty or post-thrombotic rescue angioplasty) should receive ReoPro, initiated after formal sheath introduction. In North America this has led to rates of usage of between 50–80% of all cases. In mainland Europe and in the UK in particular, ReoPro tends to be reserved for those lesions thought to be at risk (poor stent deployment, stent thrombosis, refractory acute coronary syndrome with unfavourable lesion characteristics, multiple stents, non-reflow, rescue angioplasty, for example. Current usage ranges from <10% to 40%.

Recent assessment of the data by the National Institute of Clinical Excellence (NICE) in which ReoPro use for all PCI was supported is likely to lead to a major expansion in its use.

There are concerns that there is little benefit in routine 'cold' PCI and further direct studies are planned. With widespread use, the cost benefit will still (at £800 per patient) need to be proven.

ERASER. In the EPIC Trial there was a suggestion of longer-term benefit even after a short administration of ReoPro. Since one factor in the restenotic process is the intimal migration and proliferation of smooth muscle cells, the effect of ReoPro on this process was considered. Smooth muscle cells depend on a number of receptors for their function. One of these is the vit-ronectin receptor which contains the b3 chain (GPIIIa) of the platelet GPIIb–IIIa receptor. Since the 7E3 antibody binds preferentially to the GPIIIa component of this complex theoretically ReoPro might also influence smooth muscle cell function. This was tested in the ERASER trial. Patients ($n = 225$) were randomly allocated to stent plus ReoPro bolus plus infusion for 12 hours, stent plus ReoPro bolus plus infusion for 24 hours, or to stent plus placebo for 24 hours. At 6 months patients were assessed with the sensitive measure of intravascular ultrasound (IVUS) to determine in-stent volume which was found to be not significantly different between the groups. The conclusions to be drawn are either that GPIIb–IIIa receptor blockers do not have any effect on restenosis in man, or that longer exposure to higher concentrations of the drug is needed for an effect to be seen. Local delivery of the drug on stents has been advocated and is the target of intense current research.[18]

In the as yet unpublished RAPPORT trial 483 patients were randomised to undergo primary angioplasty with or without ReoPro. Again the end-point of death, MI and urgent target lesion revascularisation was reached in significantly less of the treated patients at 30 days (4.6% vs 12.0%; $p = 0.006$) and in this study continued benefit was seen up to 6 months.

Upcoming trials include GUSTO IV in which ReoPro will be tested as adjunctive therapy to thrombolytic treatment. Safety, and in particular bleeding rates, will be an important part of the evaluation in this study, especially in the light of the TLMI 9a and GUSTO II trials which assessed the antithrombin hirudin in a similar trial design. These studies were terminated early because of an excess of intracranial bleeding in the group of patients also receiving thrombolytic therapy.

Peptide antagonists: Fibrinogen binds to GPIIb–IIIa via a short sequence of amino acids in the fibrinogen a-chain; the RGD (arginine–glycine–alanine) sequence. Peptide analogues of this RGD sequence act as potent GPIIb–IIIa antagonists and one such, integrilin, has undergone a number of clinical trials.

IMPACT II study[19] Integrilin was tested in 4000 patients undergoing any intervention. The initial combined end-point incidence was 30–35% less in the treated group, but this benefit was not maintained except in those patients analysed according to protocol and receiving a low dose of the drug ($p = 0.035$). In the PURSUIT trial integrilin reduced the absolute rate of death or myocardial infarction by a small but significant amount (1.5%; $p = 0.042$).

Non-peptide mimetics: Many pharmaceutical companies have invested heavily in non-peptide GPIIb–IIIa antagonists in a search for agents with better stability, bioavailability and potential for oral administration. Two such agents, lami faban and tirofiban have been used in clinical trials, while others are in various stages of development.

RESTORE trial[20] Patients undergoing high-risk angioplasty were randomised to receive tirofiban or placebo. A significant benefit was seen at 2 days (38% reduction in combined end point $p = 0.005$), but this was less at 7 days (27% $p = 0.027$) and had become non significant at 30 days (16% difference).

Recently the PRISM and PRISM-PLUS investigators have published their findings.[21] In the PRISM study 3232 patients with unstable angina who were already receiving aspirin were randomised to either further treatment with heparin or tirofiban. The primary end-point was a composite of death, myocardial infarction or refactory ischaemia at 48 hours and was reached in 3.8% of those receiving tirofiban vs 5.6% in those receiving heparin (RR 0.67 95% CI 0.48–0.92). This overall benefit had been lost by 30 days (15.9% vs 17.1% NS) but mortality was lower (2.3% vs 3.6% $p = 0.02$) at this time. Bleeding side effects were similar in the two groups. In PRISM-PLUS 1915 patients were randomised to either tirofiban, heparin or tirofiban plus heparin for 72 hours during which time coronary angiography and angioplasty were undertaken after 48 hours if indicated. The tirofiban alone group were discontinued early because of an excess of mortality at 7 days, a result perhaps of rebound hypercoagulopathy due to discontinuation of heparin. The frequency of primary end-point at 7 days was lower in the group receiving tirofiban plus heparin compared with heparin alone (12.9% vs 17.9% RR 0.68 95% CI 0.53–0.88 $p = 0.004$) as it was at 30 days (18.5 vs 22.3% $p = 0.03$) and at 6 months (27.2% vs 32.1% $p = 0.02$). Rates of mortality and infarction were significantly less in the tirofiban plus heparin group at all time points.

These studies imply a benefit in patients treated medically, something that was also evident but less conspicuous in the CAPTURE study. However while benefit was shown prior to intervention it is clear that those who underwent intervention benefited most and a longer-term analysis of the outcome of those who did not receive angioplasty was not presented. Whether these agents reduce the need for intervention in unstable angina has still not been demonstrated.

Current concepts about the use of these agents have led to the following clinical applications. There are licences for the use of Integrilin and Aggrastat in patients suffering acute coronary syndromes. These patients with unstable angina or non-ST elevation myocardial infarction are now being administered these agents, since retrospective data, especially in those with recent onset, recurrent or rest pain, plus ECG changes plus Troponin T/I positivity appear to suffer less MACE. NICE have recently supported the use of these agents in such patients. Whether these patients should undergo coronary angioplasty even if they settle (almost certainly yes), when this should be or whether they should be transferred if necessary and undergo PCI during the GP IIb/IIIa administration (probably yes) is still being debated. If these patients do settle and have not undergone coronary angiography, the issue is when this should be done and whether further GP IIb/IIIa receptor blocker should be administered (perhaps ReoPro). Length of infusion, timing of sheath removal and place of subcutaneous heparin and when coronary angioplasty does not lead to PCI but perhaps to coronary surgery are issues that need to be resolved.

While these agents have a licence for use in non-PCI acute coronary syndromes a recently presented trial (ESPRIT) suggests a benefit for Integrilin in the setting of PCI (36% reduction in combined endpoint).

TARGET, the equivalent study with Aggrastat comparing it with ReoPro in all PCI has just been reported and demonstrates that Aggrastat is not as beneficial as ReoPro in the setting of PCI (Primary End Point at 30 days: Aggrastat, 7.55%; ReoPro, 6.01%; $p = 0.037$). This makes the management of patients with ACS interesting. Since GUSTO IV acute coronary syndrome (ACS) was negative, ReoPro will not be given to patients presenting with ACS, but Aggrastat or Integrilin will. Does one intervene during the infusion (counter to TARGET results) or change infusion (problems with platelet-receptor occupancy)? Currently such issues are unresolved.

There is likely to be a continuum with these agents being administered in patients undergoing PCI. Cost differences and the lower risk of bleeding with Integrilin and Aggrastat if, for example, a patient needed to undergo coronary surgery, may be important deciding issues about which agent is likely to be taken up. A direct head to head trial is unlikely.

Current understanding of cost effectiveness

The clinical problems with these agents, such as systemic bleeding, have been largely overcome and trials have clearly shown that in selected, high-risk patients, such as those undergoing angioplasty for unstable angina, or in the context of routine stenting, significant overall benefit may be obtained. Consistently the difference has been in the incidence of enzyme-determined acute myocardial infarction. Some argue that this is an important measure which determines future clinical outcome, but others are less convinced that an enzyme level of three times the upper limit of normal carries such a significant adverse prognosis. The extra cost to an angioplasty is about £800 per case, and true cost benefit analyses will be needed to justify the extra outlay in the use of these drugs. A cost benefit evaluation for the EPIC trial, using the figures of an absolute reduction in serious cardiovascular events and a relative reduction of 23% in ReoPro treated patients, calculated that the additional cost per patient remaining free from serious event over a 6-month period was Aus$13 012. Using a modelled analysis, the cost per additional life-year gained was Aus$5547 and the cost per additional event-free year was Aus$4285. Whether this represents value for money will need to be considered. Certainly there are data indicating that cost effectiveness may not be present in the small number of patients in whom surgery is required for failed angioplasty despite their being given ReoPro.

Recent data from Kereiakes *et al.* suggests in a retrospective analysis that ReoPro was associated with an average reduction in 6-month mortality of 4.9%. In higher risk patients this group have calculated the average cost per life-year gained to be $1243.[22] This is perhaps an over-optimistic figure. However, NICE have a brief to examine cost effectiveness as well as benefit and in supporting the use of these agents in high-risk acute coronary syndromes and in high-risk PCI have confirmed an acceptable cost/QALY; cost/event prevented argument. Current figures for cost/life year gained is between £7000 and £11 500. NICE have estimated the cost/QALY at about £12 000.

Delivering such agents with stents themselves is the logical way forward. If the beneficial findings that have clearly been shown *in vitro* and in models of stent thrombosis[23,24] with drug eluting stents can be reproduced in man then cost beneficial use of these agents may be achieved. The removal of the need for adjunctive therapy such as pre-procedure heparin and ticlopidine/clopidogrel may also be possible. The dose delivered locally may also be sufficient to influence smooth muscle cell activity through an effect on the vitronectin receptor as has been shown *in vitro*.[25] In future eluting stents, be this ReoPro, activated protein C, VEGF, taxol or other drug may render the stent truly non-thrombotic under any circumstances as well as non-restenosing.

Overview of GPIIb–IIIa receptor blockers

Glycoprotein IIb–IIIa receptor blockers have been established as having a beneficial impact on outcome in patients who undergo angioplasty in the setting of acute coronary syndrome. This has been most obvious with the antibody c7E3, although this is related to differences in the various trial designs. A number of questions still need to be addressed about the use of these agents, but it is highly likely they will play a major part in antiplatelet therapeutic strategies. Whether a reduction in enzyme-determined myocardial infarction is cost effective, or even has any true long-term benefit is less clear. Such markers of myocardial damage may be mere markers of other factors, such as lesion complexity, which determine adverse long-term outcome. The effect of such drugs in preventing the need for intervention and influencing the outcome of acute infarction will become clearer in the next 18 months. Current agents can only be given intravenously. Oral agents such as xemilofiban have been tested in combination with IV preparations and have been shown to be safe in phase II studies. Clinical trials of the oral agents have been published and in the main have been very disappointing. Some have been stopped early because of apparent adverse outcome in the treated group and others have shown no benefit over and above aspirin. The reasons are unclear, but may relate disappointingly to trial design or perhaps prothrombogenicity at incorrect dosing levels. Long-term use and reversal of bleeding complications have further added to the shelving for the time being of such agents being considered for clinical use. Further study has recently been terminated early however and while details will emerge in due course, the issue of safety will need to be assessed. Many new synthetic agents have long half-lives and while this is likely to mean prolonged inhibition of the ongoing pathological process, side effects such as severe bleeding are difficult to treat as transfused platelets are also be inhibited by the drug.

Newer approaches to antiplatelet therapy

Since the platelet is involved in a range of adhesive reactions, and can be activated by many naturally occurring agonists, other targets have been identified for antiplatelet therapy.

Inhibition of GPIb platelet adhesion: Since platelet adhesion is one of the earliest events in thrombus formation, attempts to block the attachment of platelets to the damaged subendothelium offers an attractive therapeutic route. As with GPIIb–IIIa, an abnormality of nature demonstrates the importance of this mechanism. Patients with Bernard–Soulier syndrome (BSS) lack the platelet membrane GPIb which anchors the platelet to VWF in the subendothelium and these patients have a severe bleeding tendency. Studies *in vitro* and in animal models, with Mabs to GPIb, and peptide analogues of the A-domain of VWF have proved interesting, but clinical trials of these agents are awaited.

Agonist receptor antagonists: Three agonist receptors on the platelet surface present themselves as potential targets; the ADP, thrombin and collagen receptors.

The platelet ADP receptor has not been identified, but it is known that ADP acts through a P2T-type receptor on the platelet surface and synthetic compounds, based on known P2T receptor antagonists have proved effective in animal studies and are currently entering Phase II and Phase III clinical trials.

The platelet thrombin receptor also proved elusive until a seven-transmembrane receptor was identified that acted both as a binding site for thrombin and as a substrate for proteolytic cleavage. However, despite early enthusiasm it has become clear that this receptor, though important, is not the only thrombin receptor on the platelet surface. Added to this, attempts to block the seven-transmembrane-domain thrombin receptor with antibodies, peptides or synthetic analogues have proved unsuccessful and at the present time most pharmaceutical companies have given up the search for a thrombin-receptor antagonist.

The collagen receptor.   The platelet has been reported to have at least four separate collagen receptors and until recently it has been hard to explain the need for this apparent multiplication of function. Evidence is now emerging that the functions of adhesion to collagen and signalling by collagen may be affected by different receptors; the GPIa–IIa complex serving as a key adhesive ligand for collagen while GPVI is the main receptor by which platelets are activated by collagen. Inhibitors of these receptors are in development and the investigation of their effects will prove interesting.

ANTITHROMBOTIC APPROACHES

Heparin

Peri-procedural heparin has been used since the early days of angioplasty. The only apparent 'controversy' has been whether to give 5000, 10 000 or 15 000 IU and under which circumstances to continue heparin as an infusion post-procedure. Some authors have explored the use of high dose heparin (300 U/kg) as a bolus to increase and maintain patency in the setting of primary angioplasty for acute infarction[26] and have shown such a strategy to have some impact. Others have attempted to address the problem of sheath removal and early ambulation by using low-dose heparin with smaller catheters. Thus Koch[27] evaluated 900 patients undergoing elective angioplasty and stenting given 5000 IU heparin and using 6 F size sheaths. There was no difference in femoral site complications (2.2%) when sheath removal was immediate with early (4 hour) mobilisation compared with 12 hour rest (2.3%).

Since there is a general tendency in current practice to use the glycoprotein IIb/IIIa receptor blockers such as ReoPro as a response to the case complications rather than proactively, it cannot be predicted which patients may require such agents. It was clear from the EPILOG trial that use of standard dose heparin resulted in excess bleeding compared with weight adjusted heparin. Thus it would seem sensible to give all patients weight adjusted heparin at the start of any procedure on the asumption that glycoprotein IIb/IIIa receptor blockers may be needed. The weight adjusted dose can be less than 100 IU/kg, but would be best adjusted by measurement of the ACT after a bolus of 50 or 75 IU/kg. The ACT should be in the range 200–250 seconds. Clearly weight adjusted heparin is of particular concern when interventional procedures are being undertaken in lighter patients. Once drugs such as ReoPro have been given, no further heparin should be administered.

Heparin has theoretical disadvantages as an anti-thrombotic (high inter-individual dose response, inability to act on clot-bound thrombin, need for endogenous co-factors, and inactivation by platelet factor 4 and heparinase). Drugs designed to overcome these limitations such as the direct thrombin inhibitor hirudin have not found a place in the setting of coronary intervention. Part of the problem relates to anticoagulant monitoring and partly to the narrow therapeutic window such agents have. The dose that provides additional benefit over heparin is not much lower than the dose that increases the risk of intracerebral haemorrhage.

Can antithrombotics influence restenosis?

Restenosis after angioplasty has been the subject of much scientific thought and the focus of many clinical trials. Rates of 30–40% meant that the process that involved recoil, negative remodelling and smooth muscle cell intimal hyperplasia required clear understanding and appropriate solutions. There have been over 50 trials, many involving anti-thrombotic agents, all of which failed to to show benefit, apart from the implication of benefit in the EPIC study. Stenting has undoubtbly had a major impact on restenosis, reducing the influences of recoil and negative remodelling, but restenosis still occurs within stents and is difficult to treat. Whether anti-thrombotic agents delivered with the stent will reduce the release of platelet derived growth factors and reduce local thrombus formation, which has been shown to become incorporated into the new intimal lesion, will need to be tested clinically.[28]

UNRESOLVED ISSUES

The following may be considered as unresolved issues:

1. High-risk stenting – are the currently available agents potent enough? Would drug eluting stents help?
2. Can antiplatelet/anti-thrombotic treatments impact on in-stent restenosis?
3. Will the use of antiplatelet agents such as the GP IIb/IIIa receptor blocker reduce or increase the need/rate of PCA? Will outcome in the short, medium or longer term be truly improved? How will we treat patients with ACS proceeding to PCI?
4. Will the combination of thrombolytic and GP IIb/IIIa receptor blocker increase the TIM 1 and 3 flow, reducing the need for rescue angioplasty?
5. Are 'smart stents' the next phase of PCI? Such stents, particularly those that elute growth factors such as VEGF[29] that encourage endothelial cell growth may reduce the need for systemic anti-thrombotic/antiplatelet agents. In particular the use of such stents including those that are heparinised or elute glycoprotein IIb/IIIa receptor blockers may be of particular value in conditions such as acute coronary symptoms or where there is excess endothelial loss (vascular brachytherapy).

REFERENCES

1. Gawaz M, Neumann FJ, Ott I *et al.* Role of activation-dependant platelet membrane glycoproteins in development of subacute occlusive coronary stent thrombosis. Coron Art Dis 1997;8:121–8.

2. Nyman I, Larsson H, Wallentin L. Prevention of serious cardiac events by low-dose aspirin in patients with silent myocardial ischaemia. Lancer 1992;340:497–501.

3. Antiplatelet Trialists' Collaboration. Collaborative overview of randomised trials of antiplatelet therapy–I; prevention of death, myocardial infarction, and stroke by prolonged antiplatelet therapy in various categories of patients. BMJ 1994; 308:81–106.

4. Gent M, Blakely JA, Easton *et al.* The Canadian American Ticlopidine Study (CATS) in thrombo-embolic stroke. Lancet 1989;I:1215–20.

5. Hass WK, Easton JD, Adams HP *et al.* A randomized trial comparing ticlopidine hydrochloride with aspirin for the prevention of stroke in high-risk patients. N Engl J Med 1989;321:501–507.

6. Balsano F, Rizzon P, Violi F *et al.* Antiplatlet treatment with ticlopidine in unstable angina. A controlled multicenter clinical trial. Circulation 1990;82:17–26.

7. Schomig A, Neuman FJ, Kastrati A *et al.* A randomised comparison of antiplatelet therapy after the placement of coronary stents. N Engl J Med 1996;334:1084–9.

8. Colombo A, Hall P, Nakamura S *et al.* Intracoronary stenting without anticoagulation accomplished with intravascular ultrasound guidance. Circulation 1995;1676–88.

9. Bertrand M, Legrand V, Boland J *et al.* Full anticoagulation versus ticlopidine plus aspirin after stent implantation: A randomised multicenter European trial. Circulation 1996;94:1–685 (Abstract).

10. CAPRIE Steering Committee. A randomised, blinded trial of clopidogrel versus aspirin in patients at risk of ischaemic events (CAPRIE). Lancert 1996;348:1329–39.

11. Bertrand M, Hans-Jurgen R, Urban P, Gershlick AH. Double blind study of the safety of clopidogrel with and without a loading dose in combination with aspirin compared to ticlopidine in combination with aspirin after coronary stenting. Circulation 2000;102:624–9.

12. Lincoff AM, Califf RM, Anderson KM *et al.* Evidence for prevention of death and myocardial infarction with platelet membrane glycoprotein IIb/IIIa receptor blockade by abciximab (c7E3 Fab) among patients with unstable angina undergoing percutaneous coronary revascularization. EPIC Investigators JACC 1997;30:149–56.

13. Anonymous. Platelet glycoprotein IIb/IIIa receptor blockade and low-dose heparin during percutaneous coronary revascularization. The EPILOG Investigators. New Engl J Med 1997;336:1689–96.

14. Anonymous. Randomised placebo-controlled trial of abciximab before and during coronary intervention in refractory unstable angina: the CAPTURE Study. Lancet 1997;349:1429–35.

15. Anonymous. Randomised, placebo controlled and balloon-angioplasty-controlled trial to assess the safety of coronary stenting with the use of platelet glycoprotein IIb/IIIa blockade. The EPISTENT investigators. Lancet 1998;ii:87–92.

16. Cho L, Topol EJ, Balog C *et al*. Clinical benefit of glycoprotein IIb/IIIa blockade with Abciximab is independent of gender: pooled analysis from EPIC, EPILOG and EPISTENT trials. Evaluation of 7E3 for the Prevention of ischemic complications. Evaluation in percutaneous transluminal coronary angioplasty to improve long-term outcome with Abciximab GP IIb/IIIa blockade. Evaluation of Platelet IIb/IIIa inhibitor for stent. J Am Coll Cardiol 2000;36(2):381–6.

17. Marso SP, Lincoff AM, Ellis SG *et al*. Optimizing the percutaneous interventional outcomes for patients with diabetes mellitus: results of the EPISTENT (Evaluation of platelet IIb/IIIa inhibitor for stenting trial) diabetic substudy. Circulation 1999;100(25):2477–84.

18. Aggarwal RK, Ireland DC, Azrin MA, Ezekowitz MD, De Bono D, Gershlick AH. Antithrombotic potential of polymer-coated stents eluting platelet glycoprotein IIb/IIIa receptor antibody. Circulation 1996;94:3311–17.

19. Tcheng JE. Impact of eptifibatide on early ischemic events in acute ischemic coronary syndromes: a review of the IMPACT II trial. Integrilin to minimize platelet aggregation and coronary thrombosis. Am J Cardiol 1997;80:21B–28B.

20. Tcheng JE. Glycoprotein IIb/IIIa receptor inhibitors: putting the EPIC, IMPACT II, RESTORE, and EPILOG trials into perspective. Am J Cardiol 1996;78:35–40.

21. Prism Study Investigators. Inhibitors of the platelet glycoprotein IIb/IIIa receptor with Tirofiban in unstable angina and non-Q wave infarction. N Engl J Med 1998;338:1488–98.

22. Kereiakes DJ, Obenchain RL, Barber BL *et al*. Abciximab provides cost-effective survival advantage in high volume interventional practice. Am Heart J 2000;140:603–610.

23. Baron JH, Aggrawal R, Ezekowitz MD, Azrin A, de Bono DP, Gershlick AH. Adsorption and elution of c7E3 Fab from polymer coated stents *in-vitro*. Am J Cardiol 1997;80:37S.

24. Baron JH, Aggrawal R, de Bono D, Gershlick AH. Adsorption and elution of c7E3 Fab from polymer coated stents inhibits platelet aggregation *in-vitro*. Am J Cardiol 1997;30:95 (Abstract).

25. Baron JH, Ezekowitz MD, Azrin MA, De Bono D, Gershlick AH. c7E3 Fab inhibits adhesion of smooth muscle cells to vitronectin and osteopontin: a possible way of inhibiting in stent restenosis. Am J Cardiol 1997;80:20S(Abstract).

26. Verheught FW, Liem A, Zijlstra F *et al*. High dose heparin as initial therapy before primary angioplasty for acute myocardial infarction: results of the Heparin in Early Patency (HEAP) pilot study. JACC 1998;31:289–93.

27. Koch KT, Piek JJ, de Winter RJ *et al*. Early ambulation after coronary angioplasty and stenting with six French guiding catheters and low dose heparin. Am J Cardiol 1997;80:1084–6.

28. Foo RS, Hogrieve K, Baron J *et al*. Activated protein C adsorbed on a stent reduces its thrombogenicity. Eur Heart J 1998;Suppl I:4488.

29. Swanson N, Hogref K, Joved Q, Gershlick AH. VEGF-eluting coronary stents stimulate endothelial growth *in vitro*. J Submicrosc Cytol Pathol 2000; 32(3)419:BO87.

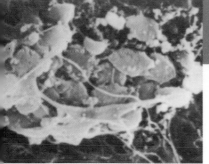

6

Intra-coronary stenting

E. JOHN PERRINS

KEY POINTS

■ Stents are a landmark technology and are used in the majority of percutaneous interventions (PCI).

■ Modern stents are both radially strong and conformable.

■ Balloon expandable slotted tube stents predominate.

■ Stents are available pre-mounted on balloons with a wide variety of diameters and lengths.

■ Stents reduce restenosis and reintervention in PCI.

■ Stents reduce acute complications of conventional balloon angioplasty and reduce the need for emergency bypass surgery.

■ Bifurcations, long diffuse lesions and small vessels have higher restenosis rates.

■ In-stent restenosis is difficult to treat.

INTRODUCTION

The development and widespread use of coronary stents has probably been the single most significant advance in the field of interventional cardiology over the last 10 years. So much so that the use of a stent at the time of coronary artery dilatation is now carried out in more than 70% of all intra-coronary angioplasty procedures and so, in many ways, coronary angioplasty has become coronary stenting. Despite this coronary stenting is still perceived as a relatively immature technology; there is still very significant and important debate concerning its exact role and there is a proliferation of stent designs, stent technologies and stent coatings which continue to challenge the interventional cardiologist to try and utilise them to their best ability. The increased cost of stenting represents financial challenges that have been taken up to a greater or lesser extent in different health-care systems and countries. The UK, as in so many other things, tends to lag behind other developed countries in this regard.

The fundamental principle of coronary stenting is that a mechanical scaffold will be placed at the site of the treated segment of the coronary artery. The scaffold increases the radial strength of the vessel wall thereby preventing elastic recoil. In addition by pressing the intima firmly against the media of the arterial wall, it will tend to prevent disruption of the plaque or dissected flaps from proliferating or expanding and may cause more rapid healing at the site of the intervention. Equally the stent itself will introduce new properties into the treated segment of artery. It will alter the fundamental elasticity of that vessel and the stent itself may induce subsequent biological changes, for example intimal hyperplasia, which may to some extent undo the initial advantages of placing the stent in the first place (restenosis).

Fundamental challenges in stenting

- The actual mechanical design of the stent itself.
- The problem of physically delivering the stent to the coronary artery in question.
- Expanding the stent to its proper dimensions.
- Ensuring that the stent is evenly and properly applied to the intimal surface of the vessel.
- The ensuing biological response to the stent itself.

The rapid growth of stenting in the UK is illustrated by Figure 6.1.

HISTORICAL OVERVIEW

Although the widespread use of stents is a relatively recent phenomenon in the world of percutaneous coronary intervention (PCI) the concept of using a device to maintain the lumen goes right back to the originators of

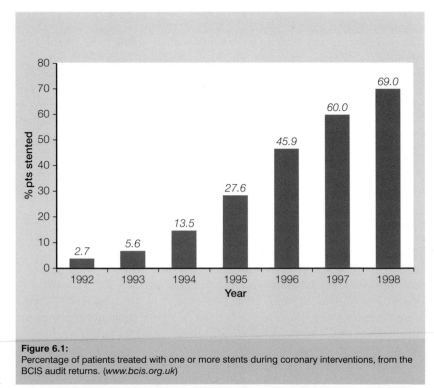

Figure 6.1:
Percentage of patients treated with one or more stents during coronary interventions, from the BCIS audit returns. (*www.bcis.org.uk*)

angioplasty itself. Charles Dotter who originally described the use of progressive dilating devices to push through and create an opening in occluded peripheral vessels, also proposed in 1964 that a silastic supporting device might be placed in an artery following such a procedure to maintain patency.[1] Dotter and Judkins were also first to coin the term 'stent' to describe an intra-vascular implant in a peripheral artery in 1969. The origin of the word stent itself is obscure, but may be related to the work of a dentist, Charles Thomas Stent, who developed a material for taking dental impressions. In 1977 Grünzig made his first description of balloon coronary angioplasty, and the subsequent rapid interest and growth of that technique caused the concept of stenting to be put into the background. In 1983 Dotter and colleagues described the use of transcatheter placement of nitinol coil stents into canine arteries.[2] Shortly after, Maas and colleagues described the use of steel springs as a stenting device.[3] In 1985 Palmaz and colleagues hit upon the idea of using an angioplasty balloon to assist in the deployment of a stent in the peripheral arteries. They came up with the entirely novel concept of using a balloon to expand the stent within the coronary arteries; the technique that has now become more or less the de facto technique for intra-coronary stenting. In 1987 Palmaz and Schatz described the implantation of balloon expandable stents in the canine coronary circulation.[4] Between 1986 and 1988 a number of initial implantations of both balloon expandable and self-expanding (Wallstent) were reported in humans. All of the early stent experience was plagued by problems of thrombosis of the stent after placement, and the difficulty of manipulating relatively rigid and bulky stent devices into the appropriate part of the coronary circulation.

While these early attempts at developing coronary stent devices were taking place, it was apparent from the wider application of simple balloon angioplasty that this technique was not without its problems. In particular the problems of vessel dissection, acute closure and restenosis were starting to become a major limitation in the application of angioplasty. It was apparent to many of the pioneering investigators at that time that stenting might well provide a partial solution to all of these problems. In the early 1990s when the balloon expandable Palmaz–Schatz stent was the most practical and proven of the available devices, two seminal studies were commenced: the Benenstent in Europe and the Stress Study in North America.[5,6] These two randomised controlled studies focused on the use of coronary stenting in the single discrete lesion and looked specifically at restenosis rates compared with simple balloon angioplasty. Both studies showed a very important reduction in restenosis (Benenstent: 22% stent, 32% balloon. Stress: 32% stent, 42% balloon.) These trials although they have been extensively analysed and criticised, triggered an explosion in stenting which has continued unabated.

There have, of course, been numerous highly significant developments since Benestent and Stress were published. Antonio Colombo[7] is widely regarded as having recognised that one of the fundamental problems with stent placement (particularly with the Palmaz–Schatz stent) was failure to completely expand all of the stent when placed in the coronary vessel. He proposed the technique of high pressure stent deployment, initially with the thought of over-expanding the stent, but subsequently realising, particularly with ultrasound, that the stents simply required a high pressure to completely expand them.

Although many stents are now manufactured claiming to require lower deployment pressures, most operators still deploy stents with pressures in the region of 10–16 atmospheres in the deploying balloon. The recognition that antiplatelet agents reduce subacute stent thrombosis, in particular the early use of ticlopidine, further opened the way to widespread stent usage. Controlled trials[8] showing that warfarin actually added nothing and possibly increased complications in elective stenting allowed the abandonment of warfarin with marked reduction in femoral arterial closure complications. Of course the subsequent development of closure devices has largely eliminated these problems. Intravascular ultrasound has allowed us to fully appreciate the difficulties of actually estimating the proper diameter of the intra-coronary vessel, the adequacy of deployed stent expansion and the importance of covering all of the at risk lesion. Most significant of all has been the technological development carried out by the stent manufacturers in producing balloon expandable stents that have a low profile, high flexibility and which are easy to use.

STENT DESIGN

Most articles on coronary stenting describe the various stent designs available at the time of writing the book or chapter. In my view all this does is uniquely date the text as stent design and development is progressing so rapidly that even in the relatively short time it has taken to produce this book any such information may be out of date. However, it is fair to say that the balloon expandable stent currently reigns supreme and as nearly all of the balloon expandable stents share common design features I will concentrate on these. Julio Palmaz had the brilliant idea that if one took a very thin stainless steel tube and cut small longitudinal slots in that tube using a laser cutter, if the tube was then expanded by a balloon then the expanded slotted tube would become a mesh. Clearly the shape and properties of that mesh would depend entirely upon the way the tube was cut, the material from which the tube was made and the way in which the tube was expanded with the balloon. As with so many good ideas, he initially found it difficult to interest a manufacturer to produce it. Johnson & Johnson Inc. (who had had very little prior involvement with cardiac intervention) eventually listened to his suggestions and the balloon expandable stent was born. Figure 6.2 shows the appearance of a modern balloon mounted slotted tube stent in expanded and unexpanded forms.

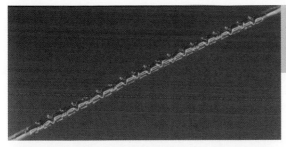

Figure 6.2a:
An unexpanded NIR stent (Boston Scientific Inc). The complex slots in the steel tube are evident.

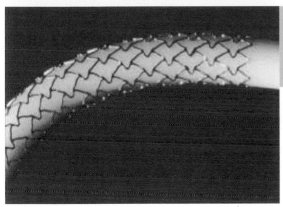

Figure 6.2b:
The same stent expanded on the balloon. The slotted tube becomes a tubular Mesh which is both radially strong and conformable.

Desirable design features for stents

- Biologically inert
- Flexible when mounted on delivery balloon
- Good radio-opacity
- Radial strength and conformable when expanded
- Smooth surface and/or coating
- Good side branch access through stent cells
- Availability of wide range of diameters and lengths
- Reduced metal or cell design for smaller vessels, increased for larger diameter vessels
- Low cost.

The design of any stent is always a trade-off between a number of desirable characteristics. The stent requires radial strength in order to prevent the collapse of the stent and to hold the wall of the stented segment of artery firmly in place. However, at the same time the stent needs to be conformable and flexible, both when it is compressed upon the delivery balloon and when it is expanded within the coronary vessel, since coronary vessels have highly complex 3D shapes. The material of the stent must be biologically inert. It is a highly desirable characteristic that the stent can be seen during its placement, by utilising X-ray screening equipment. The radio-opaqueness of the stent is therefore a vital factor when actually implanting it. The surface of the stent needs to be smooth, in order to attract as little platelet attachment as possible. In early stent designs, because of the problems of the rigidity of the slotted tube, small segments of slotted tube were linked together by articulations. This allowed the stent to bend in certain places but obviously meant that the coverage of the wall of the vessel would be incomplete at the point of articulation. Numerous clever geometric designs in the method of cutting the stainless steel tube have now resulted in stents that are both flexible, but have radial strength. The size of the associated cells in the expanded mesh is therefore not too large. Many manufacturers now produce different stents for different sizes of vessel, providing different diameters. Obviously if one stent is used for all coronary diameters, then the larger the stent is expanded the smaller the amount of vessel wall that will be covered. The stent may therefore have too much metal coverage in small vessels and too little in large vessels. Most stents are made from some form of stainless steel, although other metals have been used, particularly nitinol and tantalum. Stents have also been coated in a range of various materials, most of which have a neutral effect, although there has been some suspicion that coating the stent with gold may produce adverse consequences. More recently attention has focused on other methods of coating a stent, for example the PC coating process (Biocompatibles Inc.) and the Carmeda coating process – bonding heparin to the surface of the stent (Cordis Inc.). Obviously modifying the surface properties of the stent may eventually allow lower platelet activation and reduce the amount of intimal hyperplasia, but there is no real clinical evidence to support this. In the early days of stenting, the stent was supplied on its own and had to be crimped, usually by hand, on to an angioplasty balloon. Modern stents almost invariably consist of a stent pre-mounted on the balloon, and in fact balloons are now designed specifically to accept stents. Many stents are heat-sealed on to the balloon, so that it is almost impossible to detach the stent while the balloon is deflated.

There are many other stent designs (Fig. 6.3). Some have used coiled or twisted wire to produce expandable cells which can then be welded together to form longer stents (e.g. AVE Micro stent and GFX stents) Some are made entirely from complex coils which when expanded are similar to mesh stents (Cordis Crossflex). Others have used a steel backbone to which are attached segments which can be expanded. Finally there was the Wallstent, a lattice work of stainless steel wires which when unconstrained expand to form a tube. The device is held in its collapsed state by a sheath which when withdrawn allows the stent to self-expand. Although still used in larger peripheral vessels, the wallstent is rarely used in the coronary circulation today.

Covered stents

All the stents discussed so far are various kinds of meshes which have holes in them. Covered stents aim to totally cover the intimal surface of the treated vessel in a manner similar to a tube graft. The only current device is the Jomed covered stent which consists of a thin tube of polythene sandwiched between two conventional slotted tube stents. As the stent is expanded the polythene stretches and forms a tube graft. There is uncertainty as to whether the covered stents will offer advantages over conventional stents; they are more difficult to deploy and expand due to their thickness. They do have a unique place however in the treatment of coronary perforation and in the exclusion of coronary aneurysms.

TECHNIQUE OF STENT DEPLOYMENT

The technique of stent deployment is relatively simple in theory! Following conventional arterial access ordinary guiding catheters are used and a guidewire, usually 0.14, is used to cross the target lesion. Until relatively recently pre-dilatation of the target lesion was always required

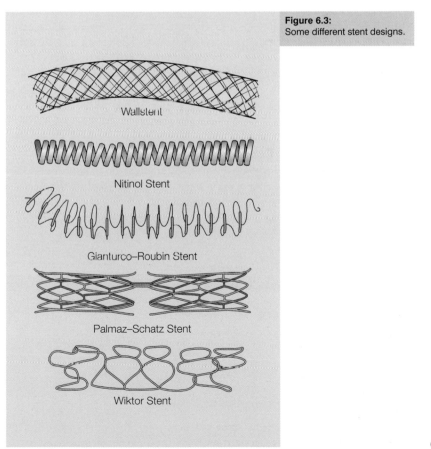

Figure 6.3:
Some different stent designs.

Wallstent

Nitinol Stent

Gianturco–Roubin Stent

Palmaz–Schatz Stent

Wiktor Stent

as the stent was too bulky to pass directly across the narrow vessel. However, in the last 2–3 years balloon mounted stents have become significantly lower in profile and have increased flexibility to allow direct crossing of the undilated lesion in a high proportion of cases, so called primary or direct stenting. Once the stent is positioned satisfactorily the balloon is inflated and generally the stent deployed at a pressure somewhere in the region of 10–16 atmospheres. Most modern stent deployment balloons allow a high enough pressure to be used so that the deploying balloon can carry out the final deployment of the stent. In addition stents are now mounted on balloons whose length is matched to that of the stent, removing the risk of either end of the deploying balloon damaging the unstented vessel wall when expanded to high pressure. However, for many reasons post-inflation of the stent may sometimes be required, often with a shorter balloon at even higher pressures. The wire is then withdrawn, the groin closed and the patient generally discharged the following day. Periprocedural heparin is generally considered to be essential; most centres will monitor KCT although this is not always universal, and with the use of or increasing use of GPIIb/IIIa inhibitors such as Reo-Pro, weight-adjusted heparin is more commonly used. Powerful antiplatelet drugs such as ticlopidine or more recently clopidogrel are universally prescribed following stent deployment. Some centres will only use aspirin, particularly in larger stented segments, but the majority of centres, particularly in the UK, will use aspirin and clopidogrel. There is no absolute agreement either on the duration of treatment required with antiplatelet drugs or on the doses, but the use of 75 mg clopidogrel and 300 mg aspirin for at least 2 weeks and often 4 weeks following the procedure is common, and most patients will be maintained on aspirin at lower doses indefinitely unless they are hypersensitive to it. Warfarin is generally not used in the context of coronary stenting nowadays. Several controlled trials suggested that it may actually increase the rate of complication, but in patients who are already established on warfarin for some other reason, then the operator has to take in individual patient considerations as to whether to continue warfarin during the first few weeks of the procedure.

GENERAL INDICATIONS FOR STENTING

The clinical selection of patients for intervention is covered elsewhere in this book. Stents are placed in the following situations:

■ Bail-out

■ Elective with pre-dilatation

■ Elective without pre-dilatation.

■ Following a preceding device therapy (e.g. after rotablator).

In the early days of stenting stent placement for bail-out indications after unsatisfactory or unsuccessful balloon angioplasty or other device

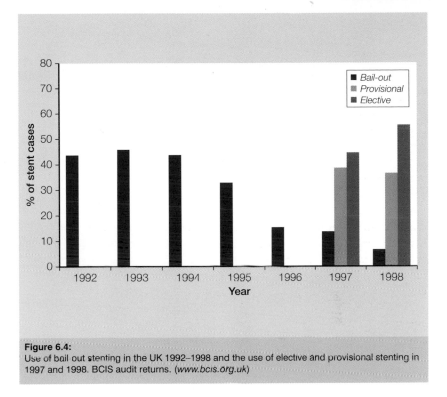

Figure 6.4:
Use of bail out stenting in the UK 1992–1998 and the use of elective and provisional stenting in 1997 and 1998. BCIS audit returns. (*www.bcis.org.uk*)

intervention was the primary indication. However following the realisation that elective stenting reduced restenosis, bail-out stenting is now uncommon (Fig. 6.4). There is still discussion as to whether provisional stenting should be carried out. However particularly with primary stenting (see below) it is unquestionably quicker and cheaper to perform primary stenting electively rather than provisional stenting (i.e. balloon angioplasty first and only stent if angiographic result is unsatisfactory).

Figure 6.5a–e illustrates a primary stent procedure using only one balloon mounted stent and no additional balloons or other devices.

PERI-PROCEDURAL COMPLICATIONS OF STENTING

Procedural complications primarily relate to whether it is possible to deliver a stent to the intended site in the coronary artery. As operators started to use stenting in more complex coronary arteries, the limitations of the mechanical properties of the stent–balloon combination sometimes led to the situation where the unexpanded stent could not be taken forward to the desired place, requiring an attempt at withdrawing the stent balloon or deploying the stent in an unwanted area. Withdrawal of the undeployed stent on the balloon used to represent a considerable risk of the stent being pulled off the balloon and being left unexpanded, but

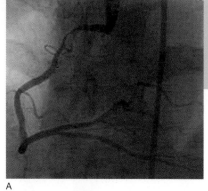

A

Figure 6.5:
These five angio frames show a primary stent procedure to the right coronary vessel in a patient with unstable angina. The lesion is crossed with a 014 wire and a Cordis Velocity 3.5 mm × 23 mm stent. The final result is excellent. Procedure time 8.5 minutes!

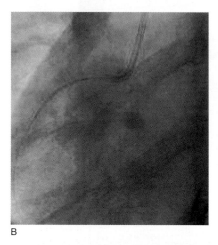

B

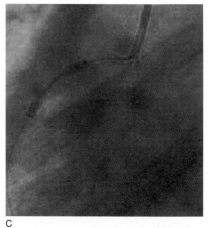

C

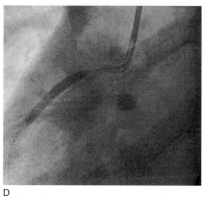

D

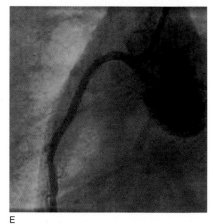

E

left within the coronary circulation. This is now a very rare complication as most stents, if they have been applied to the balloon by the manufacturer, are very resistant to being loosened in this way. However, there are many operator errors which can still allow this to occur, for example if the balloon has been inflated at any time during the procedure, the stent may have been loosened. If the balloon is left on negative pressure during deployment (the routine for balloon angioplasty) the balloon may loosen from the stent sufficiently for it to come off the balloon. Occasionally when a stent is withdrawn back into a guiding catheter, the edge of the catheter will lift up the back of the stent and then strip it off the balloon as the balloon is withdrawn. The importance of screening the balloon and stent whenever the balloon and stent are moved together cannot be emphasised enough but particularly during withdrawal. It is vital to ensure that the tip of the guide catheter and the stent are as coaxial as possible during withdrawal. Even when the stent balloon is not being intentionally withdrawn it may move between the time at which the stent was in the right position and the time at which the balloon is actually inflated. It is very important to continue to screen at the time of the inflation.

Under-expansion of the stent

The second major group of procedural complications relate to inability or failure to deploy the stent adequately, even though it may be in the right place. Routine use of relatively high pressure balloon expansion together with more compliant stent designs have made this complication less common, but adequate expansion of the stent is fundamentally predicated by having selected a stent of the correct diameter for the lumen of the vessel. Also, the routine use of quantitative coronary angiography (QCA) is still to be highly recommended to ensure proper selection of stent size as long as it is carried out and calibrated properly. Strict attention to the appearance of the stent following deployment in more than one projection remains vital to assessing whether the stent is actually deployed both completely and at the right diameter. As mentioned earlier in this chapter under-deployment of the stent is one of the fundamental causes of subacute stent thrombosis and unquestionably contributes to a higher restenosis rate.

Edge dissections

Stenting fundamentally reduces the risk of dissection at the point at which the stent is placed. However, sometimes a dissection will propagate from the end of the stent. Most commonly this is a distal edge dissection. If there is only a very small shelf or irregularity at the end of the stent then it may not be necessary to do anything further, but it is very important to observe the lesion for a minute or two if nothing else is done. However, in the author's experience one commonly ends up having to place another stent at the outflow of the first. Although intravascular ultrasound is well described as a way of helping to manage these kinds of complication, the fact that it is not used routinely generally leads operators to place another stent. Anterograde dissection is much less common but potentially very serious, because if a dissection propagates proximally towards the ostium of the stented vessel there is the risk of involvement of the main stem or another major proximal side branch. It is easy for the operator to miss proximal problems related to the stent. It should also be remembered that it is possible to dissect the proximal vessel during the passage of a stent, particularly if that stent passage has been difficult. Prompt stenting of the affected proximal segment of the vessel is essential and may be life saving. Proximal dissections can sometimes involve the wall of the aorta itself.

Side branches

Obviously whenever a stent is placed over the ostium of a side branch unpredictable consequences may occur. If the side branches are relatively small and there is clearly good angiographic flow down the side branch, then experience has shown that no further attention to that side branch is required. However, often a side branch may appear nipped or may even disappear when a stent is expanded across it. Most modern stents will allow the passage of a wire through the mesh into a side branch which can then generally be dilated and even stented itself. As soon as the operator moves into that realm he has to face up to the techniques and limitations of bifurcation stenting which will be discussed in a later section.

Vessel rupture

Vessel rupture during stenting itself is relatively rare although obviously it may occur, particularly during pre-dilatation. Occasionally if a lesion is resistant to dilatation and very high pressure is required, a balloon rupture may still cause a vessel perforation despite a stent having been placed. Stenting may, of course, be a life saving maneouvre when vessel rupture has occurred for other reasons and the covered stent is particularly useful in that rare but very dramatic situation. Inflation of a standard angioplasty balloon in the vessel proximal to the perforation will often prevent major bleeding into the pericardium.

Distal embolisation

Significant embolisation of material following a stent expansion in a stable chronic atheromatous plaque is very rare. However, as stenting is used more and more both in acute unstable syndromes and in myocardial infarction, stents are increasingly being used in situations where embolisation may occur. It is the author's personal experience that in this situation primary or direct stenting comes into its own as the balloon and stent can be placed directly across a soft friable lesion and the stent expanded and deployed with a single balloon dilatation. Embolisation often occurs if post-dilatation of such a stent is then attempted. It is the author's opinion that post-dilatation should not be carried out on stents in these acute and friable lesions. This is particularly important in the context of acute myocardial infarction or where stents are being placed in bulky friable vein grafts. The management of embolisation is difficult, and Reo-Pro would generally be considered to be mandatory unless there were some fundamental contraindication to its use. Intra-coronary nitrates and particularly intra-coronary verapamil may help to combat the no reflow situation that occurs. More recently devices are becoming available which may catch embolic material in particular high-risk situations (e.g. Cordis Angioguard).

POST-PROCEDURAL COMPLICATIONS

By far away the most important complication in the early days of stenting was subacute stent thrombosis with abrupt closure of the vessel, usually within the first 7–14 days of stent placement. Modern antiplatelet treatment, high pressure ballooning and adequate stent to vessel sizing have largely eliminated this problem; in modern practice subacute stent thrombosis rates are well below 1%. Paradoxically it is now so rare that it may be missed altogether if a patient re-presents. Curiously if a subacute stent thrombosis does occur, simple ballooning of the stent together with heparin or Reo-Pro generally results in an excellent angiographic appearance and repeated subacute thrombosis seems to be virtually non-existent. Presumably it all relates to the mechanics of the initial stent dilatation.

Restenosis

Restenosis remains a fundamental complication of any percutaneous intervention and although stenting fundamentally reduces restenosis, it does not by any stretch of the imagination eliminate it. It is difficult to get a true perspective as to what the clinical impact of restenosis is. It is well known that angiographic restenosis rates are higher than clinical restenosis rates – a consistent feature in nearly all interventional trials. Clearly there is a fundamental difference between a restenosis and representation following interventional procedure. Within the UK at least restenosis appears to be being treated in between 7–10% of patients. The treatment of restenosis is a complex topic and in my view fundamentally relates to the context in which the original intervention was done, in particular whether additional moderate or perhaps more severe disease is still present in other vessels. Coronary artery bypass grafting is an excellent treatment for restenosis and it is essential that patients are offered surgical revascularisation if it is clearly the most appropriate option. All known methods of treating restenosis themselves result in a higher rate of further restenosis. In the author's view diffuse disease in long stents should always been treated by surgery unless there is a contraindication. Focal restenosis may well be susceptible either to balloon inflation, cutting balloon inflation or restenting. Because the material within the stent in a restenotic lesion is smooth and rubbery it is often the case that if a balloon is inflated within a restenosed stent the balloon prolapses either antero-gradely or distally and does not expand the material. Repeated attempts to expand the stent in this situation can lead to catastrophic damage to the vessel; if migration of the balloon is occurring prompt restenting is the treatment of choice as the stent is able to engage the intimable hyperplasia and can then be deployed without migration of the balloon. Similarly the blades in the cutting balloon will cut into the intimal hyperplasia, generally allowing dilatation of the segment without balloon migration. Unfortunately it may be difficult to place the cutting balloon in the stented segment due to its rigidity and it may be difficult to obtain a good match of the length of cutting balloon to the length of restenotic segment. There has been a lot of focus on the use of radiation both for the treatment of restenosis and for its prevention and this is covered elsewhere in this book.

STENTING IN LESION SUBSETS

Small vessels

All of the randomised trials of stenting vs balloon angioplasty have shown a fundamental relationship between vessel size and restenosis. As vessel size gets smaller restenosis becomes more common. These data relate to stents which have not specifically been designed for small vessels. Newer designs allowing less wall coverage and with improved surface coatings may allow small vessel stenting with similar results to larger vessels, but clinical trial results are not yet available. Small vessel stenting probably relates to the use of stents in vessels between 2.25 and 2.75 mm internal diameter. Whether any intervention at all is justified in vessels smaller than 2 mm is not known.

At the moment it is hard to justify the use of stents in an elective scenario for small vessels. However, because small vessels are frequently involved in interventional procedures and are certainly no less likely to suffer complications of dissection than larger vessels it is often necessary to stent smaller vessels. It is important to attain the largest possible lumen size in these situations and the availability of quarter sized balloons, particularly 2.75 mm balloons, is important but not always recognised.

Left main stem

The left main stem used to be an absolute contraindication to angioplasty or stenting and although in general terms surgery should always be offered, there are many circumstances where surgery may be high-risk or impossible. There have been a number of studies presented of elective stenting in the left main stem scenario, particularly in elderly patients, and although these appear to be successful the short-term data suggest a considerably higher mortality in the region of 5–8%. One or two series have produced much better results, and it is likely that left main stem disease will be eventually treated by stents, particularly when there is a discrete lesion not involving the bifurcation. However at the time of writing there is currently no acceptable indication for elective stenting of the left main stem other than where surgery is impossible or inappropriate.

Saphenous bypass grafts

The management of the diseased bypass graft is a difficult problem for everybody treating patients who have been revascularised. The graft is frequently diffusely diseased, may have friable material within it and often is of large diameter which may stretch the mechanical properties of stents to their limits. It should be remembered that nearly all of the longitudinal studies of stenting and angioplasty in vein grafts show a consistently higher restenosis rate, and perhaps much more importantly, a very significant chronic occlusion rate in the graft within 2 years of the procedure. With current technologies, stenting of a bypass graft cannot really be considered to be a definitive treatment. Careful attention should always be paid to the native vessels, because if it is possible to revascularise the native vessel to which the graft is attached, this is generally a better procedure to carry out and is likely to have a better long-term outcome. There is no convincing evidence that the use of Reo-Pro reduces the risk of complications from graft angioplasty other than where thrombus is clearly present. The newer thrombus collecting devices (Angioguard) although interesting are not yet proven. I believe primary stenting offers a fundamental advantage in the treatment of the bypass graft since by avoiding pre-dilatation and then placing the stent with one inflation, the risk of embolisation seems to be reduced. Therefore, primary stenting should be employed wherever possible in the saphenous vein graft.

Ostial lesions

Treatment of ostial lesions either of grafts or the right coronary artery is made simpler by stenting but the restenosis rates are significantly higher than in the body of the vessel. It can be very difficult to accurately size the ostium without intravascular ultrasound. Placement of the stent right up to the ostium can be difficult and careful guide catheter selection and positioning is required. It is very easy to miss the first 2–3 mm of the vessel with subsequent restenosis. The use of a longer stent (18 mm or greater) even in short discrete ostial lesions may be helpful as it allows easier positioning and decreases the chance of the stent moving during deployment. High pressures are required in the ostium but dissection of the main aortic wall is possible.

Bifurcation lesions

The treatment of coronary bifurcations remains the most technically challenging and contentious area of intervention. All current routine treatments have higher restenosis and adverse event rates than for lesions in the body of the vessel. This applies as much to stenting as to other device technologies discussed elsewhere in this book. Coronary bifurcations are a heterogeneous collection of anatomical variations and different strategies are employed according to whether both limbs are involved, the angulation the proximal segment, etc. The presence of significant bifurcation disease, particularly at the left anterior descending (LAD)/diagonal position, mandates a careful consideration of the benefits of coronary artery bypass grafting. If other adverse factors such as diabetes are present then surgery has to be the strategy of first choice. A detailed discussion of bifurcation stenting is beyond the scope of this chapter.

BIFURCATION STENTING – SUMMARY

- There is a steep learning curve.

- The use of two guidewires and simultaneous inflation of both pre-dilating and post-deployment balloons is associated with improved results.

- Primary stenting is currently not possible.

- Larger lumen guide catheters are helpful.

- Stent the most important (generally larger) vessel first.

- Culotte stenting (where both stents are in the proximal segment as well as in each limb) is widely advocated but early clinical results are uncertain.

- Wrapping of the two guidewires either in the guide catheter or in the proximal vessel can produce catastrophic 'jamming' of the two balloons or stents.

- A bifurcation restenosis is even more difficult to treat than the original lesion.

Long lesions

Stents are now generally available in a variety of lengths up to 40 mm. Longer lesions may require more aggressive pre-dilatation and the use of support wires may facilitate stent passage. Longer stented segments are probably associated with higher rates of in-stent restenosis. Very careful attention needs to be paid to adequate stent expansion. Post-dilatation to high pressure is more commonly needed and it is vital to taper the stent if the reference diameter at the start of the lesion is more than 0.5 mm of the distal lesion. Calcified long lesions are particularly likely to have some areas of poor stent expansion. Ideally intravascular ultrasound should be used in this situation to optimise deployment.

STENTING IN CLINICAL SUBSETS

Stents have been shown to improve outcomes, not only when treating patients with stable angina, but also when treating unstable coronary syndromes, acute myocardial infarction and shock. Stents can now be

placed very quickly, often without pre-dilatation. The reduction of ischaemia during the procedure and the certainty that the vessel will remain open after the stent is placed dominate the acute clinical procedure. Stents should be used in all acute procedures with vessel size 2.5 mm or greater. There is considerable evidence that Reo-Pro (abciximab) is indicated prior to acute interventions for unstable angina. It produces both early and late mortality benefits, particularly in high-risk cases and diabetics. Trials in acute MI show an additional benefit to stenting compared to balloon alone and GP2a3b inhibitors add further benefit.

FUTURE DIRECTIONS

Stenting will continue to dominate PCI for some years to come. It is likely that primary or direct stenting will increase and formal clinical trials are under way. New aggressive stent coating technologies will probably be shown to have advantages, particularly in smaller vessels. There is still very active research into the area of bioabsorbable stents; they may ultimately be an even better method of local drug delivery than coated stents. Innovative devices will eventually allow better treatment of bifurcation and main stem disease. Restenosis will remain a clinical and technological challenge.

REFERENCES

1. Dotter CT, Judkins MP. Transluminal treatment of arteriosclerotic obstruction. Circulation 1964;30:654–70.

2. Dotter CT, Buschman PAC, McKinney MK, Rosch J. Transluminal expandable nitinol coil stent grafting. Radiology 1983;147:259–60.

3. Maas D, Zollikofer CL, Largiader F, Senning A. Radiological follow-up of transluminally inserted vascular endoprostheses: an experimental study using expanding spirals. Radiology 1984;152:659–63.

4. Schatz RA, Palmaz JC, Tio FO, Garcia F, Garcia O, Reuter SR. Balloon expandable intra-coronary stents in the adult dog. Circulation 1987;76:450–57.

5. Serruys PW, De Jaegre P, Kiemeneij F et al. for the Benestent study group. A comparison of balloon-expandable stent implantation with balloon angioplasty in patients with coronary artery disease. New Engl J Med 1994;331:489–95.

6. Fischman DL, Leon MB, Baim DS et al. for the Stent Restenosis Study Investigators. A randomised comparison of coronary stent placement and balloon angioplasty in the treatment of coronary artery disease.

7. Colombo A, Hall P, Nakamura S et al. Intra-coronary stenting without anticoagulation accomplished with intravascular ultrasound guidance. Circulation 1995;91:1676–88.

8. Schomig A, Neuman FJ, Kastrati A et al. A randomised comparison of antiplatelet and anticoagulant therapy after placement of Intra-coronary stents. N Engl J Med 1996;334:1084–9.

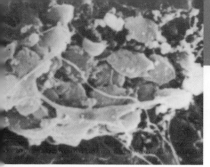

7

Complications of angioplasty

DAVID SMITH

KEY POINTS
- All complications are caused by the operation, but some by the operator!
- Meticulous technique is mandatory.
- Acute vessel closure is the commonest cause of serious morbidity and mortality.
- GpIIb/IIIa inhibitors and stents significantly reduce the incidence of acute vessel closure.
- Coronary perforation, embolisation and infection are very rare.
- Despite advances in technology and technique the requirement for emergency coronary artery bypass grafting has not fallen (1–2% in the UK).
- The arterial access site remains a major potential cause of morbidity.

Any aspect of an angioplasty procedure that prolongs the procedure time or detracts from the well-being of the patient can be considered a complication. Some seem more important than others, but often it is from an apparently trivial slip that a cascade of events ensues, spiralling down towards disaster. Major complications are those that cause vessel closure with subsequent myocardial ischaemia, infarction and possibly death yet they may be caused by a brief lapse of concentration – many a main stem has been dissected with a guide catheter by the casual and abrupt withdrawal of a balloon catheter causing the guide suddenly to be deeply engaged. There is no room for bravado and no place for the slap-dash; attention to detail is everything. Whatever the complication, it is the responsibility of the operator.

GENERAL PRINCIPLES TO AVOID COMPLICATIONS
There are some general principles of angioplasty that in broad terms might be applied to any technical procedure in an attempt to prevent a 'botch up'. What follows is not an exhaustive manual of how to do an angioplasty, but a short list of guiding principles employed to avoid disaster.

Preparation
Prepare appropriately for the case with:

- **Adequate assessment of the angiogram.** Study the lesions carefully, their length, extent of calcification, tortuosity and relationship to branches. Consider the route to the lesion, the distance from the ostium and the bends involved and consider the involvement of side branches, the nature of the distal vessel and the extent and origin of collaterals. Use all views for your assessment. If you are not sure take another picture.

■ **Sound procedural strategy.** Based on the assessment of the angiogram select the appropriate guide catheter, wire and balloon diameter and length. Use quantitative coronary angiography (QCA) to help. Plan what you will do after you have used them, e.g. change up for a bigger balloon, change wires for a stiffer wire. Run through the planned procedure using 'what if' scenarios e.g. 'what if it dissects back to …?' 'What if I need a stent then which one? How long? How big?' Make sure you have the appropriate equipment available to treat them.

■ **Adequate preparation of the patient.** Check intravenous access, state of hydration, state of sedation, state of oxygenation if sedated, extent of anticoagulation (activated clotting time (ACT), aspirin dosage and/or ticlopidine).

Execution

During the procedure attention to detail is everything.

■ Take great care with the arterial puncture – one hole is all that is required!

■ *Never* pull, push, inflate or deflate anything without fluoroscopy.

■ Make sure your guide catheter support is good at the start – if not change it.

■ Instrumentation in the coronary artery should be done gently and carefully – steer the wire, ease the wire, coax the wire – *don't shove it*!

■ Remember the catheter system is a co-axial system; movements of the elements are interdependent, therefore all elements need to be controlled at once. Pay attention to the guide catheter and wire tips even when the action has moved to positioning the balloon or deploying the stent.

■ Remember you are working in three dimensions – take advantage of different views to check the position of branches, wires, balloons, stents, etc.

■ When it is not going according to plan stay calm. Do not lose your temper. If you cannot think what to do next ask someone else.

Post-procedure

Aftercare of the patient is very important. Particular attention should be paid to:

■ The arterial puncture site – many a fine piece of coronary work has been ruined by poor care of the arterial puncture site leading to hypotension and subsequent stent thrombosis.

■ Control of systemic blood pressure – not too high, not too low.

■ Appropriate anticoagulation and antiplatelet treatment.

Although adherence to the above guidelines will limit the likelihood of complications, it will not eradicate them. Those that occur however are likely to be the result of the biological response to the angioplasty process and not the result of operator technique.

COMPLICATIONS

Angioplasty necessitates the introduction into the coronary circulation of thrombogenic instruments with the intention of causing vessel wall injury. Dissection of the vessel and exposure of subintimal prothrombotic tissues are essential components of this process. It is therefore not surprising that dissection, thrombosis, subintimal haematoma and spasm are the major contributing factors to the most important of angioplasty complications, acute vessel closure.

Acute vessel closure

Acute closure may be defined as occlusion of the coronary artery occurring during or after the procedure with consequent electrocardiographic and haemodynamic instability. It is the most common cause of peri-procedural myocardial infarction, referral for emergency coronary artery bypass grafting (CABG) and death.

Frequency

Acute closure occurs in anything from 2% to 13.5% of balloon angioplasty with the majority of reported series suggesting at least 5% established closure and 3% impending closure.[1,2] The majority of abrupt closure occurs in the laboratory, but a significant proportion occurs afterwards within the first 6 hours. Acute closure is rare after 6 hours and very unlikely after 24 hours.

Predictors of acute closure

Clinical predictors are insulin-dependent diabetes mellitus, female sex and unstable angina. Lesion characteristics that predict acute closure are those of very severe stenosis, long lesions (at least twice the luminal diameter), ulcerated lesions, branch point lesions and lesions on a bend of more the 45 degrees. Lesion characteristics have been classified on the basis of angiographic morphology[3] into types A, B1, B2 and C according to risk of failure and risk of acute closure. Lesions of the B2 (more than one B characteristic) and C categories are at high risk of dissection and acute closure.

Predictors of death with acute closure

Acute closure may or may not produce fatal haemodynamic collapse but is more likely to do so in the following circumstances: females, the elderly (> 65), those with left main disease, triple vessel disease and/or left ventricle ejection fraction < 30%. Any vessel closure that results in an acute loss of function of 40% of the myocardium is likely to result in cardiogenic shock and death.

Causes

The role of dissection The major component to acute closure is the initial dissection caused by the balloon inflation. Some post-mortem and intravascular ultrasound studies have demonstrated, not surprisingly, that dissection occurs in nearly 100% of cases, but unfortunately contrast angiography is a relatively insensitive technique for demonstrating it. Angiographic appearances of dissection have been classified into six categories A to F[4] associated with an increasing likelihood of major in-hospital complications from C (persisting extraluminal contrast) 10% risk, D (spiral dissections) 30% risk, E (new persistent intraluminal filling defects) 40% risk to F (occlusive dissection) 70% risk.

The role of thrombus (See Chapter 5) Despite some popular misconceptions it should be noted that it is not possible to identify accurately the material composition of an angiographic filling defect on the angiogram. Dissection flaps can mimic the appearance of thrombus and vice versa while the contribution made by spasm to an angiographic 'train smash' should never be underestimated. Given that the collagens exposed by intimal disruption are highly thrombogenic it can be assumed that any acute closure involving dissection also involves thrombus. Adequate pre-medication with anti-thrombotic agents such as aspirin, ticlopidine or clopidogrel and appropriate procedural anticoagulation with heparin will help limit thrombus formation but not preclude it. Once established it may be successfully treated with intra-coronary thrombolytics such as urokinase or t-PA, although this practice has largely been superceded by the advent of intravenous platelet GP IIb/IIIa receptor blockers such as abciximab that have a surprisingly rapid acute effect on thrombus. These potent antiplatelet agents are probably best applied in the prevention of acute thrombus in high-risk cases by being prescribed in the 24 to 48 hours before angioplasty. Thrombus is more likely to become the dominant problem in acute closure when a stent has been deployed, since almost all available stents are made of thrombotic materials. Although type D, E and F dissections can occur both proximal and distal to a newly deployed stent, acute closure of a stented lesion is more likely to be caused by acute thrombosis. It may respond well to mechanical disruption with balloon inflation with concomitant use of IIb/IIIa blockers.

No reflow No reflow is phenomenon of no antegrade flow in the coronary artery following apparently successful lesion dilatation and in the absence of identifiable dissection, obstruction or distal vessel 'cut off' suggestive of distal embolisation. The exact mechanism of this phenomenon is unknown, but appears to be related to the distal microcirculatory dysfunction. While it may occur during any angioplasty it is more likely to occur in relation to angioplasty in the setting of acute myocardial infarction (seven times more likely) or unstable angina rather than elective procedures although it is more likely in cases of vein graft angioplasty and stenting, particularly of bulky lesions. These circumstances have major disruption of the vessel wall as a common factor and this supports the two theoretical causes, namely a local humoral effect on the distal vessel or a microembolic effect in the distal microcirculation. The fact that intra-coronary Verapamil can be very successful as treatment (dose 100–600 µg) favours the former theory. The immediate clinical consequences may be the same as for any acute closure with haemodynamic collapse. Bradycardia requiring pacing may ensue, particularly with right coronary intervention. However support of the rhythm and circulation (pacing, intra-aortic balloon pumping, etc) for a period often results in spontaneous restoration of antegrade flow.

Spasm and recoil Spasm of the dilated segment is a common feature and responds to intra-coronary nitroglycerin (100–300 µg) while recoil is not abolished by nitrates and may take up to 3 months to disappear. Theories abound as to the cause of elastic recoil. Contributing factors are the abnormal vascular autoregulation that occurs in response to a sudden change in shear stress, an imbalance between the production of EDRF (endothelium derived relaxing factor) and endothelin (endothelial derived constricting factor) and sympathetic activation. The recoil may take a week or more to recover while adjustments of the coronary flow may take up to 3 months.

Coronary perforation
Coronary perforation is a rare complication with balloon angioplasty with rates of approximately 0.1%. However the later technologies, which are inherently more aggressive, such as directional atherectomy, excimer laser angioplasty and less commonly rotablation, have all led to an increase in perforation rates of up to 10% in some circumstances (see Chapters 10, 11 and 12) Even stents, which act as a vessel wall scaffold and may be used to treat perforation, can at times cause perforation especially if the 'bigger is better' therefore 'biggest is best' approach is used and the stent is over dilated (see Chapter 6)

Acute sequelae
The majority of coronary perforations do not lead to haemoperiocardium and pericardial tamponade, but it is a possibility and pericardiocentesis or emergency surgery and repair of the vessel may be required. Alternative means of managing uncomplicated perforations range from using long inflations with a perfusion balloon catheter, the deployment of a stent or more recently the use of a covered stent (two stents sandwiching a layer of dacron between them). The covered stent is probably the best option.

Late sequelae
Small perforations that appear haemodynamically stable and are safely left may in time result in pseudoaneurysm formation with its own potential complications of rupture and distal embolisation.

Stent complications
The advent of stents and their increasingly widespread use has undoubtedly provided a huge improvement in intravascular intervention, but at the same time it has brought to the practice of angioplasty a plethora of new complications. It is worth considering these under a separate heading and in some detail since the use of stents seems set to increase.

Stent mounting

Stents may be self-expanding or balloon expandable. Most fall into the latter group. Originally balloon expandable stents were 'bare' stents being mounted by hand and crimped onto the dilating balloon just prior to delivery; many stents can still be used this way, but most also come as ready balloon mounted with no operator crimping required. This has reduced the likelihood of complications associated with hand crimping such as dropping the stent on the catheter laboratory floor – a simple but expensive complication – or inadequate crimping such that the stent profile remains too large. As a result the stent can be damaged, displaced or dislodged particularly when passing into or out of the guiding catheter system. The lifting of one strut of the leading edge of the stent as it is introduced into the guiding catheter can go unnoticed until the stent will not easily exit the guide, traverse the proximal coronary section or cross the lesion. The stent may be displaced a millimetre or two inadvertently in the same manner which may then result in malposition of the stent when it is deployed. Poor crimping can result in complete dislodging of the stent such that it is lost from the balloon altogether. This can also occur with balloon mounted stents although it is less common.

Stent embolisation

This term is used to describe the loss of the stent from the delivery system. The dislodging may occur at the guide catheter tip, when traversing the coronary artery proximal to the lesion or in the lesion itself.

If the guide choice and stability are not good the guide will be displaced from the coronary ostium as the stent exits the guide and meets resistance in the coronary artery. The stent cannot be pushed on because there is no backup. Either the guide can be advanced over the stent or the stent can be withdrawn into the guide until a better guide position is found. Either manoeuvre may cause stent displacement and embolisation. This complication is avoided by choosing appropriate equipment: a low profile balloon-mounted stent that is well attached to the balloon, a guide catheter that will fit snugly and provide back-up and possibly a stiffer wire that will help to straighten bends in the coronary artery and reduce resistance. But whatever difficulties are encountered with equipment choice the most important means of avoiding this complication is to take great care with the manipulations as the stent exits or re-enters the guide. Manoeuvring of the guide catheter will often straighten the guide tip to allow the stent and its delivery catheter to become co-axial and permit uneventful passage in either direction.

Unnoticed proximal coronary lesions or calcification can cause the stent to be held up or displaced as it traverses the artery towards the target lesion. A different angiographic view or intra-coronary ultrasound (ICUS) of this section may reveal the problem and appropriate adjustment to the strategy may be made. If the hold-up can be overcome by force alone – often possible if the guide is secure – there is a considerable risk of damage to that section of coronary artery and it should be inspected carefully afterwards and treated if necessary to pre-empt any occlusive dissection.

Hold-up at the lesion may also cause displacement or embolisation of the stent especially if it is not securely mounted. Adequate predilation is the key. Often high pressures are required to disrupt the plaque sufficiently to allow the stent through and for the passage to be sufficiently easy that fine adjustments to the position of the stent are possible prior to deployment.

Embolisation of the stent within the coronary artery can be a lot more problematic than if it is lost in the wider circulation when in general they rarely cause problems. Nevertheless strenuous efforts at stent retrieval should be made. If the stent is lost in the coronary artery but is still on the guidewire, retrieval can often be achieved with a very low profile balloon inflated enough to secure the stent which can then be withdrawn. The stent can either be secured by the balloon being inflated within it, a method that still may cause problems as the stent will not be very securely attached to the balloon, or brought to a position on the balloon catheter shaft proximal to the balloon so that when the balloon is slightly inflated the stent is secure and cannot come off the balloon catheter. If withdrawal of an embolised stent is not possible, the stent may be deployed where it is. If the stent is lost from the wire a second wire and balloon may be passed alongside and the stent crushed into the side wall of the coronary artery. Other means of retrieving stents include snares which may be fashioned from long wires doubled over and introduced into a 5 or 6 F catheter or specifically designed devices which are available on the market.

Recrossing stents

Recrossing stents is a potentially complicated procedure which needs to be performed with great care. It may be necessary to recross a deployed stent if lesions beyond require treating. When sequential lesions are being treated it may be necessary to treat the proximal lesions first in order to gain access to the distal ones. Sometimes distal lesions only become apparent after deploying the first stent such as in acutely occluded (primary angioplasty) or chronically occluded arteries. It may also be necessary to treat a dissection that occurs distal to the stent. Even if the wire is still in place across the proximal stent passage of a balloon or second stent may be held up. This particularly occurs if the stent has not been fully deployed and there is a protruding strut, but even if full deployment has been achieved hold-up may occur and it is especially likely to occur at a bend. The proximal left anterior descending and proximal right coronaries are frequently at an angle of greater then 90 degrees to the tip of the guide catheter and stents in these positions pose a problem. Part of the reason is that the guidewire naturally assumes a position on the outside of the arterial bend and thus lies firmly against the stent (this is particularly the case with the stiffer wires) and it is relatively easy for the tip of a balloon catheter or the strut of a passing stent to catch. Various manipulations however may allow passage. The wire may be withdrawn until the more floppy section is in place within the stent or a very small inflation of the balloon catheter may provide enough of a buffer to keep the balloon/stent away from the wall of the artery.

Inadequate stent deployment

Intravascular ultrasound examinations of deployed stents have revealed that often despite excellent angiographic appearances the stent is not fully deployed. The balloon on which the stent is mounted may have a nominal pressure of six atmospheres, in other words at six atmospheres the balloon reaches its nominal dimensions, but this pressure may not be enough to expand the entire stent adequately. The remaining protruding strut or struts may be responsible for early restenosis. In an attempt to circumvent this problem very high pressures may be used and specific high pressure non-compliant balloons have been developed for this purpose. However high pressure inflations increase the risk of balloon rupture.

Balloon rupture

Balloon rupture may occur with or without stents and may result from rough handling of the balloon before introducing it into the guide catheter or during manual mounting of a stent. It may also result from the lesion characteristics if, for example, there is jagged calcification. It is recognised by spontaneous reduction in inflation pressure, by release of contrast in the vessel during inflation and by blood appearing in the balloon catheter when negative pressure is applied. With the advent of high pressure inflations the incidence of balloon rupture has probably increased and may be as high as 5–6% of stent deployments. Most commonly the rupture is a pinhole perforation, but it is this that probably causes the most dangerous consequence of balloon rupture namely dissection. The very high pressures in the balloon force a tiny but powerful jet of contrast into the vessel wall causing the dissection. Sudden explosive bursting of a balloon has been known to cause vessel perforation. Other consequences of balloon rupture include air embolism and trapping of the burst balloon when it becomes enmeshed in a partially deployed stent. Balloon rupture is best avoided by careful handling of balloon and stent and by using only specifically designed balloons to attain high pressures. If it does occur it is important to monitor and treat any complications and, if a stent is involved, to return with another balloon to ensure full deployment of the stent.

Myocardial enzyme release

Although abrupt vessel closure may lead to acute infarction with associated ECG changes of Q waves it is quite common for there to be a measured rise in creatine kinase (CK) release without any apparent ECG abnormalities in an otherwise uncomplicated procedure. This may be as frequent as 5–30% of angioplasty procedures. It is not clear exactly why this occurs but it may result from inadvertent small side branch occlusion and it does appear to be related to total balloon inflation time. Despite mechanisms not being fully elucidated studies have clearly demonstrated that such a CK rise is associated with increased mortality and later cardiac morbidity and as a result the following recommendations have been made.[5] The CK should be measured at 8 and 16 hours post-procedure and if there is a threefold or more rise in the level the patient should be treated as for myocardial infarction. Elevations less than this threshold should be noted and the patient monitored carefully. The use of CK or CK-MB as a marker of myocardial necrosis is not without its problems and may be superseded by the use of other markers such as the Troponins but for the time being it is a useful marker of increased post-procedural risk

Bleeding complications

Bleeding is a very important complication of angioplasty that can impact in a number of ways to cause serious morbidity or death. Hypotension stemming directly from hypovolaemia or indirectly from the vaso-vagal reaction to haematoma may result in cerebral or myocardial ischaemia or induce thrombosis in the otherwise successfully treated artery. Haematomata also provide a site for infection.

Bleeding complications tend to be noticed after the procedure but blood loss may be occurring during the procedure from the catheters during equipment exchanges and during blood sampling both of which should be kept to a minimum. Care should also be taken to ensure that only one puncture of the femoral artery is made and that haemostasis of any additional punctures is achieved before proceeding with the angioplasty.

Bleeding may occur at the arterial puncture site, at a distant accidental puncture site or spontaneously at a remote site, for example intracerebral or retroperitoneal due to heavy anticoagulation.

Local haemorrhage

Large local haemorrhage, enough to require transfusion, is not uncommon and may occur in as many as 10% of patients. The patients characteristics associated with bleeding are age, female sex, diabetes, hypertension and obesity. The procedural characteristics are those involving devices that require larger catheters such as directional atherectomy, rotational atherectomy and the use of intra-aortic balloon pumping. An independent predictor of haemorrhage is the use of post-procedural heparin. The site of such bleeds is usually the arterial puncture site and can normally be controlled with manual compression. Clamping devices such as the Femostop may be used, but need to be applied carefully by experienced staff to be effective. It is important to catch haemorrhage early before a large haematoma has developed as compression can become difficult and ineffective once there is a large boggy mass. This especially applies to clamping devices. No confidence should be placed in the use of sandbags as effective compression devices.

Retroperitoneal haemorrhage

Bleeding into the retroperitoneal area is not obvious and a high index of suspicion is required to make the diagnosis. Unexplained hypotension and hypovolaemia should be investigated aggressively and, if no cause is found, attributed to retroperitoneal haemorrhage until proved otherwise. The diagnosis can be confirmed with abdominal ultrasound or computed tomography (CT) examination. Retroperitoneal haemorrhage is dangerous and can readily and rapidly lead to shock and therefore requires early treatment. Anticoagulation should be stopped and reversed if necessary with protamine and fresh frozen plasma despite the risk of acute coronary closure in certain patients. Hypovolaemia should be promptly corrected. Surgical intervention is rarely indicated.

Anticoagulants and bleeding

Heavy anticoagulation regimens during angioplasty make haemorrhage from any site more likely. The use of warfarin as routine anticoagulation for patients with stents has largely stopped but antiplatelet agents are used with increasing frequency. The combination of aspirin, ticlopidine and procedural heparin increase the risks of gastrointestinal and intracerebral bleeding. The use of platelet GP IIb/IIIa receptor blockers such as abxicimab (ReoPro) is also increasing and while the benefit in terms of coronary patency is clear there are more bleeding problems such as pericardial haemorrhage and gastrointestinal bleeding. Abxicimab, like heparin, has also been reported to cause profound thrombocytopaenia compounding potential bleeding complications.

Arterial complications

Pseudoaneurysm

The most common arterial complication is a femoral artery pseudoaneurysm. This has been reported to occur in up to 9% of cases, but the incidence depends very much on how hard you look. The diagnosis can be made by noting the presence of a tender pulsatile femoral arterial swelling with a bruit. The diagnosis can be confirmed with colour flow doppler examination which may pick up clinically undetectable pseudoaneurysms. Pseudoaneurysms may resolve spontaneously particularly in patients who are not anticoagulated but they may increase in size especially in anticoagulated patients. Increased painful swelling may compress the femoral nerve and may rupture and they should therefore be treated. Surgical repair has been largely superseded by doppler guided compression repair which has a reported success rate of 84%.[6]

Arteriovenous fistulae

Arteriovenous fistulae occur most commonly when both the artery and vein of the same side have been cannulated. This is particularly the case if the vein runs superficial to the artery. Most heal spontaneously but are also amenable to compression treatment as for pseudoaneurysm. In cases where a femoral venous cannula is required as well as an arterial one, anteriovenous fistulae are avoided if the puncture sites are made 1 cm or more apart.

Thrombosis and embolism

Both thrombosis of the femoral artery and distal embolisation are relatively rare comprising 4–6% of vascular complications. They are readily recognised providing appropriate observations are made and they are readily treated with surgical intervention unless the distal embolism is small in which case a conservative approach with systemic heparin will suffice. They are more commonly associated with cases involving the use of the intra-aortic balloon pump in which case the balloon should be removed.

Infection

Infection from diagnostic cardiac catheterisation from the femoral route is extremely rare. Despite sterile equipment and a sterile technique it is almost certainly the brevity of the procedure that accounts for this. Coronary angioplasty on the other hand may involve the femoral sheath remaining *in situ* for long periods and in the presence of some local haematoma. Nevertheless significant infections secondary to angioplasty-related bacteraemia is still rare occurring in approximately 0.2% of cases. Even then the infection tends to be local causing a septic endarteritis most commonly with a *S. aureus*. Unlike diagnostic catheterisation or previously practiced angioplasty current coronary intervention frequently involves leaving foreign bodies in the patient. Stenting practice is nearly 100% of cases in some centres and the use of arterial closure devices such as the Angioseal is increasing. The potential for causing systemic infection should not be overlooked and a scrupulous sterile technique should always be employed.

REFERENCES

1. Ferguson JJ, Barasch E, Wilson JM *et al*. The relation of clinical outcome to dissection and thrombus formation during coronary angioplasty. J Invas Cardiol 1995;7:10.

2. Detre KM, Holmes DR, Holubkov R *et al*. Incidence and consequences of peri-procedural occlusion: The 1985/1986 NHLBI PTCA Registry: Circulation 1990;82:739–50.

3. ACC/AHA task force on assessment of diagnostic and therapeutic procedures. Guideline for percutaneous transluminal coronary angioplasty. J Am Coll Cardiol 1988;12:529.

4. Huber MS, Mooney JF Madison J *et al*. Use of a morphological classification to predict clinical outcome after dissection from coronary angioplasty. Am J Cardiol 1991;68:467–71.

5. Califf RM, Adelmeguiid AE, Kuntz RE *et al*. Myonecrosis after revascularisation procedures. JACC 1998:31241–51.

6. Schaub F, Theiss W, Busch R *et al*. Management of 219 consecutive cases of post-catheterisation pseudoaneurysm. JACC 1997;30:670–75.

Section Two

Devices

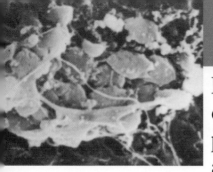

8

Physiological assessment of coronary stenosis: pressure wire and allied technologies

MICHAEL CUSACK AND SIMON REDWOOD

KEY POINTS

- Coronary angiography frequently underestimates the true significance of coronary stenoses, even where quantitative coronary angiography (QCA) is used.

- Intra-coronary data derived by both the pressure and the doppler wire systems have been shown to correlate well with both non-invasive ischaemia detection and the presence of disease found on intravascular ultrasound (IVUS) examination.

- Following coronary intervention the Myocardial Fractional flow reserve (FFRmyo) and the relative coronary flow velocity reserve (rCVR) to a lesser extent can determine whether a satisfactory physiological result has been obtained.

- Coronary intervention may be safely deferred for intermediate stenoses where the FFRmyo or CVR suggest that the lesion is not physiological significant.

- A physiologically guided approach to coronary intervention may reduce rates of coronary stenting whilst giving comparable event rates on follow-up which may be attractive economically and lead to a reduction in the burden of in-stent restenosis.

INTRODUCTION

The limitations of coronary angiography to assess the functional significance of coronary stenoses have been recognised for more than 20 years.[1] Large intra- and inter-observer variability occurs when coronary angiograms are interpreted which accounts for the frequent dissociation between clinical and angiographic findings. Morphological assessment of coronary lesions does not necessarily reflect the impairment of flow by the stenosis. This may occur as the resistance of a coronary stenosis will vary in relation to the fourth power of the luminal radius. Thus a relatively small change in vessel radius, beyond angiographic resolution, may result in a significant alteration in the resistance to flow.

As a result, measurements of coronary flow and pressure have been introduced to improve the functional evaluation of coronary stenoses and interventions.[2] Technical progress has permitted intra-coronary measurements to be made using wires with the same dimensions as those of conventional angioplasty guidewires (0.014 inches in diameter) increasing their ease of application in the catheter laboratory.

This chapter will review the physiological background of both coronary flow and pressure measurement, and will focus on the application of these techniques for diagnostic and therapeutic catheterisation.

PRESSURE MEASUREMENT

Blood flow within the coronary vessels is greatly dependent on the haemodynamic status of the patient and may demonstrate significant variations between individual recordings. To overcome this problem the concept of coronary pressure derived myocardial fractional flow reserve (FFRmyo) has been developed. FFRmyo is defined as the maximum myocardial blood flow in the presence of a stenosis expressed as a proportion of the theoretical maximum flow in the absence of any stenosis (Fig. 8.1).

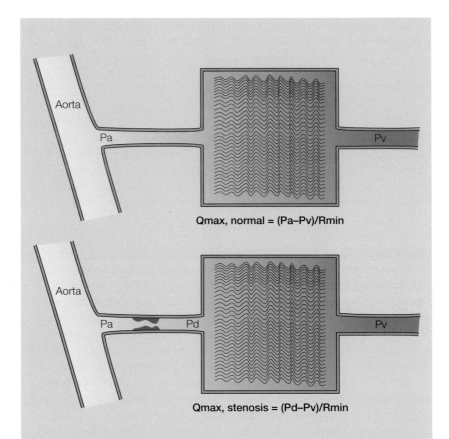

$$Q_{max,\ normal} = (P_a - P_v)/R_{min}$$

$$Q_{max,\ stenosis} = (P_d - P_v)/R_{min}$$

Figure 8.1:
Schematic representation of a coronary artery and vascular bed. Myocardial blood flow is equal to the perfusion pressure across the myocardium divided by its resistance. At maximum hyperaemia, resistance to flow (R_{min}) is minimal and constant. Maximum flow in the diseased vessel may therefore be expressed as a ratio to that of a normal vessel, i.e. one without a pressure drop, by the equation:

$$FFRmyo = (P_d - P_v)/(P_a - P_v)$$

AO, aorta; P_a, P_d and P_v mean aortic, distal coronary and central venous pressure; $Q_{max,\ normal}$, theoretical maximal achievable myocardial flow if the artery were normal; $Q_{max,\ stenosis}$, maximal achievable flow in the presence of a stenosis. Adapted from Pijls and De Bruyne.[22]

For accurate calculation of the FFRmyo, a steady state of maximal hyperaemia is required to maintain myocardial resistance at a constant minimal level. In submaximal hyperaemia the FFRmyo will be artificially high and the severity of the stenosis underestimated. During maximal hyperaemia, any changes in the measured pressure that are recorded equate to alterations in blood flow within the coronary vessel. The standard means for inducing hyperaemia is by the administration of adenosine. This is typically infused intravenously for 2 to 3 minutes (140 μg/kg/min infused via the femoral vein), though some operators give it as an intra-coronary bolus dose.[3] Intra-coronary injections of papaverine have also been used.[3] The distal coronary, aortic and right atrial (RA) pressures are then measured simultaneously via the pressure wire, guide catheter and RA catheter respectively, and the FFRmyo calculated (Fig. 8.1).

As measurement of FFRmyo is expressed as a ratio of the proximal to distal coronary pressure within the same vessel, the possible confounding effect of microvascular disease and the contribution of distal collateral vessels is eliminated. Likewise, it is independent of changes in patient haemodynamics, such as heart rate, blood pressure and myocardial contractility.[4] As a normal reference vessel is not required, FFRmyo may be used in multivessel disease. It may also be used to assess the cumulative effect on coronary flow of sequential lesions within a single vessel (Fig. 8.2).

The procedure

There are currently two available systems, both based on a high-fidelity sensor tipped guidewire. A third system based on a fluid filled guidewire is under development.[5] All of these are 0.014 inch wires with the sensor area located 3 cm proximal to the wire tip. With improvements in the performance of these wires they may be used as a first line guidewire during angioplasty.

Before the wire is introduced into the coronary tree the patient is heparinised. Once the guiding catheter is in the coronary ostium, the pressure wire is passed to the catheter tip, where it is calibrated against the pressure transduced from the guiding catheter. The pressure wire is then passed across the lesion to be studied. Maximal hyperaemia is induced and the FFRmyo calculated. As the pressure transducer is 3 cm proximal to the tip of the wire, once the wire has crossed the stenosis the sensor can be pulled back and re-advanced across the stenosis, while the wire tip remains distal to the lesion.

Application of pressure measurement

The primary indication for the use of coronary pressure measurement is to determine whether a coronary stenosis is flow limiting and as a result is responsible for myocardial ischaemia. It is now well established that an FFRmyo below 0.75, in those with normal left ventricular function, is functionally significant and has been found to correlate well with the

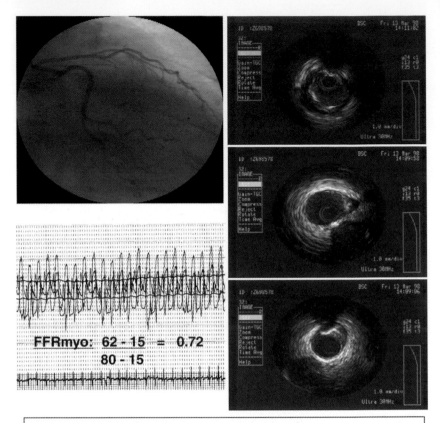

$$FFRmyo: \frac{62 - 15}{80 - 15} = 0.72$$

QCA: *Mid LAD*: MLD 1.33 mm, DS 39%, AS 64%
       LAD Ostium: MLD 1.67 mm, DS 34%, AS 56%
IVUS: *Mid LAD*: DS 24%, AS 42%;
      LAD Ostium: DS 13%, AS 25%; *LM Ostium*: DS 36%, AS 59%

Figure 8.2:
Left coronary system of patient with stable exertional angina and anterior wall ischaemia demonstrated on perfusion scintigraphy. No significant coronary lesion was identified on angiography. The pressure wire revealed a physiologically significant drop in FFRmyo of 0.72 in the distal left anterior descending artery (LAD) due to the combined effect of three sequential lesions – at the ostium of the left main stem (LM) and in the ostium of the LAD and its mid-segment. The patient underwent bypass grafting of the LAD and remains free of symptoms.

presence of ischaemia on perfusion scintigraphy, stress echocardiography and exercise testing.[4,6,7]

Thus measurement of FFRmyo may be used to determine the significance of intermediate lesions. Retrospective and prospective work from the DEFER study has demonstrated that lesions with an FFRmyo greater than 0.75 may be left untreated without any increase in subsequent events on follow-up.[6,8,9]

A further use of pressure measurement is to determine the precise location of the lesion under assessment by defining the point at which the measured pressure 'steps-up' during pull-back of the wire. A particular area where this has been applied is in the assessment of ostial coronary lesions which may be missed by conventional angiography.

In addition, measurement of the FFRmyo can provide important prognostic information following coronary intervention. An FFRmyo of less than 0.75 implies that the result of the intervention is physiologically unacceptable and would be associated with myocardial ischaemia. An FFRmyo of greater than 0.9 following balloon angioplasty without stenting, has been found to be associated with repeat intervention rates at 6, 12 and 24 months of 12%, 12% and 15% respectively.[10] Where the FFRmyo following angioplasty was less than 0.9 the rates of reintervention at these time points were 24%, 28% and 30%.[10] Therefore even where a satisfactory angiographic appearance has been achieved following angioplasty, obstruction to flow detectable physiologically is associated with an unfavourable outcome, which may be improved by stent implantation.

Where a vessel has been stented there should be no residual pressure drop across the stent once it has been fully deployed. When compared to intravascular ultrasound (IVUS), an FFRmyo across a stent of 0.94 or higher was found to correlate strongly with optimal stent deployment as determined by IVUS.[11] The concordance rate between FFRmyo and IVUS was over 90% in this study. In contrast, quantitative coronary angiography (QCA) showed a low concordance rate with IVUS and FFRmyo of 48% and 46% respectively.[11]

SUMMARY

Clearly the pressure wire can supply information both to guide the initial decision to intervene and also can determine whether the intervention itself has been successful. The technique is easily employed and the FFRmyo is a robust physiological measure of the effect of any given stenosis within the coronary arteries. Though there have been more than 30 000 cases worldwide employing the pressure wire, it is unlikely that this technique will see large-scale use while the wires themselves remain substantially more expensive than standard guidewires. As a result, their use is likely to remain principally for the assessment of angiographically intermediate lesions.

FLOW MEASUREMENT

Similar advances in guidewire technology to those seen with the pressure wires have made it possible to measure flow within the coronary arteries using 0.014 inch wires.

In the presence of an obstruction to flow within a coronary artery, the downstream microvascular resistance typically falls to maintain a satisfactory regional basal blood flow to meet metabolic demands. This resting dilatation of the microvascular bed results in a reduction in the capacity for further dilatation above baseline and reduces the potential maximal flow reserve that is available (Fig. 8.3). Thus any subsequent hyperaemic stimulus or increase in myocardial oxygen demand results in a smaller absolute increase in blood flow distal to a stenosis compared to that which would be found in a region without a stenosis present.

Unlike the flow characteristics observed in most arterial beds, coronary blood flow has a distinct phasic pattern. Blood flow is significantly higher in diastole than in systole. This reduction in flow during systole is the result of the contraction of the heart.[12] The contribution of the systolic component of flow has been found to be increased relative to the diastolic component distal to a coronary stenosis.[13] Thus the ratio of distal diastolic to systolic flow velocity encountered in normal vessels differs from that found in those with a significant stenosis. However the application of this finding to the assessment of the haemodynamic significance of coronary stenoses is limited by the differing patterns of flow found in the right and left coronary systems. Also the ratio is sensitive to changes in the contractility of the heart.

As a result of these limitations, doppler derived coronary flow velocity reserve (CVR) has been used to represent the physiological effect of coronary artery stenoses. The CVR is defined as the potential capacity for

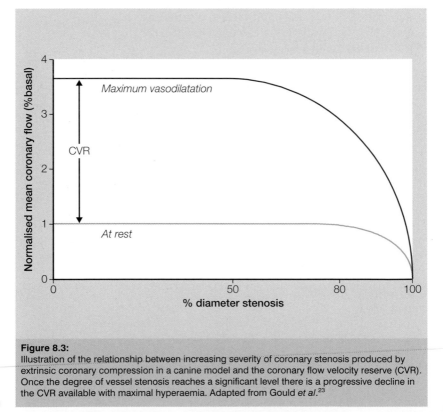

Figure 8.3:
Illustration of the relationship between increasing severity of coronary stenosis produced by extrinsic coronary compression in a canine model and the coronary flow velocity reserve (CVR). Once the degree of vessel stenosis reaches a significant level there is a progressive decline in the CVR available with maximal hyperaemia. Adapted from Gould et al.[23]

increased blood flow within both the epicardial coronary vessel and the microvasculature above the resting level (Fig. 8.3). A value of 2.7 ± 0.6 is typically found for CVR among adults with angiographically normal vessels.[14] This figure appears relatively constant between myocardial regions, even in cardiac transplants. A CVR of less than 2.0 has been found to correspond to the presence of myocardial ischaemia determined by perfusion scanning, stress echocardiography, or exercise testing.[15] However, in the absence of epicardial coronary disease the CVR may be abnormal when there is disease of the microvasculature.[16] This is typically seen in diabetes mellitus, as a result of ischaemic injury or due to the presence of left ventricular hypertrophy. In the presence of these conditions, the significance of epicardial disease may be overestimated by measurement of CVR alone. Therefore when the possibility of microvascular disease exists, the CVR is determined also in a normal reference vessel ($CVR_{reference}$). The coronary flow velocity reserve in the vessel under investigation may then be expressed as a proportion of that found in the reference vessel:

$$rCVR = CVR_{target}/CVR_{reference}$$

The normal value of rCVR is typically greater than 0.8.[14] As with measurement of the FFRmyo, the rCVR is believed to be lesion specific, having removed the contribution of the microvasculature. Both FFRmyo and rCVR have been shown to correlate well with one another across a range of lesion types.[17] In a similar way to measurement of FFRmyo, the rCVR prior to intervention has been found to bear a strong relationship to the percent area stenosis determined by IVUS.[17] However, immediately following coronary intervention the relationship between rCVR and IVUS measurements becomes less robust.[18] (in contrast to the strong relationship between FFRmyo and IVUS).

The procedure

Intra-coronary flow velocity is measured with a 0.014 inch guidewire, which has a piezoelectric ultrasound transducer at its tip. Flow is sampled at approximately 5 mm from the tip of the wire, the ultrasound beam being approximately 2 mm wide at this point. Ideally the wire tip should be positioned axially within the artery. Though when the wire is not placed axially within the coronary artery, meaningful data may still be obtained. Flow is then recorded both at rest and following the induction of hyperaemia (see Fig. 8.4). This is typically induced by an intra-coronary bolus injection of adenosine, nitrates or papaverine. The mean flow velocity is calculated by dividing the peak velocity by two, assuming that a full flow velocity profile envelope has been obtained. The CVR is determined as:

$$CVR = \frac{\text{Mean flow velocity at hyperaemia}}{\text{Mean flow velocity at rest}}$$

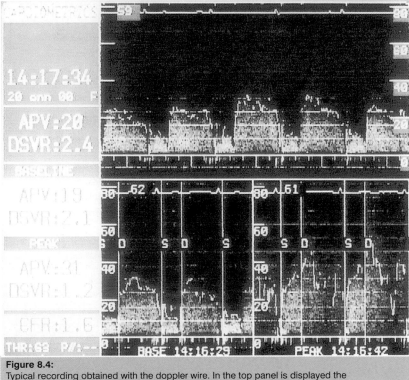

Figure 8.4:
Typical recording obtained with the doppler wire. In the top panel is displayed the instantaneous doppler recording. The lower right panel shows the peak flow recorded at hyperaemia and the lower left panel shows the peak flow at baseline. The calculated CVR of 1.6 is displayed on the left of the image.

Where rCVR is to be measured, this process is repeated in the reference vessel.

Application of flow measurement

The doppler guidewire has similar characteristics to that of a normal angioplasty guidewire and like the pressure wire systems may be used as a first line wire during percutaneous transluminal coronary angioplasty (PTCA). Again, like the pressure wire, the most common clinical application of the doppler wire is in determining the physiological significance of intermediate coronary artery lesions when contemplating intervention.

The DEBATE I study (Doppler Endpoints Balloon Angioplasty Trial Europe) has shown that a CVR of less than 2.5 following angioplasty combined with a residual percentage diameter stenosis of more than 35% on IVUS correlated with clinical recurrence and need for reintervention at 6 months.[19] Where a CVR of more than 2.5 was achieved with a satisfactory angiographic result (DS <35%), there was an angiographic restenosis rate and target vessel revascularisation rate of 16% at 6 months follow-up.[19] These later findings are not dissimilar from those that have been observed with the pressure wire. Improvement in the CVR may however, not be immediate and on long-term follow-up of patients with an initially impaired CVR following angioplasty, the CVR is frequently seen to return to normal.[18] It has been suggested that this relates to delayed recovery of autoregulation in the microvascular bed following the removal of an upstream stenosis. When a coronary stent is deployed however, the CVR is more frequently found to normalise in approximately 80% of patients.[20] As stenting results in a larger, more uniform lumen it may be that this late recovery in CVR after angioplasty relates in part to remodelling of the vessel lumen during follow-up.

Coronary intervention may be safely deferred where the CVR is greater than 2.0. In a study by Ferrari et al. 70 patients with intermediate coronary lesions and an indication for PTCA due to stable angina and/or ischaemia on non-invasive testing underwent study with the doppler wire.[21] Patients with a CVR of less than 2.0 underwent PTCA and in those in whom it was greater than 2.0 the intervention was deferred. During 15 ± 6 months follow-up, a major adverse cardiac event rate (MACE) of 33.3% was observed among the patients who had undergone PTCA compared with 9.1% in those in whom it had been deferred. However, only 40% of the patients in the non-PTCA group were free of angina on stress at follow-up compared with 53% of patients in the PTCA group.

SUMMARY

Measurement of CVR may provide important information on the physiological effects of coronary stenoses. Unlike measurement of FFRmyo, the ratio of flow reserve may indicate the contribution of microvascular disease to the impairment of coronary blood flow. However, this same microvascular disease is the major limitation to assessing the effect of a stenosis using the absolute CVR. The calculated ratio of CVR (rCVR) addresses this limitation, though it requires there to be a normal reference vessel and makes assumptions as to the uniformity of the myocardium supplied by both the reference and the stenosed vessel. In those with a previous myocardial infarction, the degree of microvascular impairment found may not be uniform. The performance of accurate flow recording is dependent upon a satisfactory position of the wire within the vessel. Poor positioning of the wire may result in considerable variation in the results obtained and represents a further limitation of this technique. In these circumstances the pressure wire may provide the more reliable data.

ONGOING INVESTIGATION

Both techniques described above provided detailed information as to how successful a coronary intervention has been in treating a given stenosis. It is already clear that normalising flow within a coronary vessel during coronary intervention reduces the subsequent event rates related to that intervention. Three multicentre trials are evaluating whether a physiologically guided approach to intervention will produce similar outcomes to those obtained by mandatory elective stenting of all lesions (DESTINI-CFR, DEBATE II and FROST). Early results from these studies indicate that although there was a cross-over rate to stenting of 40–50% in the physiologically guided groups the event rates at 6 months are comparable between the two groups. If these findings are confirmed, it is possible that the cost savings afforded by a significant reduction in the rates of vessel stenting may result in an increase in the use of this technology.

REFERENCES

1. Topol EJ, Nissen SE. Our preoccupation with coronary luminology: the dissociation between clinical and angiographic findings in ischaemic heart disease. Circulation 1995;92:2333–42.

2. Gould KL, Lipscomb K, Hamilton GW. Physiologic basis for assessing critical coronary stenosis. Instantaneous flow response and regional distribution during coronary hyperemia as measures of coronary flow reserve. Am J Cardiol 1974;33:87–94.

3. Pijls NH, De Bruyne B (eds) Maximum hyperemic stimuli. In: Coronary pressure. Dortrecht: Kluwer Academic Publishers, 1997, pp.96–104.

4. Pijls NH, Van Gelder B, Van der Voort P et al. Fractional flow reserve. A useful index to evaluate the influence of an epicardial coronary stenosis on myocardial blood flow. Circulation 1995;92(11):3183–93.

5. Pijls NHJ, Kern MJ, Yock PG, De Bruyne B. Practice and potential pitfalls of coronary pressure measurement. Cathet Cardiovasc Interven 2000;49:1–16.

6. Pijls NH, de Bruyne B, Peels K et al. Measurement of fractional flow reserve to assess the functional severity of coronary-artery stenoses. N Engl J Med 1996;334(26):1703–8.

7. Wilson RF. Assessing the severity of coronary artery stenoses. N Engl J Med 1996;334:1735–7.

8. Bech GJ, de Bruyne B, Bonnier HJ et al. Long-term follow-up after deferral of percutaneous transluminal coronary angioplasty of intermediate stenosis on the basis of coronary pressure measurement. J Am Coll Cardiol 1998;31(4):841–7.

9. Bech GJW, Pijls NHJ, De Bruyne B et al. Deferral versus performance of PTCA based on coronary pressure derived fractional flow reserve: the DEFER study. [Abstract] Eur Heart J 1999;20:(Abstract Suppl.) 371.

10. Bech GJW, Pijls NHJ, De Bruyne B et al. Usefulness of fractional flow reserve to predict clinical outcome after balloon angioplasty. Circulation 1999;99:883–8.

11. Hanekamp CEE, Koolen JJ, Pijls NHJ, Michels HR, Bonnier HJRM. Comparison of quantitative coronary angiography, intravascular ultrasound, and coronary pressure measurement to assess optimum stent deployment. Circulation 1999;99:1015–21.

12. Sabistorn DC Jr, Gregg DE. Effect of cardiac contraction on coronary blood flow. Circulation 1957;15:14–23.

13. Goto M, Flynn AE, Doucette JW et al. Effect of intra-coronary nitroglycerin administration on phasic pattern and transmural distribution of flow during coronary artery stenosis. Circulation 1992;85(6):2296–304.

14. Kern MJ, Bach RG, Mechem CJ et al. Variations in normal coronary vasodilatory reserve stratified by artery, gender, heart transplantation and coronary artery disease. [Abstract] J Am Coll Cardiol 1996;28:(5)1154–60.

15. Heller LI, Cates C, Popma J et al. Intra-coronary Doppler assessment of moderate coronary artery disease: comparison with 201TI imaging and coronary angiography. FACTS Study Group. Circulation 1997;96(2):484–90.

16. Strauer BE. The significance of coronary reserve in clinical heart disease. J Am Coll Cardiol 1990;15(4):775–83.

17. Baumgart D, Haude M, George G et al. Improved assessment of coronary stenosis severity using the relative flow velocity reserve. Circulation 1998;98(1):40–6.

18. van Liebergen RAM, Pick JJ, Koch KT, de Winter RJ, Lie, KI. Immediate and long-term effect of balloon angioplasty or stent implantation on the absolute and relative coronary blood flow velocity reserve. Circulation 1998;98(20):2133–40.

19. Serruys PW, Di Mario C, Piek J et al. Prognostic value of intra-coronary flow velocity and diameter stenosis in assessing the short- and long-term outcomes of coronary balloon angioplasty: the DEBATE Study (Doppler Endpoints Balloon Angioplasty Trial Europe). Circulation 1997;96(10):3369–77.

20. Kern MJ, Dupouy P, Drury JH et al. Role of coronary artery lumen enlargement in improving coronary blood flow after balloon angioplasty and stenting: a combined intravascular ultrasound Doppler flow and imaging study. J Am Coll Cardiol 1997;29(7):1520–7.

21. Ferrari M, Schnell B, Werner GS, Figulla HR. Safety of deferring angioplasty in patients with normal coronary flow velocity reserve. J Am Coll Cardiol 1999;33(1):82–7.

22. Pijls NH, De Bruyne B. Coronary pressure measurement and fractional flow reserve. Heart 1998;80:539–42.

23. Gould KL, Lipscomb K. Effects of coronary stenoses on coronary flow reserve and resistance. Am J Cardiol 1974;34:48–55.

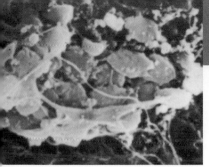

9

Which device for which lesion?

SIMON REDWOOD

KEY POINTS

■ Lesion characteristics are associated with both acute and long-term outcome.

■ Despite improvements in angioplasty practice, there is still value in adopting a lesion-specific approach to percutaneous intervention.

■ Rotational atherectomy can be useful in the presence of severe superficial calcification and for diffuse stent restenosis.

■ Thrombus-containing lesions and vein graft interventions are associated with a higher risk of distal embolisation.

■ Chronic total occlusions are the commonest single cause of failure in percutaneous intervention.

INTRODUCTION

Since the early days of angioplasty, it has been known that certain lesion characteristics are associated with worse acute and long-term results. Angiographic characteristics influencing outcome have been summarised by the American College of Cardiology/American Heart Association (ACC/AHA) Task Force (Table 9.1)[1] and have been shown in numerous reports to be predictive of outcome following balloon angioplasty (Table 9.2) and stent placement.[2]

With the widespread use of stents (currently >70% of cases in many centres) and improvements in their design and profile, the predictive value of individual lesion characteristics has declined, but there is still value in adopting a lesion-specific approach to angioplasty practice.[3,4] Bearing this in mind, this chapter will concentrate on some of the situations where individual lesion characteristics still influence decision making during angioplasty and will summarise some of the alternative approaches for individual lesions that may improve both short and long-term outcome following percutaneous intervention, including situations where stents might best be avoided.

LONG LESIONS

Progressive lesion length is inversely related not only to acute success but also to late restenosis. This powerful relationship is reflected in the ACC/AHA lesion classification; a lesion of >20 mm in length, even in the absence of other adverse characteristics, would be classified as type C. This relationship between length and restenosis holds true for stent implantation as well as balloon angioplasty. For this reason, many try not **107**

TABLE 9.1 – MODIFIED ACC/AHA LESION CLASSIFICATION

TYPE A LESIONS (MINIMALLY COMPLEX)

Discrete (length <10 mm)
Concentric
Readily accessible
Non-angulated segment (<45°)
Smooth contour
Little or no calcification
Less than totally occlusive
Not ostial in location
No major side branch involvement
Absence of thrombus

TYPE B LESIONS (MODERATELY COMPLEX)*

Tubular (length 10 to 20 mm)
Eccentric
Moderate tortuosity of proximal segment
Moderately angulated segment (45 to 90°)
Irregular contour
Moderate or heavy calcification
Total occlusions <3 months old
Ostial in location
Bifurcation lesions requiring double wire
Some thrombus present

TYPE C LESIONS (SEVERELY COMPLEX)

Diffuse (length >20 mm)
Excessive tortuosity of proximal segment
Extremely angulated segments (>90°)
Total occlusions >3 months old and/or bridging collaterals
Inability to protect major side-branches
Degenerated vein grafts with friable lesions

*Type B lesions are divided into type B1 (one B characteristic) and type B2 (two or more B characteristics).

TABLE 9.2 – OUTCOME ACCORDING TO ACC/AHA LESION CLASSIFICATION FOLLOWING BALLOON ANGIOPLASTY

TYPE	SUCCESS (%)	MAJOR ISCHAEMIC COMPLICATION (%)	% OF TOTAL LESIONS
A	92	2	29
B1	84	4	34
B2	76	10	27
C	61	21	11

to deploy long or multiple stents – not only may the restenosis rate be high, but it may also make subsequent grafting difficult.

Several approaches have been tried. For balloon angioplasty, it is generally accepted that it is important to select a balloon that is longer than the lesion. Although this has not been tested in a randomised fashion, several studies have found that long balloons yield superior results compared with 20 mm balloons. Overlapping the balloon across the whole length of the diseased segment appears to lower the dissection rate, avoids multiple inflations and may afford superior conformability around bends. When faced with a tapering lesion, it is safer to size the balloon according to the distal reference or alternatively, if available, use a tapered long balloon.

Debulking may have a role in long lesions, particularly when trying to avoid stenting. In general, directional coronary atherectomy (DCA) does not have a role in long lesions. The excimer laser provides results similar to long balloons, but trials of laser debulking prior to stenting are not available. Rotational atherectomy can be particularly useful (especially with associated calcification). A common approach would be to perform balloon angioplasty (with or without prior debulking) and if the patient re-presents with restenosis, perform stenting at that time.

CALCIFIED LESIONS

Calcification is detected on intravascular ultrasound in up to 80% of patients, and is widely accepted as a risk factor for increased complications, and for reduced acute success. The increased pressures required for dilatation of the lesion are associated with dissections, which tend to occur at the transition between the calcified plaque and more 'normal' vessel wall.

When calcification is detected on fluoroscopy, intravascular ultrasound is extremely useful to guide the approach to angioplasty. If the calcification is deep, and in the absence of superficial calcium, generally good expansion can be achieved with a balloon and/or stent particularly if the deep calcification is not circumferential; in this case it is useful to select a balloon that can withstand high inflation pressures. However, in the presence of superficial calcification, particularly if more than two quadrants (i.e. > 180 degrees) are involved, then adequate expansion can often not be achieved. In this case, the Rotablator has a particularly useful role in being able to break up and debulk the calcification. Different operators employ different techniques – either a single-burr (using a small burr, for example 1.75 or 2.0 mm) or stepped-burr approach can be used with the final burr-to-artery ratio not more than 0.7 to 0.8 with short ablation runs and minimal rpm drop, prior to adjunctive balloon angioplasty with or without stent implantation. In general, although both have been tried, neither the excimer laser nor directional atherectomy have a role in the management of calcified lesions.

ECCENTRICITY/IRREGULARITY

Although there is controversy as to whether eccentric lesions are associated with adverse outcome and an increased risk of restenosis, most interventionists approach them with a degree of caution. The compliance of the relatively disease-free portion is much higher than the adjacent atherosclerotic plaque, and luminal improvement following balloon angioplasty is produced largely by stretching of the disease-free portion of   **109** the vessel wall. This over-stretching can have several potential consequences: (i) early elastic recoil may lead to a suboptimal acute result; (ii) large intimal dissections can occur at the interface between the plaque and the non-diseased wall; and (iii) enhanced smooth muscle cell migration and proliferation resulting in enhanced late restenosis.

It is because of these limitations that interventionists have attempted alternative approaches to eccentric lesions. If eccentricity is the only 'adverse' lesion characteristic and it is mild to moderate, it is probably not associated with adverse outcome following angioplasty with or without stent implantation. However, lesions which are highly eccentric do have an increased risk of dissection and acute vessel closure. Directional atherectomy has declined in use and is limited to few centres in the UK, however bulky eccentric proximal lesions remain one of the few situations where DCA may still have a role. Use of this device may be associated with an increased risk of creatine kinase release, which may in turn be associated with an increased risk of late events. Its use is largely confined to proximal discrete lesions in large (>3 mm) vessels with little proximal or distal tortuosity. An alternative approach would be to debulk the lesion using an eccentric laser catheter. However, this is also not in widespread use and evidence for its superiority compared to balloon angioplasty is lacking. In general, rotational atherectomy does not have a role for eccentric lesions in the absence of co-existent lesion calcification.

With the widespread availability of stents, many would simply deploy a stent without prior debulking, however preliminary data suggest very low restenosis rates with a combination of optimal debulking using DCA followed by stent deployment.[5]

ANGULATED LESIONS

The risk of dissection of angulated lesions is approximately twice that of straight lesions, and angulation is also associated with higher restenosis rates. For these reasons, stents are usually deployed in angulated lesions. It is important to choose a flexible stent with good vessel conformability and either to perform 'direct' stenting, that is without pre-dilatation, or to pre-dilate with a small balloon in order to minimise the risk of dissection.

BIFURCATION LESIONS

There have been numerous classifications proposed for dividing bifurcation lesions according to whether angiographic appearances of the plaque are proximal to, at, or distal to the bifurcation and whether the side branch is also involved in the lesion. Although these can be helpful for describing the results of studies, they are not particularly helpful in clinical practice. Essentially, a lesion can be described as bifurcation if there is a greater than 50% stenosis involving both the parent vessel and the ostium of its side branch.

Angioplasty of bifurcation lesions remains technically challenging primarily because of the risk of side-branch closure, most commonly because of a 'snow-plough' effect. Balloon angioplasty, even using 'kissing balloons' results in a relatively low success rate, high complication rates and a high restenosis rate. For these reasons, debulking (using directional or rotational atherectomy) with or without stenting was frequently used, and there is some evidence of its superiority compared with balloon angioplasty.[6] Most would now deploy stents without prior debulking.

Many approaches have been tried for stent deployment to bifurcation lesions. A 'kissing stent' technique has been described, analogous to the kissing balloon technique, although this is rarely used now. Other approaches recently described include the 'Y' technique, the 'T' technique, the 'Culotte' technique, the 'inverted Y' (or 'V') technique, the 'monoclonal antibody' technique and the use of specific bifurcation stents (and probably many others!).

The 'Y' technique involves simultaneous deployment of stents at the ostia of both branches followed by a third stent deployed in the main vessel just proximal to the side branch. The 'T' technique involves deploying a stent in the main vessel and inserting a second stent into the side branch through the struts of the first stent. The 'Culotte' technique involves placing a stent in the main vessel into the side branch. A wire is then passed into the main vessel (through the stent) and a second stent is placed from the main vessel across the bifurcation with the proximal overlap of the two stents. One bifurcation stent system uses a very similar principle (Jomed UK Ltd) – it involves two separate stents, each with half metal coverage on the proximal half of the stent, thus when the two are deployed, the three 'limbs' have the same metal coverage (Fig. 9.1). Other bifurcation stent systems involve a 'trouser' stent mounted on a bifurcating balloon inserted over two wires.

Although these variations are all technically challenging and interesting, data to support their use are lacking. In fact, one interesting study divided patients according to whether a 'simple' or a 'complex' approach was used.[7] The simple approach consisted of deployment of a stent in the main vessel across the bifurcation and subsequent angioplasty of the side branch through the stent struts using either a fixed wire balloon or a low profile monorail balloon. The complex approach consisted of deployment of one stent at the ostium of the side branch and complete reconstruction of the entire bifurcation with additional implantation of one or two stents in the main vessel. Acute success was similar in the two groups (~90%). However, major cardiac events at long-term follow-up were higher with the complex approach (56% vs 25%).

Having tried several of these techniques, until further data are available our approach is as follows. Both branches of the bifurcation are wired. Generally, a wire is passed down the most difficult looking branch first; this is to minimise the two wires wrapping around each other. If the side branch has a significant stenosis, a balloon (matched to the side branch distal reference) is inflated. Next, a stent is deployed in the main vessel across the side branch (and trapping the side branch wire). If there

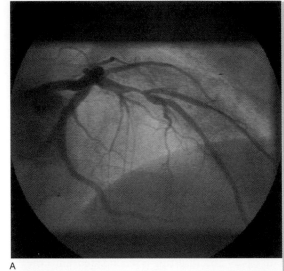

A

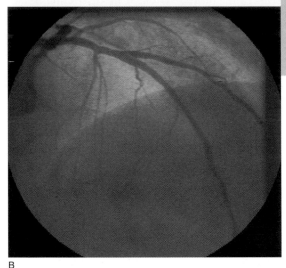

B

Figure 9.1:
(a) A right anterior oblique cranial view demonstrating a severe lesion in the proximal and mid left anterior descending involving the first diagonal branch. Following pre-dilatation, the diagonal wire was removed. The first stent was deployed in the LAD at 12 atmospheres, crossing the origin of the first diagonal. The diagonal branch was then re-crossed with the wire, and the LAD wire removed. The second stent was positioned across the ostium of the first diagonal and deployed at 12 atmospheres. The wire in the diagonal was then removed, and the LAD was recrossed with a wire and the LAD was post dilated at 12 atmospheres. (b) No residual stenosis in either the LAD or the first diagonal. The has patient remained asymptomatic, with a negative exercise test, at 6 months follow-up.

is no significant stenosis in the side branch, no further treatment is necessary; the side branch wire can be easily removed. If the side branch has an ostial stenosis, a third wire is passed into this branch using the trapped side branch wire as a guide, following which this first wire is removed. Further inflations are made using this last wire through the stent struts, if necessary using a new low profile balloon. Frequently, 'kissing balloon' inflations are required to optimise the final angiographic (and long-term) result, particulary if a stent has been deployed in the side branch.

THROMBUS-CONTAINING LESIONS

In the setting of the acute coronary syndromes, thrombus is usually present, even if it is not angiographically evident. It is, of course, also usually present in the setting of acute occlusion following angioplasty or stent implantation. The importance of the presence of thrombus has been well documented.[8] Despite pre-treatment with antiplatelet agents and intra-procedural heparin, the risk of acute occlusion and/or distal embolisation is high.

The first important consideration is to optimise the antiplatelet/anticoagulant approach to these patients, ideally prior to intervention. All patients should be on aspirin and, if stent implantation is considered, clopidogrel. There are mounting data to support the use of glycoprotein IIb/IIIa antagonists in patients with unstable angina, particularly in the setting of percutaneous intervention.[9,10] At present, abciximab (ReoPro) is the only agent licensed for use in the setting of percutaneous intervention although eptifibatide (Integrilin) and tirofiban (Aggrastat) are likely to be licensed soon. Ideally these agents should be given at the start of the procedure (or before) and not as 'rescue'. The main factor limiting their use is cost, such that ReoPro is currently only used in approximately 5% of cases in the UK. However, it is these high risk patients who derive particular benefit and their use must be considered in the presence of thrombus. In general, thrombolysis (intravenous or intra-coronary), hirudin, hirulog or dextran have little role in current angioplasty practice.

The next consideration is to optimise the results of angioplasty. Balloon angioplasty of a thrombus-containing lesion almost invariably results in distal embolisation. Several alternative approaches have therefore been tried. One would be to give the patient ReoPro (above) and to delay the angioplasty for several hours. Although data specifically supporting this approach are lacking, the benefit of these agents in patients with unstable angina is magnified in those undergoing percutaneous intervention, and dramatic results can occur (see Fig. 9.2).

There are several thrombus removal devices available. One of the first was transluminal extraction catheter (TEC). This device is a motor-driven cutting device, which is designed to excise and aspirate atherosclerotic plaque and thrombus. It requires a 10.5 F arterial sheath and although this is rarely used now, it can be of use in long thrombotic vein graft lesions. More recent devices include ultrasound thrombolysis, thrombectomy catheters (for example the Possis device and the Rescue system), and the X-Sizer thrombus removal device.

Having reduced the thrombus burden, stent implantation is usually indicated. A major potential pitfall is distal embolisation at the time of balloon inflation and/or stent deployment. For this reason, self expanding stents with a high metal-to-artery ratio (for example the Wallstent) or a covered stent (for example the JoMed Stent Graft) may be associated with less distal embolisation.

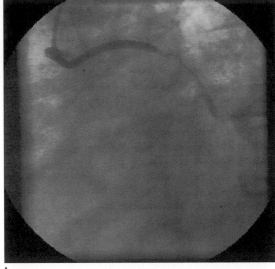

Figure 9.2:
(a) A recent occlusion in a saphenous vein graft to an obtuse marginal vessel with TIMI 0 flow and no opacification of the distal vessel. The patient was started on ReoPro and the angioplasty procedure delayed for 1 hour. Repeat angiography (b) revealed TIMI 3 flow and a large thrombus containing lesion in the mid-portion of the vein graft. Subsequent angioplasty was performed with debulking of the lesion using a 2.0 mm eccentric laser catheter and deployment of two 47 mm Wallstents.

A

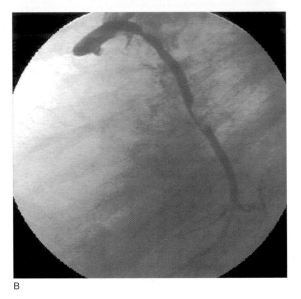

B

SAPHENOUS VEIN GRAFT LESIONS (FOCAL AND DIFFUSE)

Saphenous vein graft lesions deserve special mention. Vein grafts have an approximately 50% 10 year patency rate, and re-do bypass surgery has a much higher morbidity and mortality compared to first-time surgery. For these reasons, angioplasty may have a particular role in treating vein graft lesions. The pathology of degenerated vein grafts differs from native atherosclerosis, and it is generally accepted that restenosis rates are higher and the process tends not to be limited to the first 6 months after the procedure. Many of the considerations are similar to thrombus-containing lesions – particularly the higher risk of distal embolisation; vein graft disease tends to be much more friable than native atherosclerosis or restenotic lesions (some liken it to toothpaste or cream cheese!). Great care must therefore be taken – unfortunately it is all too common for distal embolisation to result in complete vessel occlusion with resulting myocardial infarction. In addition, as mentioned above, if the patient requires emergency surgery, the risks are much higher than in the setting of a first time operation.

Several approaches to reducing distal embolisation have been attempted. Recently, distal protection devices have been developed, and these are currently undergoing extensive development and testing in clinical trials. Broadly speaking, these devices aim to capture atherosclerotic material and thrombus that is 'released' from the lesion treated, thus preventing (or at least reducing) distal embolisation. Two such devices are the Angioguard and the PercuSurge device. The Angioguard emboli capture guidewire system (Cordis/Johnson & Johnson) consists of a polyurethane filter basket with 100 μm pores attached to a 0.014 inch guidewire, which allows continuous perfusion while ensuring effective capture of microemboli. The filter basket is deployed, the lesion is treated and the basket is re-captured with the embolic material. The PercuSurge device consists of a guidewire incorporating a 5.5-mm long balloon near its distal tip.[11] This is inflated distal to the lesion, the lesion is treated and an aspiration catheter is advanced over the wire, particulate debris is aspirated and the balloon deflated. Trials are ongoing comparing this with more conventional approaches, but preliminary data are promising.

The next consideration is whether or not to debulk the lesion. In our experience, the excimer laser can be useful to create a channel large enough to pass a stent across the lesion thus reducing the risk of distal embolisation, but is infrequently used in current practice. In the setting of an acute coronary syndrome, or where thrombus is evident angiographically, IIb/IIIa antagonists and one of the thrombectomy systems should be considered (see above). As for thrombus-containing lesions, high metal-to-artery ratio stents, or covered stents, should be considered. One problem of treating saphenous vein grafts is that not only is target lesion revascularisation high, but so is target vessel revascularisation. In other words, lesions often develop in other parts of the vein graft. Because of this, our approach is, in the presence of a degenerated vein graft, to stent the whole graft rather than just the lesion, although if the lesion is very focal and the rest of the graft is angiographically completely normal then just the lesion is treated.

RESTENOTIC LESIONS

Following balloon angioplasty, 'clinical' restenosis (i.e. target lesion revascularisation) occurs in anything up to 30% of cases depending on many factors, including final MLD (minimum lumen diameter), length and location of lesion, etc. Clearly, if a patient re-presents with symptoms and restenosis then, if further intervention is considered, stent implantation is usually indicated unless the vessel is too small. The main problem is how to deal with in-stent restenosis which, with the widespread and increasing use of stents, is becoming an increasing management problem.

Several approaches to repeat intervention for in-stent restenosis have been attempted and a detailed description of them is clearly outside the scope of this chapter. Briefly, if the restenosis is focal then balloon angioplasty using a non-compliant balloon matched to the reference vessel has reasonable results. However, if the restenosis is diffuse, the results of repeat balloon dilatation are very poor – with repeat restenosis rates up to 80%. For this reason, alternative approaches have been sought. In our experience, restenotic stents are frequently under-deployed. For this reason, intravascular ultrasound is very useful to determine stent and reference vessel size and to optimise subsequent treatment. One of the stimuli for neo-intimal proliferation is medial and adventitial stretch. With this in mind, debulking the tissue may have a role.[12,13] Trials are currently underway comparing both the excimer laser and the Rotablator with balloon angioplasty in this setting. Essentially, the approach is to remove as much tissue as possible, using either a 2.0 mm excimer laser catheter or a 2.38 mm Rotablator burr with multiple passes, followed by balloon angioplasty using a non-compliant balloon matched to the reference vessel. Although not widely available as yet, intra-coronary brachytherapy is the only technique that has convincingly been shown to reduce the late loss index following angioplasty and is likely to have an increasing role in the treatment of in-stent restenosis in the future.

CHRONIC TOTAL OCCLUSIONS

In most published series, the single commonest cause of failure in angioplasty is the presence of a total occlusion, in other words, inability to cross with a wire. If you can cross with a wire, you can usually succeed. The likelihood of success is dependent on many factors including the duration of the occlusion (low success if >6 months; best if within 4 weeks), the length of the occlusion, the presence of bridging collaterals (a bad sign), a side branch at the site of the occlusion (another bad sign) and a 'funnel' into the occlusion (a good sign). Other factors that should be taken into account are the viability of the myocardium served by the occluded vessel, the extent of the patients' symptoms, the presence of contralateral collaterals, etc. It must be remembered that trying to reopen an occluded vessel is not without risk – for example, guide catheter trauma can occur, and the wire can perforate or cause a distal dissection resulting in closure of collaterals and subsequent myocardial infarction.

This is one situation where guide catheter choice is extremely important – adequate back-up is essential. For example, for right coronary lesions, consider a hockeystick, AL1 or similar guide; for the left coronary, consider a Voda, EBU, XB or similar guide. In general, Judkins guides do not provide adequate support. Initial guidewire choice depends on personal preference. Again, adequate support is essential. Our approach is to use either a Terumo Crosswire, a Magnum wire (with a relatively atraumatic olive tip) or a Choice PT extra-support wire with back-up using a Multifunctional Probing catheter. Although a balloon can be used as back-up, the Probing catheter has the advantage of having a second over-the-wire lumen that can be used for introduction of a second wire or contrast injection to confirm wire position in the distal lumen. If a second wire is introduced this way, the Crosswire can be useful as it has a hydrophilic coating over the whole length and can be 'blown off' with a syringe of water without the need of an exchange length wire. Recently, vibrational angioplasty has been developed in an attempt to improve the success in crossing occlusions.[14] Briefly, a conventional guidewire is attached to a battery-driven handheld motorised device which generates a loose reciprocal motion in the wire with a frequency of 16–100 Hz. Preliminary data suggest reasonably high procedural success, although randomised data are awaited.

If difficulty is obtained in crossing the occlusion, the use of a biplane lab can be useful, as can simultaneous bilateral injections to delineate the collaterals. Our approach is to use the laser-tipped guidewire if unable to cross using conventional wires. If dissection or dye extravasation has occurred following conventional guidewires, it is useful to wait 6 to 8 weeks before an additional attempt with the laser-tipped guidewire. In general, provided there are sufficient collaterals and biplane and bilateral injections are used, the laser can be successful in approximately 50 to 60% of occlusions refractory to conventional wires. Following successful crossing of the total occlusion, the lesion should be pre-dilated with a balloon prior to stent implantation.

The outcome of balloon angioplasty of totally occluded saphenous vein grafts is disappointing, such that many interventionists will not attempt to re-open them. As mentioned above, distal embolisation can occur resulting in myocardial infarction. Provided the occlusion is recent, our approach is to debulk the graft using the excimer laser and to deploy Wallstents covering the whole length of the graft. However, this approach is as yet unproven and is currently undergoing evaluation with late angiographic follow-up.

AORTO-OSTIAL LESIONS

Coronary intervention for aorto-ostial stenoses is associated with a lower rate of primary success and a higher rate of restenosis compared to non-ostial stenoses. These lesions are frequently calcified and fibrotic, which can result in inadequate dilatation or stent deployment. The increased acute complications can, in part, be explained by guide catheter trauma;

guide catheter placement can be extremely difficult – it needs to be stable and co-axial without deep intubation. Finally, ostial location implies a large area of myocardium at risk should acute closure occur.

For these reasons, intravascular ultrasound can be useful in determining the lesion composition (and reference vessel size). In the presence of dense fibrosis and/or calcification, the Rotablator is useful prior to stent implantation, which frequently requires high pressure deployment or post-inflation using a non-compliant balloon to high pressures. In the absence of calcification, some operators use directional atherectomy, again prior to stent implantation, although (as discussed above) the use of this device has declined.

Unprotected left main ostial stenoses are rarely attempted. If surgery is not considered an option, for whatever reason, then angioplasty can be cautiously performed.[15] Consideration should be given to the use of a balloon pump, even in the absence of impaired left ventricular function. Because of the obvious implications of subacute closure, intravascular ultrasound is useful for accurate sizing of the stent and to confirm optimal deployment with full strut apposition and the absence of edge dissections.

Isolated vein graft ostial stenoses can usually be treated with a high degree of success with stent implantation. Occasionally, these lesions are very fibrotic necessitating dubulking with the excimer laser (or directional atherectomy) prior to stent implantation.

CONCLUSIONS

With the marked improvements in angioplasty equipment, most lesions can be treated with a high degree of success. Despite the widespread use of stents, it is still useful to adopt a lesion specific approach – particular lesion subsets, in particular chronic occlusions, calcification, thrombus, vein graft disease and bifurcation lesions require particular considerations and techniques in order to optimise acute and long-term results.

REFERENCES

1. Ryan TJ, Faxon DP, Gunnar RM *et al*. Guidelines for percutaneous transluminal coronary angioplasty. A report of the American College of Cardiology/American Heart Association task force on assessment of diagnostic and therapeutic cardiovascular procedures (subcommittee on percutaneous transluminal coronary angioplasty). Circulation 1988;78:486–502.

2. Kastrati A, Schomig A, Elezi S *et al*. Prognostic value of the modified American College of Cardiology/American Heart Association stenosis morphology classification for long-term angiographic and clinical outcome after coronary stent placement. Circulation 1999;100:1285–90.

3. Ellis SG, Guetta V, Miller D, Whitlow PL, Topol EJ. Relation between lesion characteristics and risk with percutaneous intervention in the stent and glycoprotein IIb/IIIa era. Circulation 1999;100:1971–6.

4. Zaacks SM, Allen JE, Calvin JE *et al*. Value of the American College of Cardiology/American Heart Association stenosis morphology classification for coronary interventions in the late 1990s. Am J Cardiol 1988;82:43–9.

5. Moussa I, Moses J, Di Mario C *et al*. Stenting after optimal lesion debulking (SOLD) registry. Circulation 1998;98:1604–1609.

6. Dauerman HL, Higgins PJ, Sparano AM *et al*. Mechanical debulking versus balloon angioplasty for the treatment of true bifurcation lesions. J Am Coll Cardiol 1998;32:1845–52.

7. Pan M, Suarez de Lezo J, Medina A *et al*. Simple and complex stent strategies for bifurcated coronary arterial stenosis involving the side branch origin. Am J Cardiol 1999;83:1320–25.

8. Waxman S, Sassower MA, Mittleman MA *et al*. Angioscopic predictors of early adverse outcome after coronary angioplasty in patients with unstable angina and non-Q wave myocardial infarction. Circulation 1996;93:2106–13.

9. The EPIC Investigators. Use of a monoclonal antibody directed against the platelet glycoprotein IIb/IIIa receptor in high-risk coronary angioplasty. N Engl J Med 1994;330:956–61.

10. The EPILOG Investigators: Platelet glycoprotein IIb/IIIa receptor blockade and low-dose heparin during percutaneous coronary revascularization. N Engl J Med 1997;336:1689–96.

11. Webb JG, Carere RG, Virmani R *et al*. Retrieval and analysis of particulate debris after saphenous vein graft intervention. J Am Coll Cardiol 1999;34:468–75.

12. Lee S-G, Lee CW, Cheong S-S *et al*. Immediate and long-term outcomes of rotational atherectomy versus balloon angioplasty alone for treatment of diffuse in-stent restenosis. Am J Cardiol 1998;82:140–43.

13. Mehran R, Mintz GS, Satler LF *et al*. Treatment of in-stent restenosis with excimer laser coronary angioplasty. Mechanisms and results compared with PTCA alone. Circulation 1997;96:2183–9.

14. Rees MR, Michalis LK. Activated guidewire technique for the treatment of chronic coronary artery occlusion. Lancet 1995;346:943–4.

15. Park S-J, Park S-W, Hong M-K *et al*. Stenting of unprotected left main stenoses: immediate and late outcomes. J Am Coll Cardiol 1998;31:37–42.

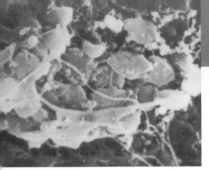

10

Rotational atherectomy

MARK DE BELDER

KEY POINTS

- Rotablation is ideal for hard, calcified or 'undilatable' lesions.

- It is technically demanding.

- Useful for debulking long diffuse disease in small vessels.

- May be the preferred treatment for diffuse in stent restenosis.

- The maximum burr size limits use in large vessels.

- Its use is not advised in saphenous vein grafts, or where angiographic evidence of dissection or thrombus.

INTRODUCTION

Rotational atherectomy (more commonly referred to as 'rotablation') is a technique which utilises a high-speed rotating diamond-coated elliptically shaped burr to ablate atheroma in the coronary or peripheral arteries (Fig. 10.1). Two to three thousand diamond microchips, 30–50 μm in diameter, are embedded in the front half of the burr. As the burr rotates, the atheromatous plaque is, in effect, emulsified. The resulting particles of atheroma (mostly 5 to 10 μm) are smaller than red cells and are washed downstream through the coronary capillary system into the coronary veins and then are removed from the circulation by the reticuloendothelial system, especially in the lung, liver and spleen.

The burrs come in a number of sizes, ranging from 1.25 to 2.50 mm in diameter. The burr is advanced along a specialised guidewire which is first positioned across the lesion of interest. The principle of action is through orthogonal displacement of friction. There is a great deal of friction in a longitudinal direction between the burr and the guidewire, but the vector

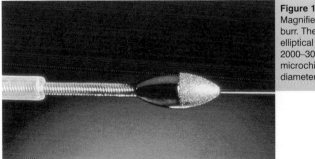

Figure 10.1:
Magnified view of a rotablator burr. The front face of the elliptical burr is studded with 2000–3000 diamond microchips, 30–50 μm in diameter.

of friction can be changed to a circumferential direction by high-speed rotation. This can be likened to removing a ring from a finger. It may be impossible to remove the ring by just pulling it straight off the finger because of the friction between the ring and skin folds. However, the ring becomes easy to remove if it is rotated as it is advanced along the finger. This orthogonal displacement of friction allows the device to be taken along tortuous vessels. The rotablator burrs are rotated at speeds of between 150 000–190 000 rpm. As larger burrs have a higher surface velocity than small ones at the same number of revolutions per second, they are used at lower rotational speeds. Trying to rotate bigger burrs at faster speeds may lead to complications, in part related to an excessive attempt at plaque ablation which can result in embolisation of large fragments and a reduction in coronary flow (see below). The cross-sectional areas of each burr are given in Table 10.1.

Another principle of operation is referred to as 'differential cutting' (Fig. 10.2). Elastic tissue deflects away from the burr whereas inelastic tissue cannot deflect and is therefore ablated. This results in ablation of

TABLE 10.1 – SIZES AND CROSS-SECTIONAL AREAS OF BURRS			
BURR DIAMETER (MM)	DIFFERENCE IN DIAMETER FROM NEXT BURR SIZE DOWN (MM)	BURR CROSS-SECTIONAL AREA CSA (MM^2)	DIFFERENCE IN CSA FROM NEXT BURR SIZE DOWN (MM^2)
1.25		1.23	
1.5	0.25	1.77	0.54
1.75	0.25	2.41	0.64
2.0	0.25	3.14	0.73
2.15	0.15	3.63	0.49
2.25	0.1	3.98	0.35
2.38	0.13	4.45	0.47
2.5	0.12	4.91	0.46

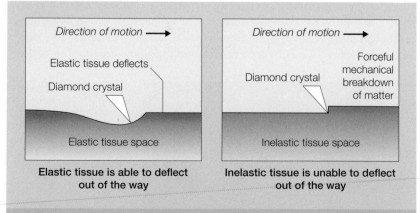

Elastic tissue is able to deflect out of the way

Inelastic tissue is unable to deflect out of the way

Figure 10.2:
Principal of 'differential cutting'.

atheromatous plaque but minimisation of injury to healthy arterial wall. In practice, especially for lesions on bends, the principle is more one of 'preferential cutting'. In other words, atheromatous plaque is the main tissue of ablation, but normal vessel wall will also be ablated in part. The technique minimises vessel wall stretch and results in a circular, smooth lumen providing ideal conditions for flow. Although developed primarily for treatment of hard or calcified plaque it has been shown to be effective also for soft plaque, but it is not a treatment for removal of thrombus.

The burr is welded to a flexible 135 cm drive shaft which is connected to a compressed air driven turbine (Fig. 10.3). The air pressure required is 90 to 100 psi. The device is activated by pressing on a foot-pedal. The speed of the device can be changed by altering the pressure and volume of compressed air entering the small turbine within the body of the operating handle. The speed is recorded by a fibre-optic cable and is constantly shown on the operating console. The drive shaft rotates within a 4.3 F Teflon sheath. This prevents the spinning shaft from causing injury, and also acts as a channel through which saline is passed as the burr is activated. The saline acts as a lubricant and heat disperser. The original stainless steel steerable 0.009 inch guidewire had a 0.017 inch tip which prevents distal embolisation of the burr in the extremely unlikely eventuality of a fracture between the burr and the drive shaft. The device should not be used with guidewires manufactured for standard angioplasty techniques.

SUMMARY

Rotablation

■ Uses a high-speed rotating burr.

■ The burr is diamond coated.

■ It rotates at 150 000–190 000 rpm.

■ The burr size is 1.25–2.50 mm in diameter.

■ Rotablation is used for ablation of atheromatous plaque.

■ It results in a smooth circular lumen.

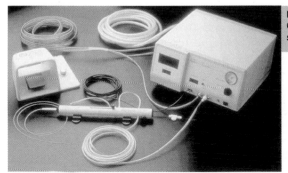

Figure 10.3:
Components of the rotablator system.

The rotablator was developed by David Auth, a physisist and engineer who initially worked on a device to remove thrombus from vessels. After early work with laser techniques, he began to investigate mechanical methods of plaque ablation. An initial design required a central aspiration tube for removal of debris but in 1983 to developed the concept of 'rotary sanding' with diamond-tipped burrs. After initial animal and human cadaver studies,[1,2] the device was used *in vivo*, first in the peripheral and then in the coronary circulation but the technique did not take off however until the early 1990s.[3-7] Initial clinical results were very favourable, especially in lesions not suited to balloon angioplasty. It is particularly suited to treat calcified lesions or lesions resistant to balloon dilatation.[8,9] After its initial release and early clinical use, a minor change to its manufacturing process resulted in a small number of major complications (including fracture of the drive shaft). The device was immediately recalled by the manufacturing company (Heart Technology), the fault identified and corrected and it was then re-released. None of the initial problems have occurred since in spite of many hundreds of thousands of patient treatments. Heart Technology has since been acquired by the Boston–Scientific–Scimed Corporation.

After initial registry data reporting high procedural success rates for complex lesion subsets, a number of randomised trials have shown that rotablation can increase the interventional success rate and reduce the complication rate compared with balloon or laser angioplasty. The most important of these has been the ERBAC (Excimer Laser, Rotational Atherectomy, and Balloon Angioplasty Comparison) study.[10] This was a single-centre study comparing rotablation with excimer laser and balloon angioplasty in complex lesion subsets. The procedural success rate was highest with rotablation (89% vs 77% vs 80%, $p = 0.0019$), although overall complications were not statistically different. Although this and other studies have shown that rotablation is advantageous in the treatment of these difficult lesions, it has not been shown to reduce restenosis.

After several years of clinical use, a number of practical considerations have resulted in minor design changes. The original guidewire had poor torque transmission, was difficult to steer, and has since been modified. With the original device, each burr and drive shaft was attached to a single operating handle. As the technique often required more than one burr, the technique became unnecessarily expensive. Now, there is a single operating handle for one case, and detachable burrs can be utilised sequentially. A number of modifications to technique have also been recommended (see below).

Although the three major techniques for atherectomy or tissue ablation all have their advantages and disadvantages, the triple helix drive shaft of the rotablator makes it much more flexible than the other two. This allows it to be used in tortuous vessels unsuitable for treatment by the other techniques. Its range of burr sizes allows it to be used safely in small vessels, but the largest burr size of 2.5 mm limits the largest final lumen area in large vessels. It is significantly less expensive than laser techniques although considerably more expensive than balloon angioplasty. Because of the expense of laser technology, many catheter laboratories limit their use of atherectomy to directional atherectomy and rotablation (and some use a fourth device, the transluminal extraction catheter – the 'TEC' device – manufactured by Interventional Technologies Inc., which is more suited to thrombus-laden lesions). Directional atherectomy is more appropriate for bulky eccentric lesions in large vessels, especially if there is a relatively straight approach to the lesion from the coronary ostium), whereas rotablation is better suited to difficult lesions in smaller vessels, especially if the lesion is downstream or in a tortuous vessel. They are thus likely to be used in different situations and are not competitive devices.

TECHNIQUE

Rotablation is probably the most difficult coronary interventional technique to master. It should not be used until an operator is extremely adept at conventional balloon and stenting techniques. It requires a much greater degree of patience and is more time-consuming than balloon angioplasty or stenting and great care has to be taken at each step of the technique. Its advantages are only seen if the technique is correctly carried out, and errors will significantly increase the complication rate.

Preparation of the patient

All patients should be on aspirin or an equivalent antiplatelet agent and heparinisation is as for any percutaneous coronary intervention. It is recommended that beta blockers are discontinued 24 hours prior to planned rotablation. The patient should be kept well hydrated and most operators give the patient a litre of intravenous saline during the procedure. Rotablation induces more angina than standard PTCA and liberal use of sedatives or opiate analgesia should be used. As this may lead to hypotension, the intravenous saline is all the more important. If the blood pressure falls below 100 mmHg, 100–300 µg aliquots of intravenous phenylephrine should be considered before or during the procedure. If the patient is bradycardic, intravenous atropine should be considered prior to starting. Although the validity of a 'vasodilator cocktail' solution is still in question, many operators use this to reduce the risk of the slow-flow phenomenon (see below). If one is to be used, the nursing staff should prepare the infusion solution prior to starting. There are a number of variations on the theme, but this author uses 5 mg glyceryl trinitrate (GTN) and 5 mg verapamil in 500 ml saline with no additional heparin.

   If the vessel to be treated is the right coronary artery or a dominant circumflex, then a temporary transvenous pacing electrode should be inserted into the right ventricle. This is because of the high incidence of bradycardia or complete heart block which occurs when treating these vessels, possibly because of an effect of microcavitation, transient haemolysis or embolisation disturbing the blood supply of the sinoatrial or atrioventricular nodes. A pacing electrode should also be used for the left anterior descending artery if a right or dominant circumflex artery is occluded. Some operators prefer to use a pacing flotation catheter with its tip in the pulmonary artery. Not only will this pace as required, but the pulmonary diastolic pressure is used to monitor ischaemia of the left ventricle.

Quantitative angiography and choice of equipment

The choice of equipment will depend on the method of rotablation to be used. In general, there are two views. The simpler method is used by many European operators and is sometimes referred to as 'facilitated angioplasty'. In this, a single medium-sized burr is used to create a channel and then balloon angioplasty is performed in conventional manner. Careful sizing of the burr is not so important. The second technique (advocated by David Auth) is used more by operators in the United States (and is often referred to as 'maximal debulking'). It is important to choose a final burr which is not too large for the vessel, and therefore most operators will use quantitative coronary angiography (QCA). Using conventional diagnostic equipment and after intra-coronary nitrates (150–300 µg GTN), QCA should be performed or intravascular ultrasound (IVUS) images acquired. The upstream reference diameter (downstream if an ostial lesion), minimal lumen diameter and lesion length should be measured. To choose the largest burr to be used, 85% of the reference diameter is calculated; the final burr will be this size or less. Most operators use a final burr:artery ratio of 0.60–0.85. The operator should then determine whether to do the case with one, two or three burrs. The difference in size of sequential burrs should be not be greater than 0.5 mm. The first burr will usually be 1.25 mm, 1.5 mm, or 1.75 mm. If the lesion is particularly complex, very calcified or long, it is better to start with the smallest burr. The size of the guiding catheter and sheath will depend on the largest burr to be used. The sizes required do not have to be committed to memory as they are available on a wall chart provided by the manufacturer. The 2.50 burr will not pass through some manufacturer's Y-connector and if this burr will be needed it is important to select appropriate equipment. Interventionists who routinely use IVUS use rotablation more frequently than those who depend primarily on angiography. IVUS reveals calcification more readily than angiography, and the extent of calcification has been shown to increase the risk of dissection with balloon angioplasty.

The choice of guide catheter is up to the operator, but in general catheters with multiple or significant bends should be avoided, as this can make it difficult getting the burr into the coronary artery. Most operators use a side-hole catheter to maximise coronary perfusion during the procedure.

Preparation prior to rotablation

The new 'Rotawire' guidewire comes in a floppy and standard form. After selecting which to use, the wire is placed across the lesion using the wire clip provided as a torquer. The 325 cm exchange length monofilament wire has a platinum spring tip. The distal part of the wire should be parked in a fairly straight part of the arterial lumen and not in a side-branch with a very angulated take-off. The system's brake prevents wire spin when the system is activated but wire spin can occur when the brake is defeated during burr withdrawal with a risk of dissection downstream of the lesion – the wire clip prevents this. The first burr should then be selected and attached to the operating handle. The fibre-optic and compressed air lines are then attached and the GTN/verapamil infusion is attached to the flush line. The whole system should be flushed through until drops appear at the rotablator burr. The burr is then fed onto the guidewire and brought up to the valve of the Y-connector. It is easier during the procedure if the operator has two assistants, one to hold the end of the wire, and one to hold the operating handle whilst the burr is being advanced. The wire clip should then be placed on the wire just distal to the advancer unit to prevent or minimise spin when the braking system is inactivated. With a technician ensuring that the flush solution is passed through the rotablator whenever it is activated, the system is started using the foot pedal, and the technician chooses the settings on the console to select the desired rotablator speed. Because of the intrinsic resistance of the system once it is in place within the coronary circulation, the speed should be set at 5000 to 10 000 rpm higher than the desired working speed. For burrs of 2 mm or less, the system should be set at about 180 000 to 190 000 rpm which will result in a speed within the coronary artery of about 175 000 to 180 000 rpm. For burrs larger than 2 mm, the speed should be set at 170 000 to 180 000 rpm, giving a working speed in the artery of about 160 000 to 165 000 rpm. Once the speed has been selected the device is turned off, and the burr is then taken up the guidewire to the coronary artery.

Rotablating

The burr should be positioned 2 mm or so upstream of the lesion. The rotablator should never be started or stopped within the lesion itself. The helical arrangement of the drive shaft acts as a spring and if the last movement prior to activation was to take the burr forward, the burr sometimes jumps forward and can lead to torsional intimal dissection. To avoid this, the burr can either be pulled back slightly before activation, or the O-ring of the Y-connector and the burr control knob on the advancer unit should be loosened to release stored energy in the drive shaft. Once everything is ready, the technician should be asked to start the GTN/verapamil infusion and the device activated using the foot-pedal. The rotablator should not be forced. Gentle pressure should be applied, keeping the rotablator passes as short as possible. In general, these should be kept down to 10 to 20 seconds but occasionally longer runs may be necessary. Between passes the burr should be brought upstream of the lesion, allowing maximal coronary perfusion. This dissipates heat, and helps wash out particulate matter. Sufficient time should be allowed between passes to allow the vessel to settle. Contrast injections can ensure that no vessel reactivity or 'slow-flow' is developing (see below). The speed should not drop by more than 5000 rpm. If the device slows more than this, heat generation is increased (a powerful stimulator of restenosis) and complications increase. Dropping the speed by more than 15 000 rpm can result in the system stalling with a high chance of torsional dissection. After the lesion has been crossed several times slightly faster 'polishing' runs are often performed. Although lesions in distal segments can be treated, the rotating burr should never be taken beyond its transition to the platinum tip as this may cut the tip off.

The burr is removed from the artery by first pressing the 'dynaglide' button on the foot-pedal which reduces the speed of the device to 60 000 to 90 000 rpm. The device is then activated whilst the brake defeat button on the operating handle is pressed, and the burr withdrawn. The wire clip is attached at this point to the end of the wire, but the wire can be looped so that the clip attaches into a space provided at the back of the advancer unit. This prevents wire spin and eases device withdrawal if there is a single operator. The burr is brought out of the Y-connector using this technique, but once out of the guide catheter, it can be easily removed from the wire without activation of the turbine. If appropriate, the next burr is connected to the operating handle and the process repeated.

Post-rotablation ballooning

There is considerable debate about the use of balloon angioplasty after rotablation. In general, in keeping with the 'Bigger is Best' rule of angioplasty, there is always a desire to maximise the lumen size at the time of a treatment, as this results in lower restenosis rates. However, it has been proposed that if rotablation is used correctly, the stimulus for neointimal proliferation should be minimised. If the internal elastic lamina remains intact, and there is minimal medial damage, then achieving a lumen of 2–2.5 mm in diameter provides adequate coronary flow reserve, abolition of angina, and hopefully no significant restenosis. David Auth has suggested that the best results would be achieved with no ballooning or, if ballooning is to be used, a slightly oversized balloon should be used at 1 atmosphere or less, achieving a satisfactory degree of plaque compression without causing deep vessel injury. Initial observational data suggested that maximal debulking with no adjunctive angioplasty may result in the lowest restenosis rates. Although a larger final lumen diameter may be achieved by using adjunctive high pressure balloon dilatation, this may result in a greater stimulus to neointimal proliferation. Conversely, the greater final lumen achieved by ballooning might accommodate future proliferation, resulting in a larger long-term luminal area. The comparative effects of 'facilitated angioplasty' and 'maximal debulking' (with little or no adjunctive ballooning) on the incidence of restenosis are being evaluated in STRATAS (Study To determine Rotablator And Transluminal Angioplasty Strategy). The potential effect of the maximal debulking/minimal ballooning technique in reducing restenosis is also being evaluated in a randomised trial comparing it with conventional balloon angioplasty in DART (Dilation vs Ablation Revascularisation Trial). Many operators acknowledge the debate, but few use just rotablation alone. However, those who want to use ballooning have modified their technique, but instead of using the method suggested by Auth, they use slightly oversized balloons at 4–6 atmospheres. Given that animal models of restenosis can be achieved with 2 atmospheres or more, this concept of a moderate reduction in balloon pressure has no scientific basis. Clearly, further research is required to identify the technique which results in the lowest restenosis rates, although these technical considerations may become irrelevant if restenosis can be prevented by intra-coronary brachytherapy. Until the results of trials are known, many operators prefer to continue with practice consistent with the 'Bigger Is Best' theory, maximising the post-procedural minimal lumen diameter.

Rotablation induces a generalised coronary spasm which takes time to wear off. In spite of the GTN/verapamil mix, the vessel is often smaller than at the end of the procedure than the size of the biggest burr used. This results in a scenario completely the opposite to standard PTCA. With PTCA, the vessel may look fine at the end of the procedure, but if one were to look the next day, the vessel would look smaller at the site of the lesion because of recoil. With rotablation, the vessel looks bigger the next day because the spasm has worn off.

Post-rotablator care
This is the same as for any percutaneous coronary intervention. Because 9 F or 10 F sheaths are often needed, an extended 8-hour bed rest after sheath removal may reduce bleeding complications from the groin.

SUMMARY

Rotablation technique:

- Is technically demanding.
- More time consuming than PTCA or stenting.
- More expensive than PTCA.
- Usually requires 9 F or 10 F guide catheters.
- Enhances procedural success for complex or calcified lesions, especially in small vessels.

LIMITATIONS AND COMPLICATIONS

Vasoreactivity

This expression can be applied to a number of scenarios:

- The patient experiences more chest pain than is expected in spite of a patent vessel.
- The vessel goes into severe spasm.
- There is a slow-flow or no-flow phenomenon.
- Fairly dramatic ECG changes occur (with or without vessel patency).

Under these circumstances, it is best to abandon rotablation, and to use balloon angioplasty with or without stenting or abciximab. If rotablation is continued there will be a much greater chance of a serious slow-flow phenomenon or even perforation. If stepping up to a larger burr had been considered, this should only be done once everything settles with liberal use of vasodilators. Even if the vessel settles however, there is still a high chance of slow-flow after the next burr.

Slow- or no-flow

This expression applies when the vessel appears to be patent, but there is no or very sluggish flow down the vessel. The incidence is low. This is probably a multifactorial phenomenon including distal embolisation (usually due to excessively aggressive rotablation, but possibly due to particles from transient haemolysis), platelet aggregation, distal spasm and microbubbles. The patient usually has transient ECG changes, a rise in cardiac enzymes, and may even develop a Q-wave infarct in spite of a patent vessel. It is of note that operators very rarely see this phenomenon with restenosis lesions, suggesting that native vessel tissue factors are important in its development. Recent work has suggested that it can be minimized by reducing the speed of rotablation. In general, the longer, more complex or more calcified the lesion the more likely it is to get a slow-flow phenomenon. It is also likely to occur in chronic occlusions or near occlusions in vessels which are well collateralised, possibly because of an increased risk of stasis beyond the lesion after rotablation. Thus, whereas collaterals make balloon angioplasty safer as a procedure, they may increase the risk of rotablation.

A number of techniques are thought to help reverse it. The coronary artery can be flushed with heparinised saline or 20 ml of the patient's own blood. Aliquots of intra-coronary GTN, verapamil, or adenosine have been suggested in order to maximally dilate the distal coronary bed. Abciximab may limit its consequences, and there is some evidence that pre-treatment with abciximab reduces the risk of slow-flow developing. Intravenous phenylephrine or dobutamine may be required to maintain arterial pressure, as slow-flow appears to be worse with hypotension. If severe, the use of an intra-aortic balloon pump should be considered. As with vessel reactivity, if it occurs early on in a planned procedure, further rotablation should be abandoned and the procedure finished with balloon angioplasty with or without stenting or abciximab.

Severe spasm

If this occurs, intra-coronary GTN, verapamil or adenosine should be used, using intravenous phenylephrine or dobutamine, if necessary, to sustain intra-aortic pressure. It can sometimes be 'broken' by a prolonged balloon inflation at low pressure.

Perforation

With careful case selection and adherence to the correct technique, this should not occur, but it has been reported in lesions with severe angulation and cases with severe 'guidewire encroachment' (see below). If it does occur, the operator should be prepared to perform emergency pericardiocentesis. Prolonged ballooning with conventional or perfusion balloons, or stenting with conventional or covered stents may seal the vessel. Reversing the heparin with protamine can be considered but if perforation occurs, a cardiothoracic surgeon should be called immediately as emergency coronary artery bypass grafting, sometimes with vascular repair, is often required.

Guidewire encroachment

This expression is used to describe a situation which might arise when a lesion is on the inner curve of a bend. When the guidewire is passed, it usually takes the outer curve. If there is a considerable bend, this might direct the burr away from the lesion and towards the opposite, relatively normal, vessel wall (Fig. 10.4). This can be a harbinger of perforation. If the bend is excessive, then rotablation should probably be avoided. If considered, however, the guidewire can be curved to suit the artery before starting the procedure. In addition, smaller burrs should be used.

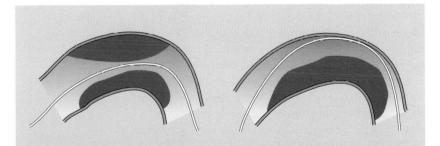

Figure 10.4:
Guidewire bias or encroachment. If a lesion on a bend is concentric, the guidewire passes through the vessel centrally and the burr is able to ablate the lesion. If, however, the lesion is predominantly on the inner curve, the wire will preferentially take the outer curve; the burr is then directed towards the outer wall and away from the plaque. Under these circumstances, there may be less tissue ablation than expected and, if extreme, there is an increased risk of perforation should excessive damage be done to the outer wall.

The avoidance of lesions with severe guidewire encroachment, a greater understanding of the limitations of rotabalation, adherence to the correct technique, the use of a vasodilatory cocktail, maintenance of blood pressure, the use of short rotablation runs, making sure that rotablator speed does not drop, and the early use of abciximab and intra-aortic balloon pumps have all probably played a role in achieving high success rates with this device whilst minimising the risk of complications.[11]

SUMMARY

Limitations and potential for complications with rotablation:

- Vaso-reactivity.

- Slow-flow or no-flow.

- Coronary spasm.

- Perforation.

- Guidewire encroachment.

- Guidewire transection.

INDICATIONS AND EXCLUSIONS

Because the rotablation technique is relatively difficult, many interventionists have elected not to use it. In the pre-stent era, the consequence of this was that some operators would choose to refer some patients with complex lesions for coronary bypass grafting rather than risk balloon angioplasty. Stents can now be used in these difficult vessels, which has increased the scope for intervention by these operators but stenting still has significant limitations, particularly in small vessels (for which stenting has not yet been shown to reduce the incidence of restenosis) or calcified vessels (in which it may be impossible to fully deploy a stent). New antiplatelet drugs (especially abciximab) have, however, led to a reduction in the complications of balloon angioplasty. The growth of rotablation has thus been limited by a reluctance to learn the technique, by the development of stents, and by new antiplatelet drugs. However, there are still some lesions which will be best treated by rotablation and, as discussed below, there is a potential role for rotablation in the treatment of in-stent restenosis, as well as a growing interest in the concept of debulking prior to stenting.

Present indications

Table 10.2 summarises those lesions conventionally considered as suitable for rotablation. Unless DART reveals a distinct advantage over balloon angioplasty, it cannot be considered the treatment of choice for relatively straightforward lesions. Thus it has perhaps been used most in calcified or resistant lesions. However, caution is required for multiple calcified lesions

TABLE 10.2 – INDICATIONS FOR ROTABLATION

Calcified lesions
Resistant lesions
Long lesions (but <25 mm in length)
Eccentric or complex lesion morphologies in small vessels
Angulated lesions
Restenosis lesions
Lesions in tapering vessels
Ostial lesions

POSSIBLE INDICATIONS

Bifurcation lesions
Graft anastomotic lesions

in tandem, as the incidence of slow-flow is increased in this situation. Although some operators have used rotablation at the same sitting as a failed angioplasty for a resistant lesion, this should be done with caution, as if an intimal dissection has occurred with the balloon but is not seen on angiography, this may lead to a major dissection using the rotablator. Under these circumstances, it may be better to bring the patient back for rotablation after 6 to 8 weeks. Although rotablation is almost certainly better for long lesions than balloon angioplasty, the incidence of slow-flow increases with length of lesion and thus lesions longer than 25 mm should probably be avoided. Difficult lesions in small vessels are ideally treated with the rotablator. Most cases treated are single vessel cases. Multivessel disease can be treated but under these circumstances it may be better to consider staging the procedure.

Although rotablation can be used with angulated lesions, the complication rate increases with the degree of angulation. The problem of guidewire encroachment should be considered and caution is required for lesions on the exit of a significant bend. Small burrs should be used for these lesions, but severely angulated lesions should probably not be treated with this technique. Considerable success has been reported in restenosis lesions especially in small vessels when stenting may not be appropriate. The rotablator technique has also been used for ostial lesions (Fig. 10.5), but it is very important for these lesions to find a guide catheter which gives co-axial support. In addition, care should be taken if there is a bend just downstream and because of the hard fibrotic nature of these lesions it is suggested that the procedure should be started with a smaller burr than might be used for other lesions. The rotablator is ideal for short lesions in tapering small vessels, when it might be difficult to find a balloon which conforms to both upstream and downstream diameters and stenting may be difficult or inadvisable. Bifurcation lesions have been treated successfully with this technique, with reports suggesting that the technique leaves a smooth lumen preserving the side-branch, but if there is significant disease at the origin of the side-branch then, as with balloon angioplasty, this may be lost secondary to spasm or a snow-plough effect

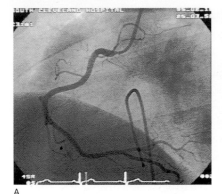

A

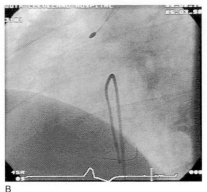

B

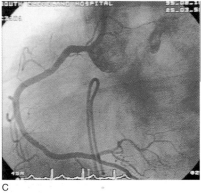

C

Figure 10.5:
Rotablator treatment of an ostial stenosis of the right coronary artery (RCA). (a) Left anterior oblique (LAO) view of the RCA before treatment. (b) During rotablation. (c) Final result after adjunctive balloon angioplasty.

on the plaque. Some success has been reported on graft anastamosis lesions but the rotablator burr should not be activated if possible until just upstream of the lesion to prevent disruption of soft plaque in the body of the graft.

Exclusions

In general, vessels not suitable for coronary bypass grafting should not be considered for rotablation. Occlusions which cannot be crossed by a guidewire cannot be treated with this technique, and the technique should only be used if the length of occlusion is relatively short, and only if it is clear that the wire is in the true distal lumen. Patients with a significantly reduced left ventricular ejection fraction should only be taken on with caution, especially if the lesion is in the last remaining vessel. The elective use of an intra-aortic balloon pump should be considered for these cases. As mentioned above, it is inappropriate to treat very long lesions with this technique. Very diffuse multivessel disease should also probably be avoided. Angiographic evidence of intraluminal thrombus is a relative contraindication, and the device is not suitable for treating unprotected left main stem lesions or lesions in the body of vein grafts. It should not be used in the presence of a visible dissection flap.

Potential indications
In-stent restenosis

Although stenting had significantly reduced the incidence of restenosis, the treatment of in-stent restenosis is difficult. Although procedural success can be high with conventional balloon angioplasty, the re-restenosis rates are high except for short focal lesions. In diffuse in-stent restenosis or proliferative restenosis extending beyond the margins of the stent, the risk of repeat restenosis may be as high as 80%. Initial experience with debulking produced more favourable results[12] (Fig. 10.6). Trial results are conflicting. The small single centre American ROSTER (ROtablator versus balloon for STEnt Restenosis) trial suggested a significant advantage for rotablation versus balloon angioplasty (clinical restenosis 20% versus 43% $p = 0.002$) but in the larger European ARTIST (Angioplasty versus Rotablation for Treatment of Intra-stent STenosis/occlusion) trial, restenosis for diffuse instent stenosis lesions was higher in the rotablator group (65% versus 51%).[13]

Rotastenting

Two observations have led to an increasing interest in the concept of debulking prior to stenting. First, rotablation has not been shown yet to

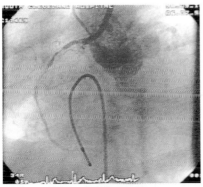
A

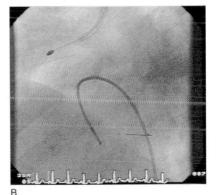
B

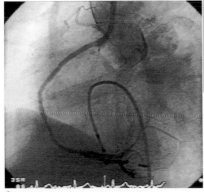
C

Figure 10.6:
Rotablator treatment of in-stent restenosis. The patient had previously been treated with two long NIR stents over the proximal and middle segments of the RCA. (a) LAO view before treatment. (b) During rotablation. (c) Final result after adjunctive balloon angioplasty.

reduce restenosis rates compared with balloon angioplasty whereas stenting has. Second, IVUS studies have shown that the greater the stent expansion, the lower the restenosis rate. Stent expansion may be limited in many vessels by the volume of plaque, and early studies suggest that removal of this plaque can result in superb angiographic results without any significant increase in complications and very low restenosis rates. This may be particularly important for small vessels. IVUS studies demonstrate that many of these vessels are actually heavily diseased large vessels. Debulking may allow successful stenting in vessels not yet considered suitable for this technique (Fig. 10.7). This is also an area under active investigation. Initial studies debulking calcified lesions prior to stent implantation have given favourable results.[14]

SUMMARY

Potentially important future role for the rotablator:

■ Debulking prior to stenting in heavily diseased, calcified or small vessels.

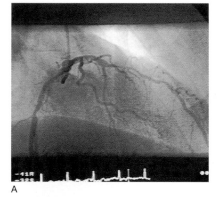

A

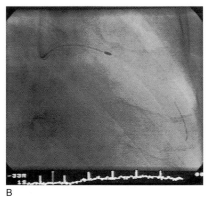

B

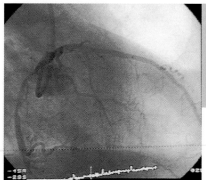

C

Figure 10.7:
Rotastenting. A lesion in a small diffusely diseased left anterior descending (LAD) artery in an 81-year-old man is first debulked by rotablation and then stented. (a) Right anterior oblique cranial view of LAD lesion before treatment. (b) During rotablation. (c) After stenting.

LEARNING THE TECHNIQUE

Not all centres use rotablation and therefore some interventional trainees will not have access to this technique during their period of training. It became very clear early in its clinical use that there is a significant learning curve for this technique. Interventionists therefore should accept a degree of training. In the United States, an interventionist can only order rotablator equipment after a formal training programme, whereas this is not required in Europe. Wherever one learns this technique, operators should avail themselves of the experience of interventionists who have been using this technique for a considerable period of time. Some trainers do not invite other interventionists to their own centre, as this inflicts the learning curve of multiple trainees on the patients of a single centre, and they prefer to travel to a learning interventionist's own centre to teach on patients carefully selected beforehand. Interventionists should not start with the most difficult cases, but learn the technique on relatively straightforward lesions which could well be treated with conventional balloon angioplasty or stenting. Short restenosis lesions are ideal lesions to start on. Only after a significant number of easy lesions are treated, when the various facets of the technique are mastered, should the more difficult lesions be treated.

It is important to maintain skills once acquired. Because most interventionists may only need this technique infrequently, it may be appropriate for the majority to refer certain cases to one or two high-volume operators who use the technique most often.

REFERENCES

1. Hansen DD, Auth DC, Vracko R, Ritchie JL. Rotational atherectomy in atherosclerotic rabbit iliac arteries. Am Heart J 1988;115:160–5.

2. Ahn SS, Auth D, Marcus DR, Moore WS. Removal of focal atheromatous lesions by angioscopically guided high-speed rotary atherectomy. Preliminary experimental observations. J Vasc Surg 1988;7:292–300.

3. Zacca NM, Raizner AE, Noon GP et al. Treatment of symptomatic peripheral atherosclerotic disease with a rotational atherectomy device. Am J Cardiol 1989;63:77–80.

4. Tierstein PS, Warth DC, Haq N et al. High speed rotational coronary atherectomy for patients with diffuse coronary artery disease. J Am Coll Cardiol 1991;18:1694–701.

5. Bertrand ME, Lablanche JM, Leroy F et al. Percutaneous transluminal coronary rotary ablation with Rotablator (European Experience). Am J Cardiol 1992;69:470–74.

6. Stertzer SH, Rosenblum J, Shaw RE et al. Coronary rotational ablation: Initial experience in 302 procedures. J Am Coll Cardiol. 1993;21:287–95.

7. Warth DC, Leon MB, O'Neill W, Zacca N, Polissar NL, Buchbinder MJ. Rotational atherectomy multicenter registry: acute results, complications and 6-month angiographic follow-up in 709 patients. Am Coll Cardiol 1994;24:641–8.

8. Brogan WC III, Popma JJ, Pichard AD et al. Rotational coronary atherectomy after unsuccessful coronary balloon angioplasty. Am J Cardiol 1993;71:794–8.

9. MacIsaac AI, Bass TA, Buchbinder M et al. High speed rotational atherectomy: outcome in calcified and noncalcified coronary artery lesions. J Am Coll Cardiol 1995;26:731–6.

10. Reifart N, Vandormael M, Krajcar M et al. Randomized comparison of angioplasty of complex coronary lesions at a single center. Excimer Laser, Rotational Atherectomy, and Balloon Angioplasty Comparison (ERBAC) Study. Circulation 1997;96:91–8.

11. Stertzer SH, Pomerantsev EV, Fitzgerald PJ et al. Effects of technique modification on immediate results of high speed rotational atherectomy in 710 procedures on 656 patients. Cathet Cardiovasc Diagn 1995;36:304–10.

12. Stone GW. Rotational atherectomy for treatment of in-stent restenosis: role of intra-coronary ultrasound guidance. Cathet Cardiovasc Diagn 1996;Suppl. 3:73–7.

13. Vom Dahl J, Dietz U, Silber S et al. on behalf of the ARTIST investigators. Angioplasty versus Rotational Atherectomy for Treatment of diffuse In-stent Restenosis: clinical and angiographic results from a randomised multicentre trial (ARTIST). J Am Coll Cardiol 2000;35:79–1 (Abstract).

14. Moussa I, Di Mario C, Moses J et al. Coronary stenting after rotational atherectomy in calcified and complex lesions. Angiographic and clinical follow-up results. Circulation 1997;96:128–36.

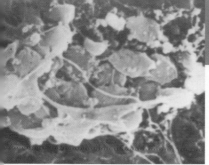

11

Directional coronary atherectomy

DAVID R. RAMSDALE

KEY POINTS

■ Directional coronary atherectomy (DCA) is ideally suited for certain lesion subsets considered unfavourable for PCTA or stenting.

■ Operator expertise is a prime determinant of success and safety.

■ It is currently used in less than 5% procedures worldwide.

■ In experienced hands acute complications are infrequent and success is high.

■ Optimal debulking is essential to reduce restenosis.

■ Debulking prior to stenting may be advantageous.

■ DCA is the only device which can retrieve tissue intact from the coronary lesion.

INTRODUCTION

Percutaneous transluminal coronary angioplasty (PTCA) is limited by a 3–5% incidence of abrupt coronary artery closure, indifferent clinical and angiographic results in complex or balloon-resistant lesions and a 25–35% incidence of restenosis occurring in the first 6 months, requiring further intervention.

Directional coronary atherectomy (DCA), involves the selective excision and retrieval of atherosclerotic material from diseased coronary arteries. By debulking such arteries it was anticipated that improved results could be obtained in lesions with complex morphology, non-dilatable lesions and those in sites associated with higher complication and restenosis rates such as ostial left anterior descending artery stenoses, bifurcation stenoses and aorta-ostial lesions. Furthermore, it was hoped that retrieval of material might help in understanding the pathology of coronary atherosclerosis and restenosis after PTCA and perhaps also result in lower restenosis rates. Some of these hopes have been realised, but not all.

HISTORY

The first successful coronary atherectomy was performed in February 1987. After the initial 50 clinical cases were performed at Sequoia Hospital, Redwood City, eleven other institutions in the USA joined a multicentre investigation in June 1988. Based on an 85% success rate and low complication rate in 1032 lesions up to November 1989, the Food and Drug Administration subsequently approved the device made by DVI (Devices for Vascular Intervention, Guidant Ltd., Santa Rosa, CA, USA) in

September 1990. The number of procedures increased dramatically and by mid-1992 more than 33 000 procedures had been carried out in over 670 centres in the USA. The Simpson AtheroCath® has since been developed and refined with the original surlyn-covered device (SCA-1) being replaced by the more streamlined SCA-EX™ device in 1992. Other devices such as the Short-Cutter, the GTO® AtheroCath, the Bantam™ and, more recently, the Flexi-Cut™ have been released for clinical use in order to overcome some of the shortcomings of the original design. Improved guiding catheters and guidewires have also helped to make the procedure more user-friendly and less daunting.

EQUIPMENT

Simpson coronary AtheroCath

The Simpson coronary atherectomy device is a coaxial over-the-wire catheter for use with a steerable 0.014 inch guidewire (Fig. 11.1). The distal portion of the device consists of a non-flexible, gold plated, stainless steel biopsy housing (17 mm long) in which lies a cup-shaped cutter. This portion has a longitudinal window of a 120 degree arc and a support PET balloon on its opposite side. Immediately distal to the housing is a tapered, flexible, stainless steel, braided nosecone that functions as a specimen collection chamber (Fig. 11.2). The braided shaft of the atherectomy catheter provides torquability – by rotation of the proximal assembly part. The proximal end of the device consists of a balloon inflation port, a distal flush port and a small lever, which is attached to the hollow drive cable that runs the length of the catheter and connects to the cutter. The 0.014 inch guidewire passes through the centre of the drive cable. A hand-held battery powered motor drive unit (MDU) connects to the proximal end and once activated spins the cutter at 2000 rpm. The cutter is advanced and retracted manually by the lever. Balloon inflation and deflation are controlled by a low-pressure indeflator attached to the balloon inflation port.

Choice of AtheroCath (Table 11.1)

The vessel size is the major factor in selecting the size of the AtheroCath® device (5 F–7 F) to use, although vessel compliance/calcification, tortuosity and accessibility, lesion/vessel angulation, lesion severity and length are similarly important. Until recently (see recent technical developments, p. 166) three devices were available (Fig. 11.3) together with a 'short-cutter'.

    The **SCA-EX**™ (5 F, 6 F, 7 F and 7 FG) is designed to address the majority of anatomical challenges. The low profile reduces the need for predilatation and the springtip nosecone improves flexibility and

trackability.

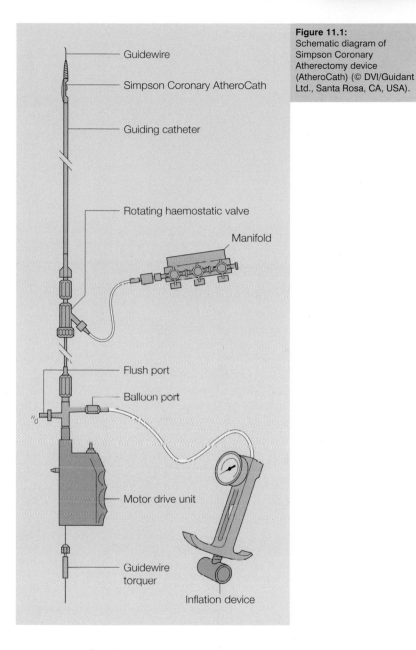

Figure 11.1:
Schematic diagram of Simpson Coronary Atherectomy device (AtheroCath) (© DVI/Guidant Ltd., Santa Rosa, CA, USA).

Guidewire

Simpson Coronary AtheroCath

Guiding catheter

Rotating haemostatic valve

Manifold

Flush port

Balloon port

Motor drive unit

Guidewire torquer

Inflation device

The **GTO® AtheroCath** (5 F, 6 F and 7 F) has a coaxial inflation lumen and a round shaft profile to allow **Greater Torque Output** and improved stability of the device within the coronary artery.

The **Bantam**™ (5 F, 6 F and 7 F) has a small shaft profile which enhances contrast visualization of the vessels during the procedure, improves trackability and of course can be used within a 8 F or 9 F Tourguide® catheter.

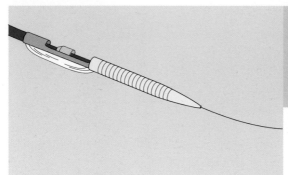

Figure 11.2:
Distal end of Simpson Coronary AtheroCath showing the flexible nose-cone, the cutter within the housing window and the balloon. (© DVI/Guidant Ltd., Santa Rosa, CA, USA).

TABLE 11.1 – CHOOSING THE ATHEROCATH

SCA-EX, GTO OR BANTAM DEVICE INDICATION	SCA-EX SHORTCUTTER INDICATION	SCA-EX 7 FG INDICATION
Most native vessels	Ostial lesions	Large native vessel
Tandem lesions	Focal (<5 mm) lesions	Aorta-ostial lesion
Distal tortuosity	Distal insertion lesions	SVGs
Tapering vessel	Acute take-offs	Calcified lesions
Distal disease beyond lesion site	Short radius turns	Bulky/long lesions

DEVICE FOR VESSEL SIZE ATHEROCATH	SIZE	VESSEL DIAMETER (MM)
SCA EX or	5 F	2.0–2.5
BANTAM	6 F	2.5–3.0
	7 F	3.0–3.5
	7 FG	3.5–4.0*
GTO	5 F	2.0–2.5
	6 F	2.5–3.1
	7 F	3.1–3.7

*7 FG is not available as Bantam.

The **Shortcutter** (5 F, 6 F and 7 F) offers 29% reduction in rigid housing length (12 mm) which widens its applications. The window is only 5 mm long and hence little tissue is retrieved per cut. It is ideal when the left anterior descending (LAD) or left circumflex (LCX) has an acute take-off, for lesions in tortuous vessel segments, distal lesions, focal and ostial lesions.

Guiding catheter

Guiding catheters must have a large internal diameter and additional stiffness in order to provide support when delivering the AtheroCath® into the coronary artery. DVI® and Tourguide® guiding catheters have soft

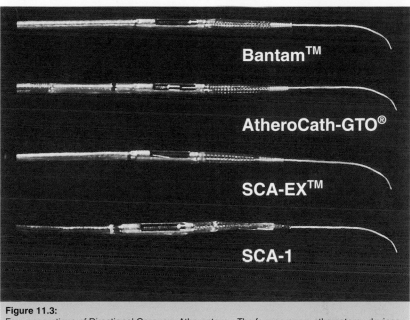

Figure 11.3:
Four generations of Directional Coronary Atherectomy. The four coronary atherectomy devices developed by DVI.

distal tips and side holes and a range of shapes and sizes are available (Fig. 11.4a–b). Compatibility between the various AtheroCaths and the guide catheters is shown in Table 11.2.

The atherectomy device is inserted into the guiding catheter through a rotating haemostatic valve (RHV).

Guidewire

A 300 cm 0.014 inch, teflon-coated, high torque, floppy guidewire is ideal but one of intermediate or standard stiffness can also be used. An 'extra support' wire (Guidant, USA) may aid delivery of the AtheroCath® into and along the coronary artery.

TABLE 11.2 – TOURGUIDE/ATHEROCATH COMPATIBILITY

	ATHEROCATH	TOURGUIDE (ID)
BANTAM	5 F	8 F (0.087″)
	6 F	9 F (0.101″)
	7 F	9 F
SCA-EX or GTO	5 F	9 F or 10 F
	6 F	9 F or 10 F
SCA-EX or GTO	7 F	10 F (0.112″)
	7 FG	10 F

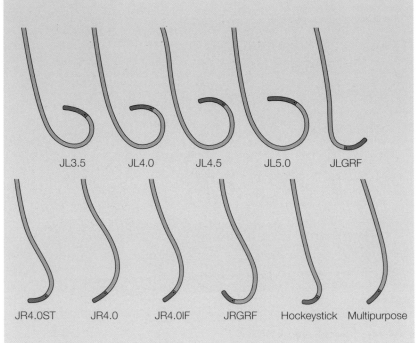

JL3.5   JL4.0   JL4.5   JL5.0   JLGRF

JR4.0ST   JR4.0   JR4.0IF   JRGRF   Hockeystick   Multipurpose

A

Figure 11.4:
(a) DVI guiding catheters (currently available). (b, opposite) Choice of guiding catheter depends on size and shape of aortic root and angle of take-off of coronary ostium or SVG.

INDICATIONS

Directional coronary atherectomy (DCA) is ideal for complex, bulky, focal, *de novo* lesions in the proximal portions of large (>2.5 mm), non-calcified, non-tortuous vessels, but the indications have expanded as the equipment has developed and more practical experience has been gained. Cases should be selected on the basis of the operator's experience, lesion location and morphology (Table 11.3).

TABLE 11.3 – IDEAL INDICATIONS FOR DCA	
VESSEL	**LESION**
Large (>2.5 mm)	Focal (<10 mm)
Non-tortuous	De novo or restenosis
LAD>RCA>LCX	Morphologically complex
Proximal/mid	– bulky concentric/eccentric
Non aorta-ostial (LAD, LCX branches)	– ulcerated, flap-like
Aorta-ostial (LM, RCA, SVG)	– local dissection
	– mild/no calcification
	– PTCA resistant
	Discrete tubular

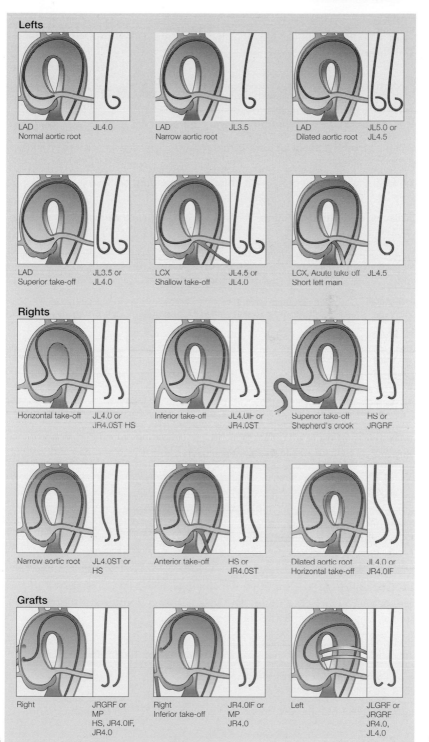

Lefts

LAD
Normal aortic root
JL4.0

LAD
Narrow aortic root
JL3.5

LAD
Dilated aortic root
JL5.0 or
JL4.5

LAD
Superior take-off
JL3.5 or
JL4.0

LCX
Shallow take-off
JL4.5 or
JL4.0

LCX, Acute take-off
Short left main
JL4.5

Rights

Horizontal take-off
JL4.0 or
JR4.0ST HS

Interior take-off
JL4.0IF or
JR4.0ST

Superior take-off
Shepherd's crook
HS or
JRGRF

Narrow aortic root
JL4.0ST or
HS

Anterior take-off
HS or
JR4.0ST

Dilated aortic root
Horizontal take-off
JL4.0 or
JR4.0IF

Grafts

Right
JRGRF or
MP
HS, JR4.0IF,
JR4.0

Right
Inferior take-off
JR4.0IF or
MP
JR4.0

Left
JLGRF or
JRGRF
JR4.0,
JL4.0

OPERATOR EXPERIENCE

Case selection guidelines for DCA have been published by DVI (Guidant) and should be adhered to.

LESION LOCATION

Lesion location is an important factor since accessibility is limited by the size, profile and rigidity of the device.

- **Left main coronary artery lesions** should only be addressed if the left main is protected by patent bypass grafts.

- **Lesions in the proximal or mid-left anterior descending coronary artery** are usually accessible unless its take-off is high or there is marked tortuosity.

- Accessibility of **circumflex lesions** depends on the angle of take-off from the left main artery. Generally, only lesions in a circumflex with a shallow take-off (<30 degrees) or a short left main should be attempted.

- **Lesions in the proximal or mid-right coronary artery (RCA)** are suitable as are more distal lesions before the crux in large, non-calcified vessels.

- **Aorta-ostial** lesions are technically demanding. Ostial left main and vein graft stenoses are easier than ostial right coronary disease but all should only be attempted by experienced operators.

- **Ostial** LAD lesions can be most effectively treated by DCA as can ostial LCX disease as long as the take-off from the left main is shallow. Ostial lesions are not ideal for PTCA because of the risk of dissection back into the left main and a high incidence of elastic recoil and restenosis. These problems can be reduced by excising tissue. It is important that a minority of the cutting window is in the left main with most being in the LAD or LCX, and that the guiding catheter is disengaged once the atherectomy device is correctly positioned in order to allow perfusion of the uninvolved vessel.

- **Bifurcation** lesions can be treated by sequential DCA in order to remove the 'shifting atheroma' seen during PTCA. Both side branches should ideally be 2.5 mm or more in diameter. The side branch should not be protected by a standard angioplasty guidewire, otherwise guidewire fracture and embolisation are possible.

- **Lesions in saphenous vein grafts (SVG)** are generally suitable as long as guiding catheter support is adequate.

LESION MORPHOLOGY

Ideal lesions for DCA are those which are ideal for PTCA (type A). However, DCA offers a higher success and lower complication rate for morphologically complex lesions (type B and C).

- **Eccentric lesions** are ideal for DCA. The window of the housing can be directed towards the eccentric plaque without damaging the 'normal' vessel wall in close proximity.

- **Lesions with complex morphology**, such as ulcerated, bulky, flap and membrane-like lesions are better treated by DCA.

- **Tough, resistant plaque** which has failed to respond to PTCA can often be removed by DCA as can restenotic lesions.

■ **Minor but potentially occlusive dissections** can also be removed by 'rescue' DCA although extensive or spiral dissections should be avoided.

■ **Mildly calcified** lesions can be excised by DCA but data suggests that procedural success is reduced and complication rates are higher.

■ **Complex** lesions with associated **thrombus**, as seen in unstable angina, can be effectively excised by DCA, but vessels containing large amounts of clot should be avoided because of an increased risk of acute closure.

■ **Saphenous vein graft (SVG)** stenoses can be effectively removed by DCA but old grafts containing friable material are not suitable. Restenosis rates are higher than in native arteries.

CONTRAINDICATIONS

Contraindications to DCA include those to PTCA and are shown in Table 11.4.

■ **Some coronary anatomy** can make DCA impossible and these include Shepherd's crook RCA, high take off LAD and LCX exiting from left main stem at >60 degree angle.

■ **Severe peripheral vascular disease** can make it impossible to deliver a suitable guiding catheter to the aortic root and marked dilatation of the ascending aorta or unfolding frequently prevents satisfactory engagement and stable alignment of the guiding catheter which is essential for success.

■ **Old, degenerated saphenous vein grafts** containing much friable, grumous material should be avoided because of the risk of embolisation.

■ **Severe tortuosity** proximal or just distal to the lesion is a contraindication to DCA because the rigid housing will not negotiate the curves and coronary dissection may result from aggressive manipulation. Even moderate tortuosity with calcification will make it difficult to advance the device through the non-compliant segments.

■ **Calcification** is a major adverse factor. The coronary artery needs to be fairly straight and compliant to allow passage of the rigid housing. Calcified lesions can usually not be excised by the current cutter.

■ **Lesions on bends** (>60 degrees) should be avoided because of the risk of dissection and perforation by deep cuts across the angle. Less severe angulated lesions can be approached with the newer, lower profile devices and the ShortCutter.

TABLE 11.4 – CONTRAINDICATIONS TO DCA	
Contraindication for PTCA	Moderate and severely calcified lesions/vessels
Shepherd's crook RCA	Large branches requiring protection
Long left main	Diffuse disease
LCX exiting left main stem at >30°*	Small vessels (<2.5 mm)
Long lesions (>20 mm)	Tortuous vessels
Distal lesions	Degenerated SVGs
Bend lesions >45°*	Dissection extensive spiral
Internal mammary arteries	Severe peripheral vascular disease

* ShortCutter takes a bend up to 60–70°.
RCA: right coronary artery; LCX: left circumflex artery; SVG: saphenous vein graft.

■ **Diffusely diseased vessels, small vessels and distal lesions** should be avoided because the large profile of the device makes advancement difficult.

■ **Excessively long** (>20 mm) lesions are unsuitable and even those of intermediate length (10–20 mm) will require multiple cuts with device position adjustment along the length of the lesion.

■ Lesions in **internal mammary arteries** are inaccessible.

PROCEDURE

Once the AtheroCath® is delivered across the lesion, the housing's window is orientated towards the main bulk of the lesion by manually torquing the AtheroCath® (Fig. 11.5a–b). The balloon is inflated to 10–15 psi (0.5–1.0 atmospheres) to support the device within the lumen. The cutter is retracted manually and the balloon further inflated to 20 psi (maximum 30 psi) thereby forcing the lesion into the window of the device. The MDU is activated and the spinning cutter advanced over 5–7 seconds using the proximal lever. Cutter advancement should be observed by fluoroscopy. Abnormal tissue protruding into the window is cut and pushed into the nosecone. The balloon is deflated. The window of the device is next directed to a different part of the lesion and the sequence of events repeated (Fig. 11.6). For concentric lesions, systematic cuts in four 90 degree

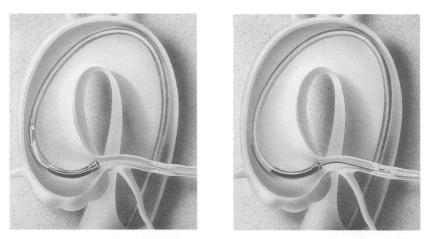

A   B

Figure 11.5:
(a) Once the guiding catheter is correctly seated, the SCA device is positioned proximal to guide curve to maintain coaxial alignment during wire placement. (b) The SCA nosecone and housing are then advanced across the lesion aided by rotation of the AtheroCath.
(© DVI/Guidant Ltd., Santa Rosa, CA, USA).

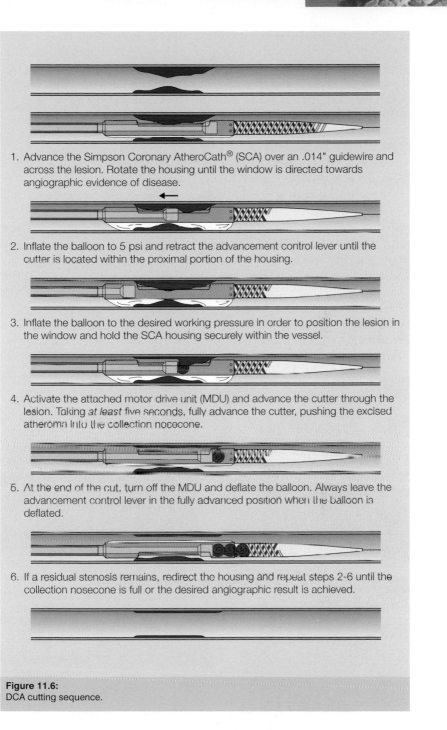

1. Advance the Simpson Coronary AtheroCath® (SCA) over an .014" guidewire and across the lesion. Rotate the housing until the window is directed towards angiographic evidence of disease.

2. Inflate the balloon to 5 psi and retract the advancement control lever until the cutter is located within the proximal portion of the housing.

3. Inflate the balloon to the desired working pressure in order to position the lesion in the window and hold the SCA housing securely within the vessel.

4. Activate the attached motor drive unit (MDU) and advance the cutter through the lesion. Taking *at least* five seconds, fully advance the cutter, pushing the excised atheroma into the collection nosecone.

5. At the end of the cut, turn off the MDU and deflate the balloon. Always leave the advancement control lever in the fully advanced position when the balloon is deflated.

6. If a residual stenosis remains, redirect the housing and repeat steps 2-6 until the collection nosecone is full or the desired angiographic result is achieved.

Figure 11.6:
DCA cutting sequence.

quadrants (or eight 45 degree sectors if possible) is usually necessary, but for eccentric lesions cuts are directed at the lesion itself. Once the angiographic appearance of the artery is acceptable (Figs 11.7 and 11.8), the catheter can be withdrawn and the chamber emptied of its specimens (Fig. 11.9). The specimens retrieved should be counted and weighed in order to provide a quantitative assessment of the degree of debulking.

Optimal endpoints
One should aim at a final residual, angiographic stenosis of <10% but as close to 0% as possible. Increasing the balloon inflation pressure to 30–40 psi during cutting may be performed before upsizing the device. Optimal endpoints also include flow around the device with contrast injection, smooth borders, absence of dissection, no distal complications, large lumen with good flow and good tissue retrieval. The best predictor of a favourable late outcome is the presence of a large lumen diameter immediately following intervention. Optimal DCA is best guided by IVUS.

Pre-dilatation
Pre-dilatation of the stenosis should not be done routinely. However, predilatation with a 2.0 mm balloon at low pressure may allow a smooth

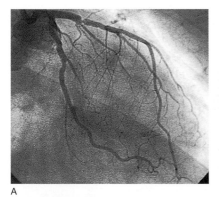

A

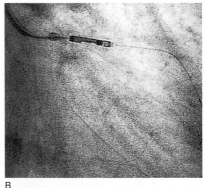

B

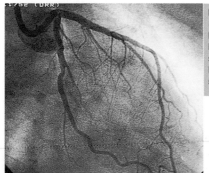

Figure 11.7:
(a) Severe balloon-resistant stenosis in proximal left anterior descending (LAD) coronary artery before DCA. (b) during DCA, with SCA across stenosis and cutter towards distal end of housing. (c) post-DCA, showing no residual stenosis.

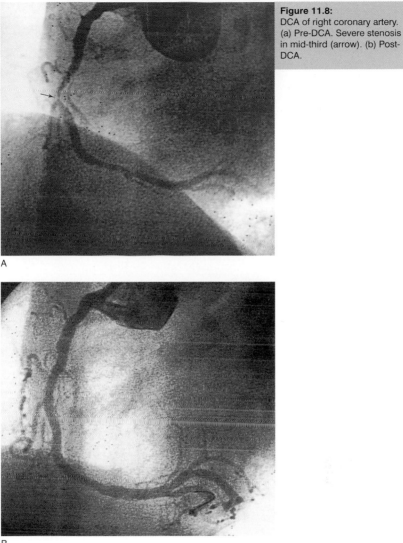

Figure 11.8:
DCA of right coronary artery.
(a) Pre-DCA. Severe stenosis in mid-third (arrow). (b) Post-DCA.

A

B

passage of the atherectomy device through severe, subtotally occluded segments, long lesions, segments of diffuse disease and heavily calcified vessels en route to a stenosis.

Adjunctive balloon dilatation after DCA

Conventional PTCA and stenting is indicated for managing unsuccessful DCA procedures and to rescue DCA-induced complications. Since it appears to be important to achieve the largest post-treatment luminal diameter safely possible, adjunctive PTCA should be performed in successful but suboptimal (>10–15% residual stenosis) DCA procedures.

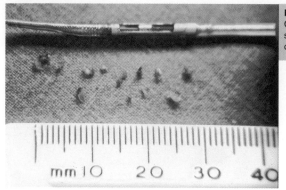

Figure 11.9:
Coronary atherectomy specimens emptied from the cutting chamber.

Most centres who have reported their results claim improved procedural success with DCA + PTCA over DCA success alone.

COMPARISON OF DCA WITH PTCA

Advantages and disadvantages of DCA compared with PTCA are shown in Table 11.5.

HISTOPATHOLOGY

The Simpson AtheroCath® has provided the unique opportunity to study vascular pathology in the living patient. Analysis of tissue removed during DCA has already helped to provide new insight and understanding of atherosclerosis, restenosis and unstable angina. It has provided samples for tissue culture, special immunological and molecular biology studies

TABLE 11.5 – ADVANTAGES AND DISADVANTAGES OF DCA

ADVANTAGES	DISADVANTAGES
Higher success/lower complication rate for – focal, eccentric plaque – bulky, ulcerated/complex lesions – resistant PTCA lesions – ostial lesions	Large guiding catheter with limited shapes Atherocath is relatively large Rigid metal housing
More predictable acute result – less frequent dissections – less abrupt closure – less residual stenosis	Confined to proximal part of non-tortuous, non-calcified, large vessels
Allows tissue removal – debulking – histology, cell culture	Need special expertise More expensive than PTCA

?Lower restenosis rates for certain subgroups, e.g. de novo, discrete, prox LAD lesions in vessels >3.0 mm, after a 7 F device with post-DCA MLD >3.0 mm aimed at developing new strategies and new pharmacological agents for treatment of these conditions.

Lesions can be classified into two major types: atherosclerotic plaque and intimal hyperplasia, although there is some overlap (Fig. 11.10). **Fibrointimal hyperplasia** is characterised by a proliferation of stellate-spindle shaped smooth muscle cells within a loose to mildly fibrotic myxoid stroma and is the commonest finding in restenosis lesions.

RESULTS

Compared with PTCA, DCA results in significantly improved post-procedure angiographic appearances due to less severe residual stenosis and a lower incidence of dissection.

DVI registry

The Investigational Device Exemption (IDE) data was collected from 12 US sites between 1988 and 1990. Data were available on 1032 lesions (838 patients in 923 procedures).

Despite using the original, higher profile and potentially more traumatic SCA-1 device, the data demonstrated an 85% primary success rate (defined as tissue removal, >20% reduction in stenosis, <50% residual

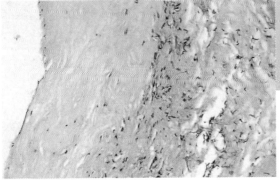

Figure 11.10:
Histopathology of DCA specimens. (a) Fibrous intimal atherosclerotic plaque. (b) Fibrointimal smooth muscle cell hyperplasia from a restenosis lesion.

A

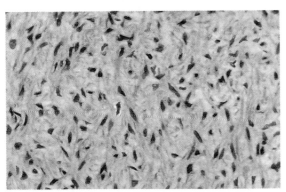

B

stenosis and no major complication) – higher in restenotic and non-calcified lesions. With adjunctive PTCA, the overall success rate was 92%. Major complications occurred in 4.9% of procedures, and included non-fatal myocardial infarction (0.9%), emergency coronary bypass surgery (CABG) (4.0%) and death (0.5%). These events were more frequent in right coronary (6.6%), de novo (6.9%) and long (>20 mm in length) lesions (10.8%). Most of the complications were due to coronary occlusion (3.9%), 80% of which occurred in the catheter laboratory and due to either local dissection (1.6%) or thrombosis (2.0%). Of these occlusions, 40% were successfully reopened by PTCA and/or thrombolytic agents.

The IDE project was expanded to a total of 25 US investigational sites before general release in October 1990. This increased the total number of patients to 1977 and the number of lesions to 2384. In this expanded cohort, the use of predilatation (25%), post-DCA dilatation (16%), DCA success (84%) and incidence of major complications (4.6%) remained largely unchanged.

Other published results

Individual centres that participated in the IDE investigation have published their own results confirming DCA to be a safe and effective procedure; some of these are shown in Table 11.6. The more experienced centres, like Sequoia Hospital, report the highest DCA success rates although all have very high procedural success rates and a low incidence of major complications. For individual operators there is likely to be a learning curve with the results improving beyond the first 50 cases.

The newer AtheroCaths are more streamlined and less traumatic and this has resulted in low complication rates (OARS, BOAT and ABACAS).

Sequoia experience

Between 1988 and 1994, 1887 DCA procedures were performed at Sequoia Hospital. A total of 2283 lesions were addressed with a DCA success rate of 91.9%, a procedural (DCA+PTCA) success of 95.6% and a major complication rate of 3.1%. The AtheroCath® was successfully placed in 95% with pre- and post-DCA dilatation being performed in 35% and 14% respectively. On average 14.8 mg of tissue was excised per case leaving an average residual stenosis of 14.4%. The mean post-DCA luminal diameter was 2.6 mm. The 7 F device (70% in 1993) resulted in more excised material (18.7 mg), less residual stenosis (10%) and a higher primary DCA success rate (95%).

Concentric and eccentric lesions had high DCA (94%) and DCA+PTCA success (96%) with a low CABG rate (1.2–2.4%). Ulcerated lesions (98%), dissections (91%) and flap lesions (95%) had similar high procedural success rates to non-complex lesions (96%). Success rates were 96% in lesions <10 mm in length, 95% if 10–20 mm long and 91% if >20 mm long. The corresponding CABG rates were 2.2%, 3.3% and 7.4%. Calcified lesions had a 93% success rate and a 4.8% CABG rate compared with 97% and 3.3% in non-calcified vessels.

TABLE 11.6 – RESULTS OF DCA: SUCCESS AND COMPLICATION RATES

CENTRE	PTS (n)	LES (n)	PROC (n)	DCA (%)	PROC (%)	QMI (%)	CABG (%)	DEATH (%)	MJR. CCM (%)	PERF (%)	OUT OF LAB CLOSURE (%)	LEG COMPLICATIONS
IDE MULTICENTER 1988–90	838	1032	923	85%	92%	0.9%	4%	0.5%	4.9%	0.6%	0.8%	1.1%
SEQUOIA HOSP												
1986–88		447		90%	94%	0.6%	3.1%	0.3%				
1986–91		1547		91%	95%	0.6%	3%	0.2%				
1988–94		2283	1,887	91.5%	95.6%	0.5%	3%	0.4%	3.1%			
MED COLL VIRGINIA 1989–92	300	427	345	95%	95%	1.7%	3.3%	0.3%	4.6%	1.2%	1.4%	2.3%
BETH ISRAEL												
1988–91	150	225		91%	98%	0%	0.5%	0%				
1993–94		132	120	84%	97%	2.3%	1.7%	0%	3.3%			
NACI REGISTRY (planned DCA)	931	1026			93.2%	1.1%	1.5%	0.6%				
WASHINGTON HOSPITAL	306		306		94.8%	0.3%	1.8%	0.6%	2.6%	0.3%	2.3%	
MAHI KANSAS CITY 1989–94	227	264			94.5	2.6%	0.8%	0.8%	4.4%	0.4%	2.6%	
MAYO CLINIC 1988–90	158	165			92%	1%	4%	3%	7%			
THORAX CENTER & UNIV. LOUVAIN 1989–91	105	113		85.7%	95.2%	4.7%	2.8%	0.9%	5.7%	0.9%	0.9%	0%
CTC LIVERPOOL	45	50	45		95.5%	0%	4.4%	0%	4.4%	0%	2.2%	0%
CHRISTIAN-ALBRECHTS UNIV. KIEL*	325	341	–		92%	1%	1.8%	0.6%	–	0%	0.6%	0.9%

* Details of data from R. Simon (personal communication).

Restenosis lesions had a higher success rate than de novo lesions. Aorta-ostial lesions had a procedural success of 95% and a CABG rate of 5.3% (5.9% left main; 8.2% RCA; 2.1% SVG). Non aorta-ostial lesions had a 93% procedural success and a 3.2% CABG rate (2.0% LAD; 13.0% LCX; 0% Diagonal). In 85 total occlusions, DCA proved successful in 91% and DCA+PTCA in 94% once the artery was recanalised and predilated. Excised tissue weighed 19.5 mg and the residual stenosis was 10%. Major complications were low.

In 312 SVG lesions (20% ostial, 78% body and 2% distal anastomosis) DCA success was 95% and DCA+PTCA success was 97%. Residual stenosis averaged 12.2% and tissue excised 17.7 mg. Dissection occurred in 8.1%. Major complications occurred in 1.8% (death 0.8%; CABG 1.6%; Q-wave myocardial infarction [MI] 0.4%). In-hospital occlusion occurred in 1%, embolism in 5.7%, CK-MB elevation in 12.7% and perforation in 1.0%.

Overall, major complications occurred in 3.2% – Q-wave MI 0.3%, CABG 3.0% and death 0.4%. Other complications include CKMB elevation 12.9%, distal embolisation 1.8%, groin repair 1.0%, stroke 0.4% and in-hospital occlusion 1.0%. Twenty-four (1.1%) patients had evidence of perforation – 11 (0.5%) perforation, 12 (0.6%) limited pseudoaneurysm and one (0.1%) A-V fistula.

Failure of DCA was due to failure to reach or cross in 53%, failure despite tissue retrieval in 29%, poor guide support in 10% and no tissue removal in 5%.

OTHER STUDIES OF DIRECTIONAL CORONARY ATHERECTOMY

As with PTCA, DCA in women tends to be associated with a higher rate of major complications compared to men (9.8% vs 2.9%).

In the elderly (>70 years), DCA has been shown to be safe and effective although significant complications may occur in 1.8–9.8% of patients. In one study, the procedural success was 98% – significantly better than PTCA (92%) and elective stenting (86%).

In protected left main coronary arteries, DCA can achieve excellent angiographic results with low procedural complication rates.

In unstable angina, despite excision of the unstable plaque material, the immediate major complication rates are probably higher in those patients with rest or post-infarction angina than in those with stable angina. In one study, abrupt closure occurred in 5% and 2.6% respectively, emergency CABG in 5% and 1.3% and in-hospital death 2% and 0% respectively. Although clinical success is very high, it is slightly lower in the group with rest/post-infarction pain (93% vs 98.7%).

DCA success in patients 1–14 days after myocardial infarction is high (92%) but major complications may be commoner than in non-MI patients (9.7% vs 2.6%; CABG 6.5% vs 1.8%; in-hospital occlusion of infarct-related artery 4.8% vs 0.8%; distal embolus 6.5% vs 1.8%). These reported outcomes were in the pre-stent era.

Although DCA has been performed successfully to both native coronary artery lesions and stenoses in SVGs via a right brachial arteriotomy, this is very difficult and should be avoided.

Angioscopy after DCA often shows highly irregular surfaces with grooves, large protrusions of atherosclerotic material and considerable luminal narrowing. Post-DCA PTCA markedly improves the angioscopic appearance producing smoother surfaces and enlarged lumina.

The short cutter was introduced for treatment of discrete lesions in tortuous vessels. One study showed that of 33 lesions treated with this device alone, DCA success rate was 73%, 85% after an additional standard device and 97% after adjunctive PTCA. Despite the use of high balloon inflation pressures, the excised tissue is significantly less than with the standard device (7.7 mg vs 17.4 mg).

CLINICAL TRIALS IN DCA

Several randomised clinical trials comparing short and long-term results of DCA and PTCA have been published. Other trials have examined the feasibility, the advantages and disadvantages of maximal debulking by optimal atherectomy.

CAVEAT I (Coronary Angioplasty vs Excisional Atherectomy Trial I)

In CAVEAT I, 1012 patients (at 35 centres) with a de novo stenosis in any major coronary artery were randomised to DCA or PTCA. Enrolment was between August 1991 to April 1992.

DCA had a greater procedural success than PTCA (82% vs 76%) and a greater angiographic success (89% vs 80%). There was no difference in in-hospital mortality between DCA (0%) and PTCA (0.4%). However, the need for emergency CABG was higher for DCA (ns) being 3.7% for DCA and 2.2% for PTCA. Myocardial infarction and abrupt closure rates were both increased in the DCA group although only non-Q wave infarcts were significantly more common after DCA (Q-wave: 2.2% DCA vs 1.0% PTCA; non-Q wave: 4.9% DCA vs 2.2% PTCA). Abrupt closure occurred in 6.8% of DCA patients and in 2.8% of PTCA patients.

Event-free survival rates at 6 months were indistinguishable (60% DCA vs 63% PTCA), but the incidence of myocardial infarction (mainly non-Q wave) was higher among the DCA group (8% vs 4%).

The frequency of angiographic restenosis after 6 months was only marginally lower with DCA (50% vs 57%). One of the limitations of this study was that the vessel size treated was relatively small and the residual stenosis after DCA relatively high (29%) – suggesting that optimal debulking was not achieved.

One year follow-up data suggests that the long-term outcome (death and MI) may be worse in the DCA group (death 2.2% for DCA vs 0.6% for PTCA), a finding possibly attributable to the doubling of periprocedural non-Q-wave MI in patients treated by DCA.

CCAT (Canadian Coronary Atherectomy Trial)

In CCAT, 274 patients at nine centres with de novo lesions >60% stenosis in the proximal LAD were randomised to DCA or PTCA. Ostial lesions were excluded. Enrolment was between July 1991 and August 1992.

In this study, the initial angiographic success was greater in the DCA than the PTCA group (98% vs 91%) but in contrast to the CAVEAT data there was no significant difference between the two groups in any of the major complications of death (0%), emergency CABG (1.4% DCA vs 4.4% PTCA), myocardial infarction (Q-wave MI: 0.7% DCA vs 0% PTCA); non-Q-wave: 3.6% DCA vs 3.7% PTCA) or abrupt closure (4.3% DCA vs 5.1% PTCA). Unfortunately residual stenosis after DCA was still 26%.

The restenosis rates were similar 6 months after DCA (46%) as after PTCA (43%). Interestingly, in CAVEAT, proximal LAD lesions had a significantly lower restenosis rate after DCA than after PTCA (51% vs 63%).

CAVEAT II (Coronary Angioplasty vs Excisional Atherectomy Trial II)

Caveat II was a randomised trial (involving 52 sites) of PTCA vs DCA in 305 patients with discrete, de novo, SVG lesions. The average age of the SVGs was over 9.5 years. Acute complications were low and similar in DCA and PTCA patients (CABG: 0% vs 1.5%; QMI: 1.6% vs 1.5%; death: 1.6% vs 1.5%) respectively.

At 6 months, there was no significant difference in restenosis rates between those undergoing DCA (45.6%) or PTCA (50.5%) and target reintervention (18.6% DCA vs 26.2% PTCA; $p = 0.09$).

Over one-year of follow-up, similar trends were present with regards to death, MI and CABG but there was a favourable trend towards fewer repeat procedures after DCA.

OARS (Optimal Atherectomy Restenosis Study)

OARS was a four centre, non-randomised study which aimed to reveal 6-month restenosis rates in patients who achieved the best possible acute DCA result. Two hundred consecutive patients recruited underwent ultrasound-assisted DCA to achieve a residual stenosis of <10% with post-dilatation by PTCA being optional if residual stenosis >10% remained despite DCA's best efforts. Enrolment began in January 1994.

Procedural success occurred in 97.5%, with major complications in 2.5% (death 0%; emergency CABG 1.0%; Q-wave MI 1.5%). Salvage stent placement was performed in 3.5% and adjunct PTCA in 87% of patients.

Quantitative coronary angiography (QCA) showed enlargement in minimal luminal diameter (MLD) from 1.18 mm to 3.16 mm reducing diameter stenosis from 64% to 7%. IVUS showed that although the luminal cross sectional area was increased from 8.2 mm^2 after DCA to 9.0 mm^2 by adjunctive PTCA, a large amount of residual plaque remained (57%).

At 6 months, the angiographic restenosis rate was 28.9%. At 12 months, target lesion revascularization was 17.8%.

BOAT (Balloon Angioplasty vs Optimal Atherectomy Trial)

BOAT's primary objective was to demonstrate if it was possible to provide larger acute results safely with DCA (acute residual stenosis <15% via QCA) compared with conventional PTCA, and that such improved acute results translated into reduced angiographic restenosis. Forty individual high volume DCA/PTCA operators randomised 1000 patients to PTCA or DCA using a 7 F device. A residual stenosis of <15% (QCA) only would suffice although post-DCA PTCA could be used to achieve this if necessary. Enrolment began in February 1994.

The data indicated that the operators were able to apply the 'optimal' DCA strategy, producing a higher lesion (99.0% vs 97.0%) and procedural success (93% vs 87.0%) than after PTCA alone. A total of 79% of patients having DCA also had adjunctive PTCA leaving a residual stenosis of 15% in comparison to 28% for those undergoing PTCA alone.

Complications were no greater after DCA (2.8%) than after PTCA (3.3%) (death: 0% vs 0.42%; emergency CABG: 1.0% vs 2.0%; Q-wave MI: 2.0% vs 1.2% although large non-Q-wave MI i.e. CK-MB >8 times normal occurred in 6.0% vs 2.0% (p = 0.002) respectively. However, the use of emergency bail-out devices was significantly less common (5.0% vs 12.0%).

The 6-month angiographic restenosis rates were 32% (DCA) and 40% (PTCA) (p = 0.016) respectively representing a 20% reduction in restenosis for patients treated with DCA.

At 12 months, the cumulative mortality was 0.6% (DCA) and 1.6% (PTCA) (p = 0.14). Moreover there was no association between mortality and post-procedure elevation of CK MB. Target vessel revascularisation rates were similar (17.1% vs 19.7%).

ABACAS (Adjunctive Balloon Angioplasty Following Coronary Atherectomy Study)

This study was designed to compare the results of IVUS-guided Optimal DCA alone vs IVUS-guided DCA followed by adjunctive PTCA. The study enrolled 214 patients in 12 centres in Japan. Despite aggressive atherectomy (residual stenosis 11–15%), very low complications were reported acutely and at 6 months.

Acute complications included death (0%), CABG (0%), Q-wave MI (0.9%) and non-Q-wave MI (1.8%).

The overall restenosis rate at 6 months was 21% (19.6% DCA alone vs 23.6% DCA+PTCA). The target lesion revascularisation (TLR) was 17% (15.2% vs 20.6%). This is the lowest restenosis rate for any DCA study and among the lowest for any study comparing restenosis rates for any interventional device.

DCA, EXCIMER LASER AND ROTABLATOR ATHERECTOMY

High-speed rotational atherectomy and excimer laser coronary atherectomy can be followed by adjunctive DCA in the treatment of calcific disease in large coronary arteries. This combined synergistic technique overcomes the limitations of each individual procedure and of simple adjunctive PTCA. Figure 11.11 shows the synergistic effects of Rotablator atherectomy and DCA for debulking a calcified, chronically occluded LAD coronary artery. Such complex procedures require careful planning.

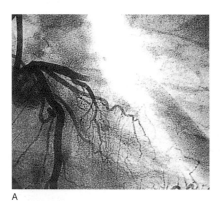

A

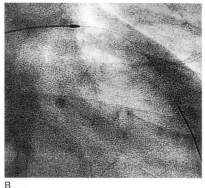

B

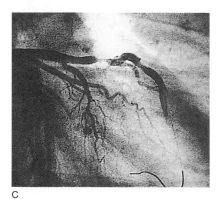

C

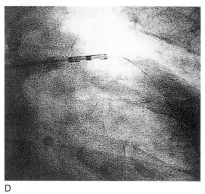

D

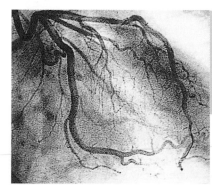

Figure 11.11:
Combined DCA and Rotablator atherectomy.
(a) Occlusion of proximal left anterior descending (LAD) coronary artery.
(b) Rotational atherectomy to reopen LAD.
(c) Residual stenosis in proximal LAD. (d) DCA using a 7 F SCA device. (e) Final result after removal of 12 specimens.

Intracoronary ultrasound is effective in assessing vessel morphology and the presence of calcification and is often helpful in deciding whether a lesion is suitable for DCA alone or whether a combined approach is required.

DCA AND CORONARY ARTERY STENTING

Debulking coronary artery plaque burden in a lesion aids more complete and concentric stent deployment and this can be demonstrated by IVUS. Stenting after DCA leads to further increase in lumenal diameter, less recoil and a reduction in residual stenosis (Fig. 11.12). Preliminary data suggest that restenosis occurs in <10% of such cases and is probably less common than after stenting alone.

The START trial in Japan is a prospective randomised trial comparing angiographic outcome and chronic vessel response assessed by serial IVUS between primary stenting ($n = 62$) and optimal DCA guided by IVUS ($n = 60$). At 6 months follow-up, aggressive DCA was associated with a larger lumen diameter and less restenosis than stenting (8.5% vs 23.0%; $p = 0.03$). The restenosis rates were 15.8% and 32.8% respectively and target vessel failure at 1 year was lower in the DCA group (18.3% vs 33.9%).

The SOLD Pilot study is a prospective study examining whether DCA prior to stenting increases lumen gain and reduces restenosis. Of the first 90 lesions in 71 patients, clinical success was high (96.0%). Complications were infrequent (CABG, MI and death occurred in one; MI in one; non-Q-wave MI in eight [11.3%]). At 6 months, angiographic restenosis occurred in 11.0% of lesions. Target lesion revascularization was needed in 7.0% of lesions.

The AMIGO trial will compare the long-term angiographic restenosis rates in 750 patients randomized to undergo either Multilink stent implantation with or without prior adjunctive DCA. The DESIRE study in Japan is also comparing restenosis rates in patients undergoing DCA prior to stenting compared to those undergoing stenting alone.

COMPLICATIONS OF DCA AND THEIR MANAGEMENT

Although DCA is safe and effective in selected cases, as with PTCA complications can occur. They are generally more common in the RCA than in the LAD or SVGs. The data below was obtained in the pre-stent era.

Death

Major complications resulting in death are infrequent, with most series showing <1%. Acute vessel closure after DCA increases the mortality risk substantially (from 0.3% to 5%).

Emergency CABG surgery

Emergency CABG surgery may be required – the majority for acute or threatened occlusion and a small number of patients for perforation. Most of these complications can now be treated by stent implantation. In the pre-stent DVI Registry, obstructive complications at the lesion site

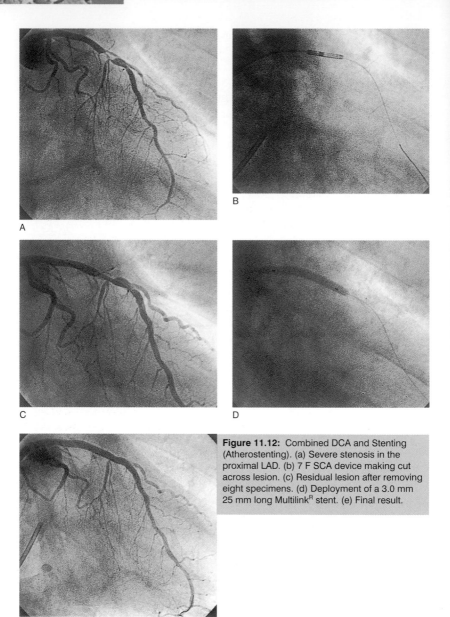

Figure 11.12: Combined DCA and Stenting (Atherostenting). (a) Severe stenosis in the proximal LAD. (b) 7 F SCA device making cut across lesion. (c) Residual lesion after removing eight specimens. (d) Deployment of a 3.0 mm 25 mm long Multilink[R] stent. (e) Final result.

accounted for 57% of cases referred for CABG, perforation (9%), guiding catheter injury (13%), device-related complications (8%), and PTCA-related complications (11%).

Acute coronary occlusion

In the DVI Multicenter Registry, acute occlusion was observed in 4.2% (out-of-lab 0.9%) i.e. 75% occurring in the cath. lab. Factors associated with abrupt closure were de novo lesions, RCA lesions, lesions with complex morphology, calcification and diffuse disease.

It is possible to deal with acute occlusion by PTCA or intracoronary stent implantation but a proportion (1.5%) will need CABG. The causes of acute occlusion are summarised in Table 11.7 and differ according to whether the occlusion is proximal to, at or beyond the lesion site.

Myocardial infarction

Acute coronary occlusion often gives rise to myocardial infarction (MI) unless it is rectified promptly. Q-wave MI occurs infrequently (0.3–2.5%) in experienced centres. However CK-MB elevation has been observed in 10% of patients undergoing DCA without any other evidence of significant myocardial ischaemia and late mortality at 3 years has been found to be worrying increased in patients who experienced significant enzyme rises. Distal embolisation of debris without angiographic evidence, prolonged ischaemia during the procedure due to device placement or small branch occlusions have been offered as possible explanations. Non-Q-wave MI occurred in 3.4% of patients in the DVI Registry.

Coronary perforation, pseudoaneurysm and ectasia

Acute consequences of deep arterial resection include coronary perforation, pseudoaneurysm formation and coronary ectasia.

Perforation occurs infrequently (0.5–1.3%). The causes are listed in Table 11.8. Appropriate case selection and technique should reduce its incidence. Although a small localised perforation can be sealed off by prolonged inflations with a perfusion balloon or by 'covered-stent' implantation and reversal of heparin, persisting significant perforations require emergency CABG without hesitation.

Pseudoaneurysm formation occurs in up to 0.5% of cases. Coronary ectasia can occur in 13% of cases.

TABLE 11.7 – CAUSES OF ACUTE CORONARY ARTERY OCCLUSION AFTER DCA
OCCLUSION PROXIMAL TO LESION
– Guide-induced dissection (RCA>LCA)
– Aggressive device manipulation (existing mild disease)
OCCLUSION AT LESION
– Failure to cross
– Salvage PTCA for failure to cross-dissection
– Device-induced dissection
– Thrombus
– Inadequate tissue removal
OCCLUSION DISTAL TO LESION
– Nosecone trauma: dissection, thrombus
– Nosecone trauma: spasm

TABLE 11.8 – CAUSES OF CORONARY ARTERY PERFORATION AFTER DCA
CASE SELECTION
– Severe angulation
– Extensive or spiral dissection
– Small vessel (<2.0 mm)
PROCEDURE
– Oversized device
– Too high balloon inflation pressure
– Incorrect device positioning
– Incorrect window orientation (very eccentric lesion)
– Cutting on spasm

Distal embolus

This complication is unusual for native coronary arteries (<1%) but may occur in 8% of SVGs when slow flow or angiographic cut-off may be evident. Most emboli occur in diffusely diseased, old vein grafts. The treatment of distal embolisation includes PTCA of vessel cut-off together with intra-coronary nitrates/calcium blocker to increase flow and reduce spasm.

Side branch occlusion

This complication can occur in up to 4% of cases due to a 'snow plough' effect. Side branches proximal or distal to the lesion have a low risk of occlusion (1.5%). The incidence is higher for those with branches exiting the diseased segment (36%) and especially those with significant ostial stenoses (45%). If the branch is of moderate size, it may be predilated before DCA in the main artery. Occluded side branches can usually be reopened by PTCA.

Arrhythmias and hypotension

In the DVI Registry, ventricular tachycardia or fibrillation complicated 0.5–1.7% of cases – similar to PTCA. Hypotension occurred in 1.8% of cases due to either ischaemia, arrhythmia, medication, perforation or tamponade as well as due to vasovagal reaction on sheath removal. Both complications should be treated aggressively to avoid a fall in coronary blood flow and treatment-site thrombosis.

Femoral artery complications

Because large arterial sheaths are often used, groin complications requiring blood transfusion (2.6%) or surgical repair (3.7%) may be higher than after PTCA.

Evidence for significant peripheral vascular disease should be sought prior to DCA. After withdrawal of the sheath, complications can be minimised by careful and prolonged haemostasis after the ACT has been shown to be normal.

■ .**Haematoma or bleeding** may occur in 1.6% of cases. Patients with hypertension, obesity or agitation have a higher incidence of haematoma because of inadequate initial haemostasis.

■ **Pseudoaneurysms of the femoral artery** may occur in 2.9% of cases and tend to develop in patients with initial significant haematoma or patients on anticoagulants following sheath removal. They can frequently be sealed off by local compression but occasionally require surgery.

■ **Arteriovenous fistulae** may occur in 0.5% of cases and may require surgical repair.

■ **Retroperitoneal haematoma** is unusual (0.3%), should be treated conservatively (bed rest, intravenous fluids and blood transfusion) and anticoagulation reversed.

■ **Femoral artery thrombosis and femoral neuropathy** are rare and should be treated surgically and conservatively respectively.

Device-specific complications

These are rare but may include guidewire fracture and entrapment, entrapment of the AtheroCath® within the coronary artery and even herniation of the cutter and fracture of the drive cable.

Contrast volume overload

Because of the large size of the guiding catheters employed during DCA, it is important especially in complex cases such as multivessel DCA or bifurcation DCA to avoid excessive contrast loading.

LATE OUTCOME AND RESTENOSIS AFTER DCA

It was originally hypothesised that debulking by DCA may reduce renarrowing by producing a large post DCA lumen, by reducing recoil and by creating a smoother, haemodynamically less turbulent surface, however restenosis remains a significant late complication.

Although data from Sequoia suggests that 74% of patients were asymptomatic or clinically improved at 6 months, 32% subsequently required treatment by CABG (14%), PTCA (4%) or repeat DCA (13%). Angiographic evidence of restenosis was observed in 42%, usually occurs within 3 months and in >90% of cases it occurs within 8 months. Few events relate to the DCA site after the first year of follow-up. The restenosis rate in native coronary arteries was 31% for primary lesions and 28% and 49% respectively for lesions treated with one or two previous PTCAs. The restenosis rates for SVGs was 53% for primary lesions and 58% and 82% respectively for lesions treated with one or two previous PTCAs.

Risk factors for increased restenosis included SVG lesions, lesion length (>10 mm), use of smaller device (6 F), smaller vessel (<3 mm), non-calcified lesions, small minimal luminal diameter (MLD) post-DCA, unstable angina, hypercholesterolaemia, hypertension, male gender, previous restenoses and short time interval after previous PTCA.

In the Netherlands, one group prospectively followed up 150 DCA procedures performed for stable and unstable angina. One and 2-year survival rates were 100% and 97% and 98% and 96% respectively. **165**

Event-free survival at 1 and 2 years was significantly lower in the unstable angina group (57% and 54%) than in the stable group (78% and 69%). Restenosis rates were 39% and 32% in the respective groups.

IVUS-guided, aggressive debulking by DCA to produce an optimal acute result is likely to result in low restenosis rates, but whether adjunctive stenting will reduce this further remains to be seen (see above).

DCA for restenosis after PTCA or previous DCA has a high success rate but a higher restenosis rate than de novo lesions. In addition, DCA can be used for restenosis after other interventional procedures such as coronary stenting and can provide insight and understanding of the ongoing pathobiology.

RECENT TECHNICAL DEVELOPMENTS

Recently, Guidant have introduced Flexi-Cut™, a low-profile (0.076″ maximum diameter of housing and shaft), more flexible atherectomy device suitable for use in 2.5–4.0 mm vessels (Fig. 11.13a). The 134 cm catheter is compatible with a 8 F guiding catheter and the custom-moulded PEBAX® balloon has a flat-bottom design to enhance stability of the housing within the vessel. The housing length is 17% less than the GTO® device and the shaft diameter has been reduced by 11% (Fig. 11.13b). The nosecone has a lower profile and a cylindrical shape and a 'dam' design at the top prevents material being extruded out of the nosecone's distal end (Fig. 11.13c). Its capacity is at least equal to that of 7 F GTO® device. The 9-mm-long cutter window has an expanded arc of 127° – improving tissue yield per cut. The ultra-hard titanium nitride-coated cutter (see Fig. 11.13a) makes cutting plaque easier and more efficient and is held in place by a bushing/cutter stem design.

A new 0.014″ guidewide, Hi-Torque Extra S'port™ has a supportive PTFE-coated distal core for smooth device delivery and a Microglide™ hydrophilic coating for reduced friction and smooth tracking (Fig. 11.13d). It provides excellent support and steerability. The 8 F Viking XT™ guiding catheter has an internal diameter of 0.087″ and provides exceptional support, flexibility and torque (Fig. 11.13e).

SUMMARY

Directional coronary atherectomy can be used in 10–15% of current interventional cases providing excellent acute results with a low complication rate especially for morphologically complex lesions which are unfavourable for PTCA. Case selection and careful technique have the major influence on the results achieved. Low restenosis rates are somewhat dependent on achieving a large post-DCA MLD and removal of a significant tissue mass. This can probably only be achieved in large (>3 mm) vessels. Post-DCA PTCA should be used to help achieve the largest MLD safely and the least residual stenosis. Combination of DCA with other techniques such as

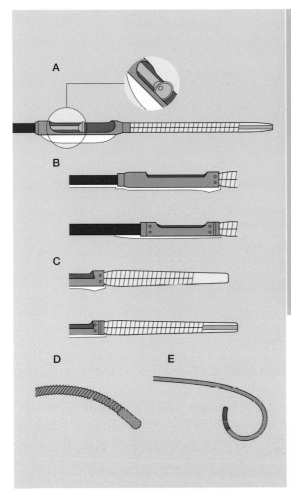

Figure 11.13:
(a) Flexi-Cut™ is the new, low-profile, more flexible atherectomy device from Guidan which is compatible with an 8 F guiding catheter. (b) The housing length is 17% less than the GTO® device and the custom-moulded PEBAX® balloon has a flat-bottom design. (c) The nosecone has a lower profile and a cylindrical shape. (d) The new 0.014″ Hi-Torque Extra-S'port™ guidewire has a supportive PTFE-coated distal core and a Microglide® coating for reduced friction and smooth tracking. (e) The 8 F Viking XT™ guiding catheter has an internal diameter of 0.087″, provides exceptional support, flexibility and torque and is available in a range of shapes including the JC shapes.

rotablator atherectomy and excimer laser atherectomy for calcific and bulky disease and as a preliminary debulking procedure prior to intracoronary stenting may improve overall early and late results.

Its use is limited by the rigid housing of the device. Currently only proximal or mid lesions in large (>2.5 mm), non-tortuous, non-calcified vessels are approachable. Intra-coronary ultrasound studies suggest that substantial plaque burden remains even after much tissue removal and a good angiographic result. The low profile, more flexible Flexi-Cut atherectomy device may make cutting plaque easier and more efficient although a combined ultrasound/AtheroCath might help to safely remove optimal amounts of plaque by improving the catheter's ability to direct the cuts more appropriately.

A major bonus of DCA is retrieval of tissue and this has already allowed study of the pathological process of atherosclerosis, unstable angina and restenosis by light and electron microscopy, cell culture experiments, cellular and molecular biology. In particular, the study of smooth muscle cell proliferation and their migratory and secretory activity has helped in the understanding of the response to arterial wall injury and the potential for locally applied agents and gene therapy to limit the phenomenon of fibrointimal hyperplasia.

FURTHER READING

Directional Coronary Atherectomy. Ramsdale DR, Grech ED. In: Grech ED, Ramsdale DR (eds). Practical Interventional Cardiology. London: Martin Dunitz 1997.

Directional Coronary Atherectomy. Hinohara T, Robertson GC, Selmon MR *et al.* J Invas Cardiol 1990;2:217–26.

Directional Coronary Atherectomy. Hinohara T, Rowe MH, Robertson GC. J Am Coll Cardiol 1991;17:1112–20.

Restenosis after Directional Coronary Atherectomy. Hinohara T, Robertson GC, Selmon MR *et al.* J Am Coll Cardiol 1992;20:623–32.

Symposium on Directional Coronary Atherectomy. Eds: Baim DS, Whitlow PL. Am J Cardiol 1993;72:1E–108E.

Case Selection Guidelines. Published by DVI (Devices for Vascular Intervention, Inc.), Redwood City, CA.

Atherectomy. Holmes Jr. DR, Garratt KN. MA: Blackwell Scientific Publications, 1992.

Directional Coronary Atherectomy. Freed MS, Safian RD. In: Freed M, Grines C (eds). Manual of interventional cardiology. Birmingham, MI: Physician's Press, 1992, pp. 275–87.

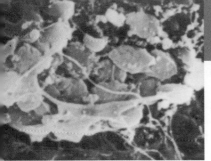

12

The use of laser in coronary intervention

PETER SCHOFIELD

KEY POINTS

- Laser guidewires have a limited application for interventional cardiology.

- Excimer laser catheters may be useful for treating coronary lesions which can be crossed with a guidewire but not with a balloon catheter.

- Laser balloon angioplasty may be useful for treating immediate vessel recoil or severe dissection. However, the introduction of coronary stents has essentially obviated the need for laser balloon angioplasty.

- Transmyocardial laser revascularisation (TMLR) improves symptoms and exercise capacity in patients with refractory angina who are not suitable for conventional revascularisation. The procedure however involves significant morbidity and mortality.

- Percutaneous myocardial revascularisation (PMR) is currently being evaluated for patients with severe angina due to disease which is not amenable to treatment by angioplasty or bypass grafting. It is likely to carry less morbidity and mortality than TMLR.

INTRODUCTION

The presence of a chronic total coronary artery occlusion continues to be a major problem for interventional cardiology. Around 10% of all attempted coronary angioplasties are performed for chronic total coronary occlusion.[1] The procedural success rate is lower for patients with chronic total occlusions who undergo coronary angioplasty when compared with patients who have stenosed, but patent, vessels. Depending to some extent on the nature of the occlusion and its duration, the success rate is usually in the order of 50–70%[2,3] – this is clearly much lower than for stenosed vessels. Failure to treat a chronic total occlusion may be due to the inability to cross the lesion with a guidewire or to inability to advance the balloon catheter across the lesion once the wire has crossed successfully. When treating a chronic total occlusion, the conventional technique uses a stiff guidewire and advancement of the balloon catheter close to the tip of the guidewire for additional rigidity. A variety of technologies have been introduced without a major improvement in the success rates. These include guidewires with olive-shaped tips, drills of various velocities, radio frequency heat applicators and laser devices. Two laser technologies will be considered further: first the laser guidewires and second the over-the-wire Excimer laser catheter.

LASER GUIDEWIRES

An Argon laser heated balltip (hot tip) guidewire has been used for the initial passage through chronic total occlusions.[4] In some cases, it has been **169** successful when conventional systems had failed. Vessel perforation is a possible complication of the technique. Further developments in hot tip recanalisation has not occurred and this technology is now rarely used.

The results of the bare Argon laser instrument Lastac are again comparable to those achieved with less costly mechanical means, although the cases undertaken may have been slightly more complex.[5] A beneficial mechanical component is undoubtedly present with these catheters which have many of the features which may be useful when treating chronic total occlusions (e.g. stiffness, bluntness). Randomised prospective trials against conventional technologies have not been carried out and this equipment now has very limited application.

EXCIMER LASER CATHETER

Excimer laser coronary angioplasty may help to solve some of the problems associated with treating chronic total occlusions. The technique requires the passage of a guidewire through the lesion, which clearly is not always possible. Once the guidewire has been advanced to the distal vessel, the Excimer laser catheter can be used to ablate tissue.

The Excimer laser system can be used with over-the-wire multifibre catheters of different diameters. Generally, the larger the diameter of the vessel being treated, the larger the diameter of the laser catheter utilised. Once the occlusion has been crossed with a conventional guidewire, the laser catheter is usually advanced to a position about 5 mm proximal to the lesion. The laser treatment is then initiated and during laser ablation the catheter is advanced slowly – at about 1 mm per second or less. Following the initial laser procedure, an acceptable angiographic result may have been achieved, or it may be necessary to sequentially increase the catheter size, or it may be necessary to use conventional angioplasty technology (i.e. balloon catheters and coronary stents). Periprocedural medications include aspirin, heparin (bolus dose), intravenous nitrate and calcium channel blockers.

In the Excimer Laser Coronary Angioplasty Registry, 172 chronic total occlusions were treated in 162 patients (10.3% of the 1569 patients entered). Once a guidewire crossed an occlusion, the overall laser success rate for treatment of chronic total occlusions was 83%. The extent of stenosis decreased from 100% to 55 ± 26%.[6] In 74% of patients, adjunctive percutaneous balloon coronary angioplasty was used after laser treatment. A final procedural success, defined as less than 50% residual stenosis and no major complication (death, myocardial infarction or coronary artery bypass grafting) was achieved in 90%. Major complications were infrequent: one death, 1.9% myocardial infarction and 1.2% requirement for emergency bypass surgery. The results suggest that Excimer laser angioplasty may be useful for treating chronic total occlusions that can be crossed with a guidewire but not with the balloon catheter. A role has also been suggested when the occlusion has been confirmed to be extremely long.[6]

Excimer laser angioplasty continues to develop, particularly as an adjunct to conventional balloon angioplasty or coronary stenting in the treatment of chronic total occlusions. The data suggest that failure of laser angioplasty occurs because of low catheter flexibility and the need for good guidewire support when treating total occlusions – once the catheter has reached the target area, the morphology of the lesion seems to be of only minor importance for the success of the procedure.[7] An alternative strategy when treating totally occluded arteries which can be crossed with a guidewire, but not the balloon catheter is to use the Rotablator system. This technology, which uses a high-speed rotational burr, produces ablation of tissue. By using burrs of increasing diameter, the lesion may be successfully treated by the rotablator technique alone. Frequently, coronary balloon angioplasty or coronary stenting are required after the initial rotablator therapy. Currently there are no randomised studies which compare Excimer laser angioplasty with Rotablator in the treatment of chronic total occlusions which can be crossed with a guidewire but not a balloon catheter.

LASER BALLOON ANGIOPLASTY

Conventional balloon coronary angioplasty improves luminal dimensions by producing fracture of the atheromatous plaque and by stretching the plaque-free wall. It is associated with dissection of the media and the formation of intimal flaps. These changes create local flow abnormalities which are associated with varying degrees of mural thrombus formation. In the vast majority of cases, dissection and thrombus formation do not result in acute vessel occlusion. During the next few months, however, the vascular reponse to injury may lead to restenosis. The aim of the laser balloon angioplasty is to create a large, smooth vascular lumen, which may lead to better short- and long-term results than conventional balloon angioplasty. In theory, this could potentially be achieved by thermal welding of dissection flaps, the elimination of vascular recoil, the elimination of coronary vasospasm, the reduction in platelet activation and the inhibition of smooth muscle cell proliferation.[8]

Laser balloon angioplasty, therefore, permits the application of heat (generated by the laser source) and pressure (by balloon inflations) to thermally weld tissue during coronary angioplasty. The system uses an Nd: YAG laser and a modified coronary balloon angioplasty catheter. The dose of laser is usually delivered over a period of around 20 seconds, which results in adventitial temperatures of between 90 and 110°C. The technique is very similar to conventional balloon angioplasty. The laser balloon catheter is positioned over a 0.014 inch guidewire. Once the balloon is in the appropriate location, it is inflated to low pressure (usually about 4 atmospheres) and the programmed laser dose is delivered over around 20 seconds. The balloon inflation is continued for an additional 20–40 seconds while the temperature of the arterial wall returns to normal. It is unusual for further balloon dilatation to be necessary in order to improve the immediate angiographic result.

Laser balloon angioplasty has been shown to be effective in the management of acute failure of balloon coronary angioplasty, due to either immediate vessel recoil or severe dissection with impaired flow ('impending closure'). Despite this early success rate, however, the late angiographic restenosis rate of laser balloon angioplasty is very similar to conventional balloon angioplasty.[8] This is despite laser balloon angioplasty producing larger vessel lumens in the acute stage. With the introduction of coronary stents, the potential role for laser balloon angioplasty seems to have been taken over. The use of coronary stents will usually solve the acute problem of vessel recoil or severe dissection resulting in threatened occlusion. In addition, coronary stents are associated with a lower angiographic restenosis rate. Therefore, there would now appear to be no role for the technique of laser balloon angioplasty.

In the vast majority of patients with angina pectoris due to coronary artery disease, successful treatment can be achieved by antianginal medication, balloon coronary angioplasty/coronary stenting, or coronary artery bypass grafting. Some patients, however, have angina refractory to medical therapy and have diffuse disease in the distal part of their coronary circulation which is not amenable to treatment by either coronary angioplasty/stenting or coronary artery bypass surgery. Such patients have often undergone several revascularisation procedures in the past. In this group of patients, who present a difficult management problem, new laser techniques have been utilised in recent years. These include transmyocardial laser revascularisation (TMLR) and percutaneous myocardial revascularisation (PMR).

TRANSMYOCARDIAL LASER REVASCULARISATION (TMLR)

This is a new technique that creates transmural channels in ischaemic myocardium using laser ablation. Before the advent of coronary angioplasty and coronary artery bypass surgery, attempts were made at direct transmyocardial revascularisation.[9,10] A variety of tubes and needles were used to create transmural channels, with limited success in terms of clinical improvement. The concept was based on the knowledge of myocardial sinusoids and the thebesian system. These communications were thought to allow the direct perfusion of the myocardium by blood from the left ventricle. Other techniques included the creation of myocardial neovascularisation by internal thoracic artery implantation directly into the myocardium.[11] In principle, TMLR incorporates the direct perfusion and neovascularisation of these other techniques. Although the exact mechanism of action of TMLR is unknown, suggestions include direct perfusion through patent channels, denervation produced by the surgical procedure and new vessel formation (angiogenesis).[12] At the moment, the most likely mechanism for symptomatic improvement seems to be angiogenesis.

The technique of TMLR is usually carried out through a left anterolateral thoracotomy. The pericardium is opened and dissected free of the heart and the area of reversible ischaemia is exposed. This is determined pre-operatively by myocardial perfusion scanning (nuclear techniques or positron emission tomography). There is no requirement for cardiopulmonary bypass. The original laser used was the high energy carbon dioxide system (The Heart Laser, PLC Medical Systems). The laser probe is placed on the surface of the heart and fired when the ventricle is maximally distended with blood and electrically quiescent. The laser energy is absorbed by the blood within the left ventricle and this produces an acoustic image analogous to steam which is readily visible on transoesophageal echocardiography. Clearly, this appearance on the echocardiogram denotes transmyocardial penetration. The channels created by the CO_2 laser are approximately 1 mm in diameter and are created in a distribution of approximately one per square centimetre (Fig. 12.1). Haemorrhage from the channel is controlled with direct finger pressure or an epicardial suture if pressure is not adequate. TMLR can also be performed using a Holmium:YAG laser or an Excimer laser.

Uncontrolled studies using the CO_2 laser have suggested an overall improvement both subjectively and objectively following TMLR. In a USA multicentre, uncontrolled phase II clinical trial, based on 200 patients, the operative mortality was 9%.[12] All patients had angina refractory to medical therapy, documented evidence of reversible ischaemia by radionuclide scanning and were untreatable by conventional forms of revascularisation. There was a significant improvement in the Canadian Cardiovascular Score (CCS) for angina at 3, 6 and 12 months following the procedure. Taking a decrease of two CCS classes as a clinically significant improvement, 75% of those assessed post-operatively achieved this. In addition, there was a significant decrease in the number of perfusion defects in the treated left ventricular wall. Patients who had at least 1 year of follow-up experienced a significant decrease in the number of admissions for angina from 2.5 per patient-year before treatment to 0.5 per patient-year in the year following surgery.

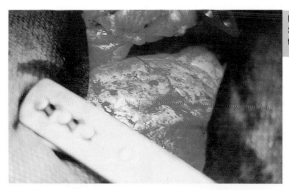

Figure 12.1:
Shows channels created at the time of TMLR surgery.

In a registry report from European and Asian centres performing TMLR using the carbon dioxide laser, the operative mortality was 9.7%.[13] Benefit in terms of improvement in exercise performance was clinically significant, but less impressive than in the USA uncontrolled study and less than benefits observed following other revascularisation procedures. Less than 50% of patients achieved an improvement of at least two angina classes compared with the 75% in the USA study. Complications of the technique include peri-operative bleeding and infection, left ventricular failure in the early post-operative period and cardiac arrhythmias – both supraventricular and ventricular.

TMLR is still a new technology which is being used more widely in Europe, the USA and Asia. It is clear that the benefits of the procedure in terms of improvements in angina and exercise tolerance will need to be sufficient to justify the peri-operative morbidity and mortality if the procedure is to become universally accepted. The results of a USA multicentre randomised controlled trial of TMLR against medical management have been submitted to the Food and Drug Administration Advisory Committee. They initially recommended non-approval for use in the USA due to the lack of a definitive explanation for the underlying mechanism, although many other well accepted techniques in clinical practice still lack full insight into the pathophysiological mechanism. In addition, there were concerns about the conduct of the trial in that the design allowed cross-over from medical therapy to TMLR and follow up data was incomplete. A follow-up submission was eventually approved. There have been two large randomised controlled trials of TMLR – one from the USA and one from the UK. The US trial randomised 198 patients to either continued medication or TMLR plus medication.[14] There was a high cross-over rate from medical therapy to TMLR and the 12-month data only includes 64 patients from the TMLR group and 23 from the control group. An improvement of at least two angina classes was found at 12 months in 72% of the TMLR group and 13% of control patients. There was an operative mortality of 3% for TMLR with no significant difference in survival at 12 months between the two groups. The results of the UK trial were less favourable.[15] In this study 188 patients with severe angina associated with coronary artery disease unsuitable for conventional revascularisation were randomised to either continued medication or TMLR plus medication. There were no cross-overs and almost complete follow-up data. At 12 months, the CCS angina score decreased by at least two classes in 25% of the TMLR patients and 4% of the control group. There was a peri-operative mortality of 5% for TMLR with no significant difference in survival at 12 months between the two groups. The morbidity associated with the TMLR procedure included wound/respiratory infection (33%) transient arrhythmia (usually atrial fibrillation) (15%) and left ventricular failure (12%). Exercise capacity measured using treadmill exercise times and 12 minutes' walk distance, was greater in the TMLR patients, although the difference between the two groups did not reach statistical significance. TMLR, therefore, seems to produce symptomatic improvement in this patient population, although an increase in exercise capacity has not been consistently demonstrated. Since the subjective improvement seems to be greater than the objective measurements, there are reservations regarding the widespread introduction of TMLR into clinical practice. It carries a peri-operative mortality of between 3% and 10% as well as a significant procedural morbidity.

PERCUTANEOUS MYOCARDIAL REVASCULARISATION (PMR)

With further developments in technology, it is now possible to perform direct myocardial laser revascularisation using a percutaneous approach. A Holmium:YAG laser has been developed in order to deliver energy directly to the endocardial surface of the left ventricular cavity (percutaneous myocardial revascularisation, CardioGenesis). Clearly, from the patient's point of view, this technique is much less invasive. It obviates the need for a general anaesthetic and thoracotomy with a consequent reduction in the length of hospital stay. Following TMLR, the mean length of stay is between 10 and 12 days, whereas patients can normally be discharged from hospital 24 to 48 hours after PMR.

With the CardioGenesis PMR system, access to the left ventricle is gained via a 9 F sheath introduced into the right femoral artery. The equipment essentially consists of a 'guiding catheter', a 'laser catheter' (which has a right angle bend towards its tip) and a 'laser fibre', which is passed through the laser catheter (Fig. 12.2). It is essential that the patient and the X-ray table do not move once the views in which to work have been selected. The two views typically selected are 40 degrees right anterior oblique and 50 degrees left anterior oblique, often with up to 10 degrees of cranial angulation. Whilst a biplane facility is preferred, the procedure can be easily carried out on single-plane equipment, although it may take slightly longer. The 'guiding catheter' is advanced to the left ventricular cavity and pre procedure left ventricular angiograms are performed in the two selected views. In addition, pre-procedure coronary

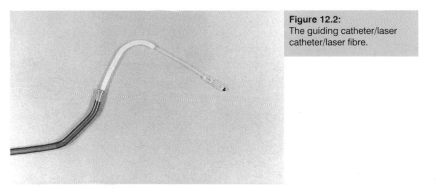

Figure 12.2:
The guiding catheter/laser catheter/laser fibre.

angiograms are usually carried out in the same projections. Both the coronary angiograms (at end-diastole) and the left ventricular angiograms (at end-diastole) are traced onto acetate sheets which have been fixed over the viewing screens (Fig. 12.3). These then act as 'maps' during the procedure. The area or areas to be treated are determined prior to the procedure using myocardial perfusion scanning. Reversible ischaemia may be present in the inferior, anterior, or lateral walls, or may involve the interventricular septum or left ventricular apex. All of these sites are accessible for treatment.

The 'laser catheter' is advanced through the 'guiding catheter' which has been positioned within the left ventricle. The 'guiding catheter' is available in a variety of curves and the one selected depends on the size and shape of the left ventricular cavity as well as the area to be treated. By manipulating the 'guiding catheter' and/or the 'laser catheter' all sites within the left ventricle can be accessed. Once in the appropriate position, the 'laser fibre' is advanced through the 'laser catheter' until there is contact with the endocardial surface of the left ventricle. This can often be felt, but can be seen as the laser catheter 'backs away' from the left ventricular wall and frequently ventricular ectopics are produced. Usually the right anterior oblique view is preferred for demonstrating contact with the anterior and inferior walls, and the left anterior oblique view for contact with the lateral and septal walls. The 'laser fibre' should be perpendicular to the left ventricular wall (Fig. 12.4). The laser is then activated, which typically produces 3 mm of penetration into the left ventricular myocardium: the 'laser fibre' is then advanced slightly and re-activated, which produces a channel of around 6 mm in total into the wall. The laser fibre is then withdrawn into the laser catheter and a new site is selected by manipulating the 'guiding catheter' and/or the 'laser

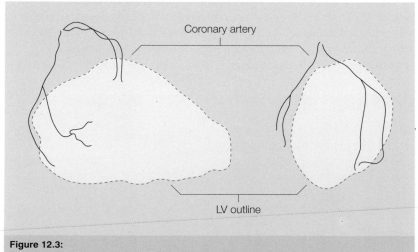

Figure 12.3:
Road map showing left ventricular (LV) outline and coronary arteries pre-procedure.

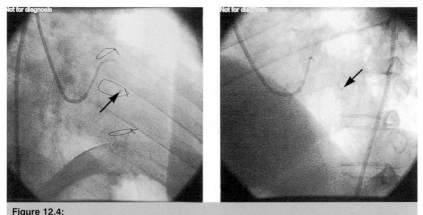

Figure 12.4:
Laser fibre against the left ventricular (LV) wall. Right anterior oblique projection (left) and left anterior oblique projection (right).

catheter'. Clearly, it is important to determine prior to the procedure that the part of the left ventricle to be treated is at least 8 mm thick, using transthoracic echocardiography, to reduce the risk of left ventricular perforation. The apex of the left ventricle is usually thinner than the rest of the ventricle, and therefore most operators will only be using one 'burst' of laser energy rather than two (i.e. only 3 mm deep channel) when treating the apical area. When a channel is created, the site is recorded by marking it on the acetate sheet in the two views. Typically, channels are created at about 1 cm intervals. When treating the anterior and inferior walls, the 'map' of channels is usually best demonstrated in the left anterior oblique view, whereas for the lateral and septal walls, the right anterior oblique view is preferred (Fig. 12.5). A total of 10–15 channels

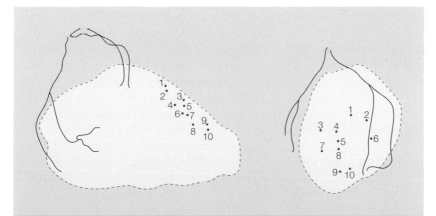

Figure 12.5:
Map of channels after procedure. Right anterior oblique projection (left). Left anterior oblique projection (right).

are typically created in each of the areas demonstrated to have evidence of reversible ischaemia (inferior, anterior, lateral or septal).

The patients are given a bolus of intravenous heparin (10 000 units) prior to the procedure. During manipulation of the 'guiding catheter' and/or 'laser catheter' it is quite common to induce ventricular ectopics, couplets or triplets and even non-sustained ventricular tachycardia. The rhythm disturbance is usually resolved by repositioning the catheters. Transient left bundle branch block can be induced during catheter manipulation. Therefore, if the patient has pre-existing right bundle branch block, it is advisable to position a temporary pacing wire prior to the procedure.

PMR is not used at the moment if there is evidence of left ventricular thrombus, if there is evidence of significant aortic stenosis or if there is severe peripheral vascular disease. The latter two exclusions produce problems of access to the left ventricular cavity. In addition, patients are unsuitable if the area intended for PMR treatment is less than 8 mm in thickness.

Recruitment for a randomised prospective trial of PMR against medical therapy, was completed in the summer of 1998. The patients included in the study had angina refractory to medical therapy, associated with coronary artery disease which was not amenable to conventional forms of revascularisation. They had evidence of reversible myocardial ischaemia on thallium scans and left ventricular ejection fractions of at least 30%. The results of this multicentre randomised prospective trial of PMR (PACIFIC trial) have recently been reported.[16] The study included 221 patients from several US sites and one UK site. The patients had angina refractory to medical therapy with disease not suitable for conventional revascularisation – 111 were randomised to medication alone and 110 to PMR and usual medication. At 6 months of follow-up there was a mean reduction of 1.4 CCS angina classes in the PMR group compared with 0.125 in the control group ($p = 0.001$). There was also a 30% increase in treadmill exercise time at 6 months in the PMR group compared with 5% in the control group, from baseline valves of a little over 400 seconds ($p < 0.001$). Noteably, there were no peri-procedural deaths in the PMR group. The morbidity associated with the procedure was also low. Of the 110 patients who underwent PMR, one developed cardiac tamponade requiring percutaneous drainage and one developed atrioventricular block which required permanent pacing. Patients can usually be discharged from hospital the day after the PMR procedure, whereas the mean hospital stay for the TMLR procedure may be up to 10 days. In an uncontrolled longitudinal study there was a significant improvement in angina class and increase in exercise time 3 months and 6 months following PMR.[17] There are several further studies of percutaneous laser revascularisation of the myocardium either planned or in progress. There are systems other than the CardioGenesis system which are being introduced. The results of the various trials of PMR are awaited with interest. If the technique is proven to be effective, then it is likely to be preferred to TMLR in patients who have no other revascularisation option, since it is much less invasive and is likely to have a lower morbidity and mortality. TMLR may, however, still have a useful role – perhaps as an adjunct to coronary artery bypass surgery. There are many patients who have obstructed coronary vessels, some of which are suitable for bypass grafting and some of which are not. In these patients a combination of bypass grafting to some territories and TMLR to other regions may be the optimal therapy. Similarly PMR may be undertaken in conjunction with coronary angioplasty/stenting in the future – for example with angioplasty/stenting of the left anterior descending artery and PMR of the inferior wall since the right coronary artery is diffusely diseased. It is likely that the use of laser myocardial revascularisation, whether TMLR or PMR, will increase in the coming years.

REFERENCES

1. Ketre K, Holubkov R, Kelsey S *et al*. Percutaneous transluminal coronary angioplasty in 1985–88 and 1977–81. The National Heart, Lung, and Blood Institute Registry. N Engl J Med 1988;318:265–70.

2. Hamm CW, Kupper W, Kuck K, Hofmann D, Bleifield W. Recanalisation of chronic, totally occluded coronary arteries by new angioplasty systems. Am J Cardiol 1990;66:1459–63.

3. Bell MR, Berger PB, Bresnahan JF, Reeder GS, Bailey KR, Holmes DR. Initial and long-term outcome of 354 patients after coronary balloon angioplasty of total coronary artery occlusions. Circulation 1992;85:1003–11.

4. Bowes RJ, Oakley GD, Fleming JS *et al*. Early clinical experience with a hot tip laser wire in patients with chronic coronary artery occlusion. J Invas Cardiol 1990;2:241–5.

5. Mast EG, Plokker HW, Ernst JM *et al*. Percutaneous recanalisation of chronic total occlusions: experience with the direct Argon laser assisted angioplasty system (LASTAC). Herz 1990;15:241–4.

6. Holmes DR, Forrester JS, Litvack F *et al*. Chronic total obstruction and short-term outcome: the Excimer laser coronary angioplasty registry experience. Mayo Clin Pro 1992;68:5–10.

7. Baumbach A, Haase K, Karsch K. Usefulness of morphologic parameters in predicting the outcome of coronary Excimer laser angioplasty. Am J Cardiol 1991;68:1310–5.

8. Safian RD, Reis GJ, Pomerantz RM. Laser balloon angioplasty: potential clinical applications. Herz 1990;15:299–306.

9. Sen PK, Udwadia TE, Kinare SG *et al*. Transmyocardial acupuncture: a new approach to myocardial revascularisation. J Thorac Cardiovasc Surg 1965;50:181–9.

10. Khazei All, Kime WP, Papadopoulous C *et al*. Myocardial canalization: a new method of myocardial revascularisation. Ann Thorac Surg 1968;6:163–71.

11. Vineberg A. Clinical and experimental studies in the treatment of coronary artery insufficiency by internal mammary artery implant. J Int Coll Surg 1954;22:503–18.

12. Horvath KA, Cohn LH, Cooley DA. Transmyocardial laser revascularisation: results of a multicentre trial with transmyocardial laser revascularisation used as sole therapy for end-stage coronary artery disease. J Thorac Cardiovasc Surg 1997;113:645–54.

13. Burns SM, Sharples ID, Tait S *et al*. The transmyocardial laser revascularisation international registry report. Eur Heart J 1999;20:31–7.

14. March RJ. Transmyocardial laser revascularisation with the CO_2 laser: one year results of a randomised controlled trial. Semin Thorac Cardiovasc Surg 1999;11:12–18.

15. Schofield PM, Sharples LD, Caine N *et al*. Transmyocardial laser revascularisation in patients with refractory angina: a randomised controlled trial. The Lancet 1999;353:519–24.

16. Oesterle SN, Yeung A, Ali N *et al*. The CardioGenesis percutaneous myocardial revascularisation (PMR) randomised trial: initial clinical results. J Am Cardiol 1999;33(2)Suppl. A:380A (Abstract).

17. Lauer B, Junghans U, Stahl F, Kluge R, Oesterle S, Schuler G. Catheter-based percutaneous myocardial laser revascularisation in patients with end-stage coronary artery disease. Eur Heart J 1998;(19 Abstract suppl.):589 (Abstract).

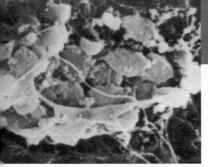

13

Cutting balloon angioplasty (CBA): technique

RAPHAEL A. PERRY

KEY POINTS
- Incisional dilatation reduces barotrauma and hoop stress and vessel wall injury.
- CBA is similar in success to POBA in and can be used in the majority of cases.
- Restenosis after CBA is lower than after POBA.
- CBA is an ideal treatment for resistant and ostial lesions effective in small vessel stenoses.
- There is emerging data that CBA may be the treatment of choice for in-stent restenosis.

INTRODUCTION

Since Adreas Grüntzig's first published series of coronary balloon angioplasty there has been an exponential rise in the complexity of coronary artery disease deemed treatable by percutaneous revascularisation. This has been enabled by the equally rapid change in the technology and number of devices available to the cardiologist. The principal driving force behind all these developments have been to conquer the two areas that have limited the application of percutaneous transluminal coronary angioplasty (PTCA), now affectionately known as POBA (plain old balloon angioplasty) namely acute vessel closure/coronary dissection and restenosis. POBA[1] increases luminal size by controlled barotrauma causing plaque rupture and vessel wall expansion. It is established that while the final angiographic result of POBA is related to the extent and force of balloon dilatation it is the extent of vessel wall trauma that determines acute vessel closure and also initiates the mechanism that when exaggerated leads to restenosis. Part of the difficulty is that the balloon frequently exerts its maximal force on the more normal parts of the vessel wall causing stretching which is prone to early recoil and damaging normal endothelium rather than cracking more organised fibrous plaque.

There is no doubt that coronary artery stenting has been the major development in coronary intervention over the last 10 years and has addressed to a significant extent the two Achilles' heels of POBA. Stenting rates are now over 70% in the majority of UK centres and the next challenge is to overcome the problem of in-stent restenosis.

The Barath cutting balloon[1] was designed specifically to address the problems of barotrauma-related complications of POBA. The device is a non-compliant balloon which when expanded has three or four longitudinally mounted microtomes on the external surface. The balloon material is folded to shield the blades and protect the vessel wall as the catheter is passed to and from the lesion. When the balloon is expanded at the site of a coronary lesion the blades produce controlled incisions into plaque rather than a random dissection. This allows the balloon barotrauma pressure to be evenly distributed and force to be applied to plaque at least as effectively as to normal parts of the vessel wall (Fig. 13.1). The reduction in hoop stress and lower pressures used to achieve an angiographically acceptable result (maximum of 6–8 atmospheres) are the main factors put forward as being likely to reduce both acute complications and restenosis.

PRACTICAL POINTS

The balloon is sized from 2.0 to 4.0 mm in quarter sizes. The deflated profile is from 0.041 to 0.046 inches, the atherotome lengths are either 10 or 15 mm and the distal shaft is 3.6 F. Clearly this is a relatively bulky device even compared with some of today's stents and in particular the 15 mm atherotome devices lack any significant flexibility. As with many interventional devices there are relative indications and contraindications which are varied in everyday use. Clear contraindications to its use are extensive vessel calcification and visible intraluminal thrombus. In practical terms excessive tortuosity and long lesions present difficulties though repeated inflations of the shorter balloon can achieve a good result. If there is difficulty crossing a lesion predilatation with a small balloon to allow passage of the cutting balloon is accepted practice. Once positioned across the lesion inflation should be undertaken slowly to reach

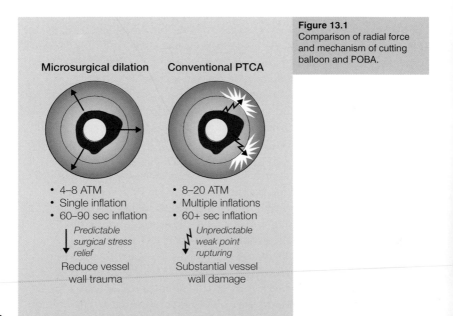

Figure 13.1
Comparison of radial force and mechanism of cutting balloon and POBA.

Microsurgical dilation

- 4–8 ATM
- Single inflation
- 60–90 sec inflation

Predictable surgical stress relief

Reduce vessel wall trauma

Conventional PTCA

- 8–20 ATM
- Multiple inflations
- 60+ sec inflation

Unpredictable weak point rupturing

Substantial vessel wall damage

6 atmospheres at 30 seconds and inflation maintained for up to 2 minutes provided patients can tolerate this. The slow unfolding of the microtomes prevents vessel damage and allows the movement of the artery to assist incision. It is important to allow full deflation to ensure involution of the microtomes prior to withdrawing the balloon. If full expansion is not achieved up to 8 atmospheres pressure may be applied. The balloon/artery ratio should be 1.2:1 and in practical terms this means using one quarter size more than the normal vessel segment. The final appearance may be 'stent-like' but up to a 30% residual stenosis is counted as an acceptable result and it is well observed that further positive remodelling takes place after initial dilatation such that follow-up angiograms not infrequently look better than the final result. Small controlled linear dissections are not uncommon and provided there is no change in the appearance over 5–10 minutes, acute vessel closure is extremely unlikely.[2]

CLINICAL DATA

There is good supporting evidence to confirm the effectiveness of cutting balloon angioplasty as a useful primary treatment of atheromatous coronary artery disease in a day-to-day setting and that the complication rates are equal to or lower than POBA with a lower restenosis rate. However since the widespread use of coronary stenting as an adjunctive or primary interventional procedure cutting balloon angioplasty has been confined to a variety of specific areas. These are principally in small vessel coronary disease, resistant or ostial lesions and more recently as a promising treatment of the burgeoning problem of in-stent restenosis.

The CUBA study examined the clinical effectiveness as a primary treatment in 304 patients randomised to CBA or POBA.[3] The average vessel size was 3 mm in both groups and there was a range of type A, B and C lesions. The acute complications were similar (major adverse cardiac event [MACE] 2% vs 3%) and there was 100% angiographic success in both groups. Stenting was avoided in general as with all studies of CBA but deemed necessary in 12% of cutting balloon patients and 8% POBA patients (NS). If the study were repeated in the light of present knowledge concerning CBA minor dissections the stenting rate would have been significantly lower. Six-month follow-up with angiography was 96% complete and showed a restenosis rate of 30% in the CBA group and 42% for POBA giving a significant relative risk in favour of CBA of 1.66. After adjusting for vessel size, location and clinical presentation the RR was 1.75 (CI 1.02–2.92, $p = 0.03$). Interestingly the benefit in restenosis for CBA was in larger vessels and in a non-left anterior descending (LAD) location.[4,5]

SMALL VESSEL PTCA

The Cutting Balloon Global Randomised Trial recruited 427 patients (495 lesions) with vessels <2.75 mm.[6] The angiographic success rate was similar **183** at 95% with a similar rate of stent implantation (6% CBA; 7% POBA). There were three perforations in the CBA group, which increased the major adverse cardiac events (MACE 3.2% vs 1.9% NS). The CAPAS study randomised 232 patients (248 lesions) with a reference diameter <3 mm all type B or C lesions.[7] The success rate was high with a stent implant rate of 6% in CBA and 11% in POBA. Angiographic follow-up was 95% complete and showed a significant reduction in restenosis after CBA (22% vs 41%; $p < 0.01$). Although there was a reduction in target vessel revascularisation after CBA this did not reach statistical significance (22% vs 29%). A further randomised trial by Ergene and colleagues[8] although small confirmed similar findings with a restenosis rate significantly lower after CBA (27% vs 47%; $p < 0.05$) and observed significantly fewer dissections after CBA. The BRIT (British Randomised Incisional Treatment) study is a randomised controlled trial of CBA vs POBA in small vessel PTCA at present ongoing which should have initial data within a year.

It would appear that CBA is safe and effective in small vessel coronary disease and it is clear that POBA has a low long-term success in these vessels. However with the advent of stents specifically designed for smaller vessels the best form of treatment to reduce the high rate of restenosis will need further evaluation. The costs of CBA are still significantly less than stenting though the costs of the latter are decreasing and repeat PTCA after CBA has a higher success than present strategies for dealing with in-stent restenosis.

The mechanism of CBA has been studied by intra-coronary ultrasound specifically in the REDUCE study which recruited 168 patients randomised to CBA and POBA.[9] As is often the case unsuspected calcification was discovered in a significant proportion of lesions (50% of CBA and 37% of POBA). It was clearly shown that in non-calcified lesions that CBA achieves significantly greater plaque compression/redistribution with lower pressures and significantly less vessel expansion than POBA. There was little difference in the ratio of vessel area, plaque area lumen area between the groups in calcified lesions. The virtual absence of vessel recoil would appear to be the significant factor in reducing the restenosis rates.

OSTIAL AND RESISTANT LESIONS

The outcome of POBA of ostial lesions at whatever site is poor. Cutting balloon angioplasty has been reported in a wide variety of both aorto-ostial lesions of SVGs and the right coronary artery and of the ostia of major branches of the coronary tree though few series have been compiled. It would seem logical that fibrotic resistant lesions would yield more readily after microsurgical dilatation and that stent deployment in such lesions would be facilitated. Muramatsu and colleagues [10] reported 37 patients undergoing CBA to ostial stenoses and compared them to a comparable group of patients having POBA with no patient being stented. The initial angiographic success rate was higher in the CBA group (95%

vs 85%)with a much higher incidence of serious dissections following
POBA 6.5% vs 0% for CBA. Angiographic restenosis occurred in 41% of
CBA patients and 53% of POBA cases. Oversizing the cutting balloon led
to a reduced restenosis rate of 31% but a higher dissection rate in POBA
patients. A small series of patients reported by Kurbaan *et al.*[11] showed
the benefits of combined cutting balloon and stenting in ostial lesions. In
these eight patients initial high pressure (18 atmospheres) ballooning led
to a modest improvement in stenosis from 82% to 68% but adjunctive
CBA left a residual stenosis of 44% which after stenting was reduced to
10%. During clinical follow-up there was no evidence of restenosis.
Combined CBA and stenting seems the most appropriate treatment for
aorto-ostial lesions and CBA alone may be the most straightforward
treatment of ostial branch lesions in an effort to reduce the difficulties of
plaque shift and concomitant bifurcation stenting.

IN-STENT RESTENOSIS

Although stenting has significantly reduced the incidence of vessel
restenosis and need for target vessel revascularisation when restenosis does
occur within a stent the rate of re-restenosis remains high with repeat
high-pressure ballooning having a recurrence rate of greater than 50%.
Intra-coronary ultrasound (ICUS) studies have shown that in-stent
restenosis is principally due to neo-intimal proliferation and hyperplasia as
there is little scope for vessel recoil after stent deployment. It was therefore
proposed that atherectomy by removing tissue would be the treatment of
choice with or without adjunctive ballooning. However there are little
data to support this and the only randomised trial of rotablation
(ARTIST) demonstrated a superior effect of POBA to rotational
atherectomy and low-pressure adjunctive ballooning for in-stent
restenosis[12].

Cutting Balloon Angioplasty has been used in in-stent restenosis with
encouraging initial results. Adamian and colleagues[13] retrospectively
reviewed 181 consecutive matched patients undergoing treatment for in-
stent restenosis using POBA rotablation (HSRA) and CBA. The final
minimal luminal diameter (MLD) was similar in all three groups with lower
MACE in the CBA group. Re-restenosis was significantly lower in the
CBA group compared to high speed rotational atherectomy (HSRA) and
POBA at 25%, 34% and 43% respectively. Although angiographic
follow-up was not complete (75% at 6 months) the target vessel
revascularisation rate was also lower at 18% vs 27% and 29% for each
group. Another series of 49 patients reported by Nakamura underwent
CBA for in-stent restenosis and had an angiographic restenosis rate of
27% with a target vessel revascularisation (TVR) rate of 18%.[14]

These promising initial results will be examined more closely in two
randomised trials at present ongoing. RESCUT (REStenosis CUTting
balloon evaluation study) and REDUCE II (Restenosis reDUction by
Cutting balloon Evaluation) should give a clear answer within 2 years. At **185**

present CBA for in-stent restenosis seems promising enough to use on a day-to-day basis and is the author's present choice of treatment for non-randomised patients.

SUMMARY

Cutting balloon angioplasty is a novel technique of incisional microsurgical dilatation combined with low-pressure ballooning. The procedure is safe and effective and although stenting is now widely used not dissimilar results can be obtained after CBA at a lesser cost. The balloon profile and flexibility limit its usefulness in a proportion of lesions and accurate sizing is essential to avoid the rare but significant problem of perforation. There are data to support CBA as a primary strategy in resistant and ostial lesions, small vessels and emerging data in in-stent restenosis. Restenosis rates in a variety of settings are lower than POBA.

REFERENCES

1. Barath P, Fishbein MC, Vari S, Forrester JS. Cutting balloon: a novel approach to percutaneous angioplasty. Am J Cardiol 1991;68:1249–52.

2. Martai V, Martin V, Carcia J, Guiteras P, Auge JM. Significance of angiographic coronary dissection after cutting balloon angioplasty. Am J Cardiol 1998;81:1349–52.

3. Mainar V, Auge JM, Dominguez J et al. Randomised comparison of cutting balloon vs conventional balloon angioplasty: final report an the in-hospital results of the CUBA study. Circulation 1997;96(8) Suppl.:1526–7.

4. Moris C, Bethencourt A, Gomez-Recio M et al. Angiographic follow-up of cutting balloon vs conventional balloon angioplasty: results of the CUBA study. JACC 1998;31(2) Suppl. A: 233A.

5. Dominguez J, Rodriguez JA, Gomez-Recio M et al. Cutting balloon vs conventional balloon angioplasty: subgroup analysis of a prospective randomised trial. JACC 1999;33(2) Suppl. A:48A;1098–41.

6. Bassand J-PL, Weiner BH et al. Efficacy and safety of cutting balloon in small coronary arteries (<2.75 mm): a report from the Cutting Balloon Randomised Trial. JACC Abs 70th sessions 1–527.

7. Izumi M, Tsuchikane E, Fumamoto F et al. One year clinical and 3-month angiographic follow-up of cutting balloon angioplasty versus plain old balloon angioplasty randomised study in small coronary artery (CAPAS). JACC 1999;33(2) Suppl. A:47;810–5.

8. Ergene O, Seyithanogula BY, Tastan A et al. Comparison of angiographic and clinical outcome after cutting balloon and conventional balloon angioplasty in vessels smaller than 3 mm in diameter: a randomized trial. J Invasive Cardiol 1998;10:70–75.

9. Okura H, Hayase M, Hosokawa H *et al*. Acute lumen gain after cutting balloon angioplasty in calcified and non calcified lesions: intravascular ultrasound analysis of the REDUCE study. JACC February 1999;33(2) Suppl. A:101A;886–3.

10. Muramatsu T, Tsukahara R, Ho M *et al*. Efficacy of cutting balloon angioplasty for lesions at the ostium of the coronary arteries. J Invas Cardiol 1999;11:201–206.

11. Kurbaan AS, Kelly PA, Sigward U. Cutting balloon angioplasty and stenting for aorto-ostial lesions. Heart 1997;77:350–52.

12. Ferguson JJ. Meeting highlights: highlights of the 21st congress of ESC. Circulation 1999;100:126–31.

13. Adamian MG, Marisco F, Brigouri C *et al*. Cutting balloon treatment for in stent restenosis, a matched comparison with conventional angioplasty and rotational atherectomy. Circulation 1999;100:1–305.

14. Nakamura M, Anzai H, Asahara T *et al*. Cutting balloon angioplasty for stent restenosis. Jpn J Intero Cardiol 1999;14:15–20.

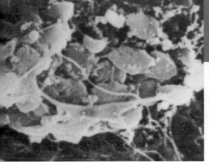

14

The X-Sizer: technique

MAN FAI SHUI

KEY POINTS

- The X-Sizer™ is a helical atherectomy/thrombectomy device that both cuts and retrieves material from the coronary artery or saphenous vein bypass grafts.

- The cutter is a single use device in a simple pack without the need of external power.

- Present models include a 1.5 mm cutter for 6 F and 2 mm cutter for 8 F guide catheters.

- Present cutters are more effective in removal of thrombus and loose or soft atheromatous plaque than for firm severe lesions.

- The device has a promising role in the treatment of acute coronary syndromes ranging from acute myocardial infarction to recent total coronary occlusions.

INTRODUCTION

The X-Sizer™ is a novel interventional catheter which has recently become available for clinical use in Europe. Originally invented as a device for drilling through chronic total occlusions, in the course of development it became clear that it could be highly effective in thrombus removal. In essence it is a spiral cutter inside a closely fitting ring at the tip of the catheter. The turn of the spiral plus additional vacuum suction enables the cut material to be removed from the artery. The catheter system has potential applications in a variety of clinical and angiographic settings such as acute thrombotic occlusions, chronic in-stent restenosis and treatment of degenerative vein grafts.

THE DEVICE

The X-Sizer™ catheter system is made up of four key elements: (i) a proprietary, helical cutter assembly; (ii) a catheter having dual, concentric lumens (the inner being formed by the torque tube, the lumen of which allows a 0.014 inch guidewire); (iii) an integral battery-powered drive module (Fig. 14.2); and (iv) connecting tubes to a pre-vacuumed bottle.

Figure 14.1 shows the one-piece system of the catheter-drive module assembly. The latter contains the motor, a 9-volt alkaline battery, and circuitry to ensure the cutter is only activated when there is sufficient vacuum in the catheter. The catheter tip (Fig. 14.2) contains an 'Archimedes-type' screw that fits inside a metal collar with only a portion of the screw protruding. The cutter rotates at 2100 rpm and the cutting action is between the screw blade and the collar. The catheter is normally used over a guidewire of exchange length to allow subsequent balloon dilatation and/or stent implantation. Current models include a 2.0 mm

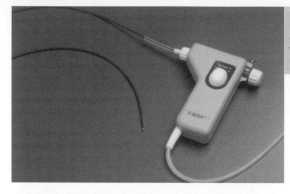

Figure 14.1:
Showing the X-Sizer™ catheter and drive module in which is housed a dry cell battery and circuitry.

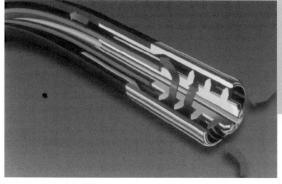

Figure 14.2:
A stylised cut-out view of the 'Archimedes-type' screw cutter in its metal collar showing how material is cut at the top and transported down the shaft of the catheter. The usual guidewire is not shown.

catheter for use with 8 F guiding catheters and a 1.5 mm catheter for use with 6 F guiding catheters. New designs including larger cutters and those with serrated cutting edges for excision of hard atheromatous plaques are under evaluation.

Preparation and use of the device

The system comes in a single sterile pack containing the catheter and its drive module, and vacuum-sealed bottles. The connecting tube from the drive unit is first joined to the vacuum bottle. The system is tested by switching on with the tip of the catheter in a bowl of saline. Once vacuum is developed in the unit, rotation starts as signified by a green light on the module. A red warning light indicates absence of vacuum and the rotation stops. The inner guidewire channel is flushed with saline and the catheter is threaded over the wire, which indicates absence of vacuum and the rotation then stops. Contrast visualisation is possible prior to and after passage of the catheter inside the vessel. The catheter tip is clearly visible on fluoroscopy. The cutter is activated as it approaches the area of obstruction. Advancement should be very slow to allow debris removal. If obstruction is felt, the catheter is withdrawn, again at a slow rate, into the guiding catheter and a check injection of contrast made. In the unusual event of the cutter stopping during forward passage, there is a reverse switch on the drive module that allows freeing of the cutter without loss of continuous aspiration of debris. During rotational cutting, blood can be seen to come through the tubing into the bottle, and an in line filter allows inspection of solid material collected. A typical procedure involves approximately 1 to 2 minutes of cutting in the course of which about 30–40 ml of blood would be aspirated into the bottle.

Comparison with other devices

There are three rotational atherectomy devices in clinical use, namely the rotablator (Boston Scientific), the transluminal extraction catheter (Interventional Technologies Inc) and the directional coronary atherectomy catheter (DCA). At first glance the X-Sizer is similar to the transluminal extraction catheters (TEC) device, except the latter is an 'open' cutter and rotates at speed, resulting in a much greater tendency to vessel trauma.[1] For this reason the use of the TEC catheter has largely been limited to vein grafts. The DCA is a cylindrical cutter inside a housing with a side opening. Repeated removal of the catheter from the patient is necessary for substantial plaque excision.[2] The device is not appropriate for thrombus removal. The rotablator is an open burr which achieves debulking by high-speed rotation.[3] Cut material is necessarily embolised distally; hence the need for very high rotational speeds to reduce particle size. Such microembolisation can still lead to temporary flow reduction and related wall motion abnormalities. Of the three devices this is the only one not able to retrieve ablated material and as such is not appropriate for the removal of intra-coronary thrombus or debulking of diffusely diseased vein grafts.

Another novel device the Angiojet, has been developed with the specific aim of removing intra-coronary thrombus.[4] This is an 'over the wire' catheter which utilises a number of high-pressure fluid jets to fragment and retrieve thrombotic material. The system requires a separate power console which generates some 20 atmospheres of fluid pressure. This is used to force saline down the catheter and emit a number of very fine jets directed back towards a collecting lumen. By a combination of the ablating force of the saline jets and the venturi effect the thrombus is fragmented into small pieces and flushed up the collecting lumen.

CLINICAL EXPERIENCE WITH THE X-SIZER™ CATHETER

Early experience with the 2.0 mm catheter has shown the ability of the catheter to negotiate vessels of moderate tortuosity. Thrombus extraction is quick, usually involving just one or two passes, and is rarely associated with any patient discomfort or even awareness of the process. The device has been used in over 300 cases in Europe in a variety of situations including acute myocardial infarction, unstable angina, and severely diseased vein grafts. Unlike other atherectomy techniques, there is minimal haemodynamic effect on heart rate and blood pressure, and no disturbance of A-V conduction has been reported. Temporary pacing wire is not required during use of the X-Sizer. Failure to reach target lesion occurred in a few instances due to the more rigid catheter construction in the first series of the device. Inability to cut through severe native vessel lesion has been observed, though passage through tight narrowings is possible, presumably depending on the tissue characteristics of the plaque. Given that this is a slow rotational cutting device, use in calcific lesion is not recommended. The current device is highly effective at removal of thrombus or any loose intra-coronary debris as found in old vein grafts. It is also able to debulk in-stent fibroelastic restenotic tissue. As with other non-balloon interventional devices, proper guide catheter choice for support and use of a high support guidewire improves access to more distal lesions. Following use of the device no special precaution is needed in subsequent balloon angioplasty or stent deployment. Adjunctive medication is the same as routine balloon angioplasty and stent procedures. At present there are no data to indicate whether the use of IIb/IIIa receptor antagonist improves clinical outcome.

THROMBECTOMY

Thrombus is the usual culprit in acute myocardial infarction, and is often seen in the setting of unstable angina.[5] Other situations include degenerate vein grafts and subacute occlusion after balloon angioplasty or stent implantation. The presence of thrombus is known to greatly increase the risk of coronary interventions.[6] Until recently operators have little choice than to proceed with balloon angioplasty followed by stent implantation. There are many drawbacks to this approach. Thrombus may be dislodged resulting in distal branch occlusion. It may be fragmented, leading to microembolisation and causing the no-reflow phenomenon. Balloon angioplasty alone may result in significant residual stenosis due to the presence of adherent thrombus. The use of stents has improved angiographic and clinical outcome. Even so, stenting in the presence of significant intra-coronary thrombus is believed to increase both the rates of subacute occlusion and subsequent restenosis.[7,8] There is therefore a need for safe removal of visible thrombus prior to angioplasty and stenting. Apart from the benefit of prompt restoration of antegrade flow and reducing the risk of distal embolisation, removal of loose thrombus allows better assessment of the culprit lesion and helps avoid wrong positioning of stents or unnecessary stenting of normal segments.

Case example

A 54-year-old man was admitted with an acute inferior infarct and treated with streptokinase with satisfactory resolution of chest pain and ST segment elevation. Two days later, reinfarction occurred and this time repeat thrombolysis with tissue plasminogen activator (tPa) had no effect. He was transferred to the tertiary centre where angiography at 4 hours after onset of symptoms showed complete occlusion of the right coronary artery near its origin (Fig. 14.3). The left coronary artery was normal. The

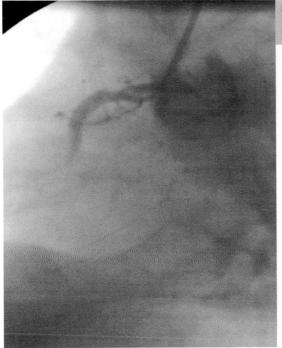

Figure 14.3:
RCA injection showing an
acute thrombotic occlusion.

occlusion was crossed using an exchange length wire with the support of a
balloon catheter but without balloon inflation. This resulted in a small
amount of antegrade flow (TIMI 1) showing a severe stenotic lesion plus
the presence of thrombotic occlusion beyond (Fig. 14.4). A 2 mm
X-Sizer was passed slowly with little force past the stenotic lesion and
then as far as the origin of the posterior descending branch. After two
passes, there was prompt antegrade flow of contrast (TIMI 3) revealing
the presence of a further stenosis after the first (Fig. 14.5). Without prior
balloon dilatation two stents were implanted one at each lesion (3.5 ×
24 mm distal and 3.5 × 15 proximal) with a good angiographic result
(Fig. 14.6). The procedure was performed with the standard dose of
heparin but not with a IIb/IIIa receptor antagonist, and clopidogrel was
prescribed as for other stent procedures. There were no adverse clinical
events and the patient was discharged home 5 days after the intervention.

DIFFUSELY DISEASED CORONARY BYPASS GRAFTS

The problems of interventions in diffusely diseased vein grafts are similar
to but more serious than intra-coronary thrombus.[9] Both macroscopic and
microscopic embolisation are common. There is often a mismatch of
vessel size between the larger graft diameter and smaller native vessels,
making any degree of embolisation more serious. Currently new devices
are under evaluation for the capture of embolised debris downstream to

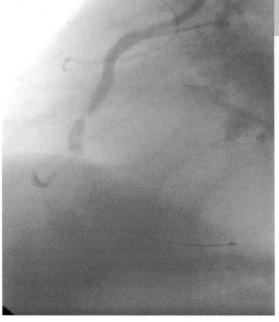

Figure 14.4:
RCA injection showing appearance after passage of the angioplasty wire.

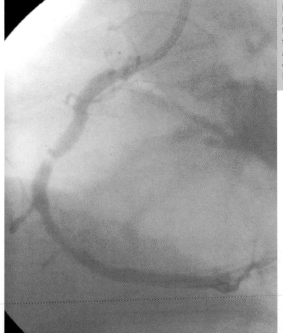

Figure 14.5:
RCA injection following two passes of the X-Sizer showing two underlying lesions: one at the site of original occlusion and a longer and less severe one a few centimetres beyond.

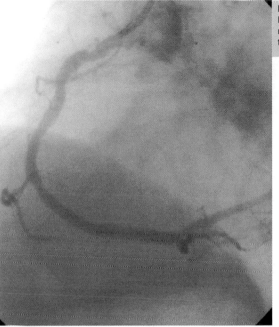

Figure 14.6:
Final angiogram showing results after implantation of two coronary stents.

the site of intervention. The X-Sizer has been used with good effect in pre-treatment of diffusely diseased segments before stent implantation. It is not possible to determine how much distal embolisation still occurs, and experience is still limited as to the effectiveness of a 2 mm cutter in grafts of 4 mm or larger. It may be that in such situations the combination of a distal capture device with plaque excision offer the best solution.

IN-STENT RESTENOSIS

The concept of debulking in in-stent stenosis has been the basis for the use of devices such as the rotablator. The X-Sizer has been used to similar effect and has the additional advantage of being able to retrieve the excised material. By debulking and enlarging the restenotic segment it has been possible to produce a good angiographic result without further stent deployment. Evidence for this approach of debulking for in-stent restenosis will obviously need to come from a randomised controlled trial against other forms of treatment.

ATHERECTOMY

Present experience with the existing cutters showed that they often cannot pass through severe native vessel stenoses. The cutter is seen to be held up at the site without necessarily causing any damage to the vessel. Occasionally very tight stenoses are crossed, possibly due to the softness of the plaque or presence of thrombus contributing to the stenosis. Nevertheless it is not recommended that the device, in its present form, be used for ordinary native disease. However, cutters with serrated edges which have the potential of excising harder tissue are currently under evaluation, and indications will therefore change accordingly.

SUMMARY

In summary, the X-Sizer™ catheter is a thrombectomy/atherectomy device which has the advantage of being simple to use without the need for a separate power console. The catheter comes as a single package with a long shelf-life. This allows immediate use with minimal preparation, an important consideration as its main use at present would seem to be for emergency thrombectomy in the setting of acute coronary occlusions. With the increasing role of direct intervention for acute myocardial infarction and early intervention for unstable angina, this seems an obvious necessity in the interventional laboratory

REFERENCES

1. Sketch MH, Phillips HR, Lee MM *et al*. Coronary Transluminal Extraction-endarterectomy. J Invas Cardiol 1991;3:13–18.

2. Hinohara T, Robertson GC, Selmon MR. Directional coronary atherectomy. J Invas Cardiol 1990:2:217–26.

3. Casterella J, Teirstein PS. Rotational coronary artherectomy. Pract Intervent Cardiol. London: Martin Dunitz, 1977.

4. Whisenant BK, Baim DS, Kuntz RE *et al*. Rheolytic thrombectomy with the Possis Angiojet: technical considerations and initial clinical experience. J Invasive Cardiol 1999;7:421–6.

5. Mizuno K, Satomura K, Miyamoto A. Angioscopic evaluation of coronary artery thrombus in acute coronary syndromes. NEJM 1992;326:287–91.

6. Grassman ED, Leya F, Johnson SA *et al*. Percutaneous transluminal coronary angioplasty for unstable angina: predictors of outcome in a multicentre study. J Thromb Thrombolysis 1994;1:73–8.

7. Fuster JS, Fishbein M, Helfant R. A paradigm for restenosis based on cell biology: clues for development of new preventive therapies. JACC 1999;17:758–69.

8. White CJ, Ramee SR, Collins TJ. Coronary thrombi increase PTCA risk. Angioscopy as a clinical tool. Circulation 1996;93:253–8.

9. Dooris M, Hoffmann M, Glazier S *et al*. Comparative results of transluminal extraction coronary atherectomy in saphenous vein graft lesions with and without thrombus. J Am Coll Cardiol 1995;25:1700–1705.

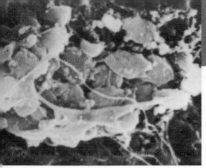

15

Transluminal extraction catheter (TEC): technique

JIM HALL

KEY POINTS
- TEC is a niche-only device.
- It is suitable for degenerate saphenous vein grafts and/or thrombus containing lesions.
- Adjunctive balloon angioplasty and/or stents are needed.

INTRODUCTION

The transluminal extraction catheter (TEC) is an atherectomy device for use in percutaneous coronary intervention (PCI) designed for front cutting and simultaneous aspiration of plaque and thrombus. TEC was developed by Interventional Technologies Inc, IVT (San Diego, CA, USA). It received FDA approval in 1992 and has been used worldwide to remove atheromatous plaque and intra-coronary thrombus in native coronary vessels and saphenous vein bypass grafts.

As with all atherectomy devices the impetus behind its development was an attempt to reduce the acute and long-term complications of PCI. Removal of plaque and thrombus may reduce the risk of distal embolisation, acute closure and peri-procedural myocardial infarction. Removal of plaque (debulking) may reduce restenosis.

DESIGN

TEC is an over the wire device which is basically a motor-driven rotating flexible tube with two stainless steel conical blades at its tip. Once in position in the coronary artery the TEC rotates rapidly and as the device is advanced the steel blades excise plaque. The rotating blades also disrupt intra-coronary thrombus. The proximal end of the TEC is connected to vacuum bottles hence aspirating and collecting the resulting debris.

The TEC is controlled by a hand-held catheter drive unit with a lever to precisely advance and retract the catheter. The rotation at 750 rpm is powered by a remote battery power source. The 30 ml vacuum bottle for simultaneous and continuous aspiration can be simply replaced with a fresh vacuum bottle when full of aspirate.

The TEC is advanced over a unique 300 cm 0.014 inch stainless steel coronary guidewire which has a radio-opaque distal 2.5 cm floppy tip ending in a 0.020 inch distal ball to prevent wire entrapment. The proximal section of the guidewire is very stiff to improve tracking of the TEC within the coronary artery. The TECs are available in 5 F to 7.5 F sizes (i.e. 1.83 mm, 2 mm, 2.17 mm, 2.33 mm and 2.5 mm).

DEPLOYMENT

The TEC is suitable for a standard femoral approach but requires 10 F guide catheters which can be a limitation in patients with severe peripheral vascular disease. The recommended IVT guide catheters give excellent support when advancing the TEC but are somewhat inflexible. Standard antiplatelet therapy and peri-procedural heparinisation regimes should be used.

Following preliminary angiography and positioning of the guide catheter the TEC guidewire is advanced across the lesion. The TEC catheter can now be advanced into the coronary artery or vein graft without rotation. The TEC should be advanced up to the beginning of the lesion, not into it, before starting the rotation. During cutting it is essential to continuously flush the guide catheter with heparinised saline to facilitate aspiration of particulate debri. Liberal use of intra-coronary GTN will minimise spasm. The TEC should start atherectomy at the beginning of the lesion (the foothills) and advance *slowly* (no more than 1 mm per second) to avoid a Dotter effect (simple mechanical stretching of the artery with plaque compression/disruption) and distal embolisation. It may not be possible to traverse the whole lesion in one pass and runs should be limited to approximately 15 seconds going 'into and out of' the lesion. The TEC should not be pushed forcibly across the lesion nor 'jump' forward since this will produce a high incidence of dissection. Some operators recommend a stepped approach with multiple catheters for particularly long or bulky lesions but this is an expensive strategy. If removing thrombus from a large vessel is probably better to use larger cutters but for most occasions the 6 F cutter is the most appropriate.

After serial passes of the catheter (usually less than four in native coronaries, but can be many more in long vein graft procedures) the TEC passes easily and maximal debulking has occurred. The device is removed leaving the guide catheter and guidewire *in situ*. Adjunctive balloon angioplasty can now be performed over the TEC guidewire aiming for a minimal residual stenosis with or without the use of stents.

There are some lesions which are unsuitable for TEC, e.g. heavily calcified lesions (rotablator better), lesions on a severe bend or with extreme eccentricity (risk of perforation), lesions which have a pre-existing dissection (risk of propagation of dissection), small vessels (< 2.5 mm) or tortuous vessels will not allow safe passage of the device. The TEC cannot be used if the lesion cannot be crossed with the guidewire.

APPLICATIONS

Experience with TEC has led to a consensus that its main niches are the treatment of degenerate saphenous vein grafts and the removal of intra-coronary thrombus. These are particular subsets of lesions for PCI which are beset with the problems of acute closure, distal embolisation and restenosis. Removing intraluminal plaque and thrombus should improve results.

Case example

This case illustrates the use of the TEC for percutaneous coronary intervention in a patient with a combination of the two main indications for TEC, i.e. an acute coronary syndrome due to thrombosis of a degenerate vein graft.

The patient was a 64-year-old diabetic man who had had coronary artery bypass grafting (CABG) 11 years previously, with saphenous vein bypass grafts (SVBG) to the left anterior descending, first diagonal, obtuse marginal, right coronary and distal circumflex arteries. He had a return of angina 6 years after surgery, but this had been controlled with medical therapy until this admission. He had a crescendo story of unstable angina pectoris requiring admission to hospital. Despite aspirin, intravenous heparin and intravenous nitrates as well as his usual oral medication he had repeated episodes of ischaemic pain at rest associated with sinus tachycardia, ST depression and on two occasions transient ST elevation infero-laterally. Diagnostic coronary angiography had shown severe native three vessel disease with mildly impaired left ventricular function. The vein grafts to diagonal and obtuse marginal were occluded. The vein graft to the left anterior descending artery was patent with good flow. The saphenous vein bypass graft to the right coronary and distal circumflex arteries was patent but with poor flow due to severe disease. There was a tight proximal stenosis and a very tight distal stenosis with associated filling defects (probable thrombus) (Fig. 15.1).

It was elected to attempt percutaneous intervention to the SVBG. In view of the diffuse disease and probable intra-coronary thrombus the SVBG was treated with TEC. A 10 F FR4 guide catheter was used and the graft crossed with the TEC guidewire. A 6 F cutter was advanced into the graft and cutting started proximally. After three preliminary proximal passes the TEC was advanced to the distal thrombus laden segment (Fig. 15.2).

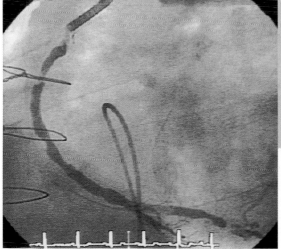

Figure 15.1:
Angiogram of saphenous vein bypass graft to the right coronary artery and distal circumflex artery taken using a TEC guide catheter. A pacing wire can be seen. The graft is severely diffusely diseased with multiple narrowings and intraluminal filling defects, with probable thrombus.

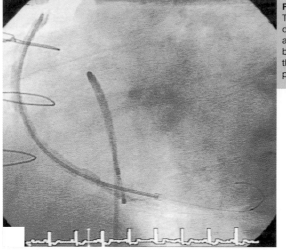

Figure 15.2:
The TEC guidewire is in the distal circumflex coronary artery. The TEC cutter is being advanced slowly through the graft to remove plaque and thrombus.

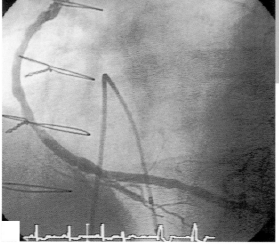

Figure 15.3:
Angiogram after multiple passages of the TEC showing improvement in the narrowings and removal of the intra-coronary filling defects.

Following a further four passes distally the TEC was withdrawn. There was considerable improvement in flow and the filling defects were no longer visible (Fig. 15.3). The procedure was completed with serial balloon dilatation along the graft. No stents were deployed. The procedure was not associated with a myocardial infarction (no Q-waves and no enzyme rise).

EVIDENCE

When TEC was developed it was hoped that it would have advantages compared with balloon angioplasty with reduced acute or chronic complications, sometimes summarised as MACE (major adverse cardiac events).[1] The acute MACE are often secondary to acute vessel closure or distal embolisation (both of which may produce death, Q-wave myocardial infarction (MI) and the need for emergency CABG). The long-term MACE relate to restenosis or reocclusion (leading to death, MI or repeat revascularisation).

Percutaneous interventions for the treatment of old SVBG are beset with acute and long-term complications. Such interventions are often undertaken in patients for whom repeat CABG would entail an excessive risk. Consequently the treatment of SVBG often represents a high-risk lesion in a high-risk patient. Not surprisingly angioplasty alone produces only moderate results, e.g. 69% procedural success and 46% restenosis.[2] The use of TEC for such lesions has been found to produce better acute results, e.g. 86% procedural success.[3] Unfortunately, distal embolisation and acute closure can still be encountered.[4]

Long-term MACE have not been found to be reduced. This is despite the hope that plaque debulking would reduce recoil and long-term restenosis (following the bigger is best principle). On the contrary a high restenosis rate has been a consistent finding.[3,4]

Further information about TEC comes from the NACI (new approaches to coronary intervention) registry. This is a voluntary registry covering 41 interventional centres which aims to evaluate several new devices (TEC, directional coronary atherectomy (DCA), rotablator, stents and laser angioplasty). Between 1990 and 1994, 331 patients had TEC treatments of 385 lesions of which 292 were in saphenous vein grafts. Adjunctive balloon angioplasty was needed in 90% of cases. There was an 86% procedural success rate but a 6.2% acute complication rate (death, Q-wave MI or emergency CABG).[5] The 1-year follow-up data show a death, MI or revascularisation rate of 51%.[5] Other data from the NACI registry examined the distal embolisation rate with TEC. This found a disappointing 8.3% distal embolisation rate, and when distal embolisation occurred it was associated with 18.5% mortality and 25.9% Q-wave MI.[6]

Hence, despite the beneficial effect of TEC compared with plain balloon angioplasty the results of SVBG interventions are still not as good as one would like. The combination of TEC with stents has been found to further improve results, with a 92% procedural success rate and a 1-year freedom from MACE of 72%.[7] Similarly the combination of TEC with abciximab has been suggested as a logical combination.[8] It may be that even with these combinations distal embolisation is not abolished and the TEC may need to be complemented with the use of other new devices, e.g. distal protection devices.

Interpretation of observational databases has some problems such as the question of comparing like with like and the inclusion in registries of operators' learning curves, etc. There are ongoing randomised studies which will help guide us in the optimal use of TEC. TOPIT (transluminal extractional atherectomy or PTCA in thrombus containing lesions) aims to determine the results of TEC in acute ischaemic syndromes in native coronary arteries. TECBEST (transluminal extraction catheter before stenting) aims to determine the results of TEC in saphenous vein bypass graft interventions. It is studies such as these and also high quality observational studies which will hopefully inform our future use of TEC.

SUMMARY

TEC is a useful addition to the armamentarium of the interventional cardiologist. Currently we are guided on its appropriate use by observational studies. It would appear to be useful for the removal of intra-coronary thrombus in the setting of acute coronary syndromes and the removal of plaque from old saphenous vein bypass grafts. The optimal interaction of this device with new devices and pharmacological treatments for the prevention of the acute and long-term complications of percutaneous intervention remains to be determined.

REFERENCES

1. Sketch MH Jr, Phillips HP, Lee M, Stack RS. Coronary transluminal extraction endarterectomy. J Invest Cardiol 1991;3:23–8.

2. Savage MP, Douglas JS Jr, Fischman DL *et al*. Stent placement compared with balloon angioplasty for obstructed coronary bypass grafts. Saphenous Vein De Novo Trial Investigators. New Engl J Med 1997;337:1124–30.

3. Twidale N, Barth CW 3rd, Kipperman RM, Bowles MH, Galichia JP. Acute results and long-term outcome of transluminal extraction catheter atherectomy for saphenous vein graft stenoses. Cathet Cardiovasc Diagn 1994;31:187–91.

4. Safian RD, Grines CL, May MA *et al*. Clinical and angiographic results of transluminal extraction catheter atherectomy in saphenous vein bypass grafts. Circulation 1994;89:302–312.

5. Sketch MH Jr, Davidson CJ, Yeh W *et al*. Predict of acute and long-term outcome with transluminal extraction atherectomy. The new approaches to coronary intervention (NACI) registry. Am J Cardiol 1997;80(10A):68K–77K.

6. Moses JW, Moussa I, Popma JJ, Sketch MH Jr, Yeh W. Risk of distal embolization and infarction with transluminal extraction atherectomy in saphenous vein grafts and native coronary arteries. NACI Investigators. New approaches to coronary interventions. Cathet Cardiovasc Intervent 1999;47(2):149–54.

7. Braden GA, Xenopoulos NP, Young T *et al*. Transluminal extraction atherectomy followed by immediate stenting for treatment of saphenous vein grafts. J Am Coll Cardiol 1997;30:657–63.

8. Sullebarger JT, Dalton RD, Nasser A, Mater FA. Adjunctive abciximab improves outcomes during recanalisation of totally occluded saphenous vein grafts using transluminal extraction atherectomy. Cathet Cardiovasc Intervent 1999;46:107–110.

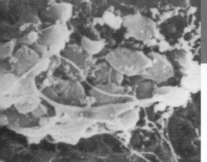

16

Intra-coronary brachytherapy

MARTYN R. THOMAS

KEY POINTS

■ Because the majority of stented coronary lesions are complex, both clinical and angiographic recurrence rates remain unacceptably high and continued research is required in the treatment of both de novo and 'in-stent' restenosis.

■ 'Brachytherapy' is the most encouraging recent advance in the prevention of restenosis following percutaneous coronary intervention. 'Brachytherapy' refers to radiation therapy with a radioactive source placed in or near to the target cell (in this context intra-coronary brachytherapy).

■ Broadly speaking two types of radiation source are currently being used for intra-coronary brachytherapy, that is those which deliver either beta or gamma radiation. Beta radiation has less problems with radiation protection but may have some disadvantages in terms of homogeneity of dosing.

■ The mechanism of action of both beta and gamma radiation is identical. Radiation disrupts DNA by strand and cross-link breakage. The target cell remains unclear but is likely to be in the adventitial layer of the coronary artery.

■ The three most important potential long-term complications of intra-coronary brachytherapy, i.e. coronary fibrosis, coronary aneurysm and tumour formation have thus far not been seen.

■ Intra-coronary brachytherapy has already been proven to reduce angiographic and clinical restenosis in animal and human randomised clinical trials both for de novo and 'in-stent' restenotic lesions.

■ The various brachytherapy systems in development differ not only in the type of radiation which is delivered (beta or gamma) but also the mechanism by which it is delivered, e.g. solid vs liquid vs gas.

■ It appears clear that there will be a therapeutic window in which radiation therapy is effective. Too low a dose appears at best ineffective and may indeed be pro-proliferative. Too high a dose may potentially lead to coronary aneurysm formation in the future due to a weakening of the vascular wall. The therapeutic dose is likely to be around 10–18 Gy at 1 mm from the endoluminal surface.

■ In order to perform intra-coronary brachytherapy within the UK currently three factors must be put in place: Ethical Committee approval, Administration of Radioactive Substances Advisory Committee (ARSAC) licence approval (usually held by a radiation oncologist) and Medical Device Agency approval of the delivery device. To fulfill these requirements a 'team' consisting of an interventional cardiologist, clinical oncologist and medical physics representative needs to be set up.

■ Intra-coronary brachytherapy may prove to be the greatest breakthrough for interventional cardiology since the coronary stent. Clearly the long-term follow-up of the pioneering work of Condado and Teirstein will be pivotal in the general acceptance of this form of treatment to the interventional community.

INTRODUCTION

The Achilles' heel of percutaneous transluminal coronary angioplasty (PTCA) has traditionally been abrupt vessel closure (occurring in 2–8%)[1] and the high incidence of restenosis (both clinical [13–16%] and angiographic [22–32%]) even for 'simple' lesions.[2,3] The early use of intra-coronary stents has greatly reduced the incidence of abrupt vessel closure during PTCA and the Stress/Benestent studies showed the benefit of this type of device in reducing both angiographic and clinical restenosis following PTCA.[2,3] However, the population of patients studied in the Stress/Benestent studies were highly selected (focal lesions < 15 mm in length, reference diameter > 3 mm, non-ostial, no thrombus, non-bifurcational, non-vein graft with elective deployment) and would account for only 15–20% of patients undergoing PTCA at our own institution.[4] The results of intra-coronary stenting in 'non-Stress/Benestent' lesions are less impressive with angiographic and clinical restenosis rates in the 30–50% range.[4,5,6] The newly produced disease process of 'in-stent restenosis' is also extremely difficult to treat. The use of simple techniques in this setting, such as re-dilatation by PTCA is associated with a recurrence rate of 50–80% especially in diffuse disease processes.[7,8] Restenosis, therefore, remains the greatest challenge to interventional cardiology, either following PTCA or intra-coronary stent insertion.

The use of radiation therapy to treat a proliferative, non-malignant disease process has been established in the treatment of keloid scars.[9] If restenosis following coronary angioplasty is considered as a similar process then the use of radiation would seem a reasonable approach in this setting.

BASIC CONCEPTS OF ANGIOPLASTY AND STENT RESTENOSIS

The pathological mechanisms of both balloon restenosis and in-stent restenosis are now well established and accepted as different.[10,11] Whereas the predominant reduction in luminal diameter at 6 months following PTCA is caused by adventitial construction (70–80%) with only a small contribution made by neointima, the reverse is true for in-stent restenosis with 90%+ of the loss of acute gain being caused by an aggressive neointima within the stented segment. The potential mechanisms for the effect of intra-coronary brachytherapy may therefore be different in these two settings.

The important measures of loss of the gain following angioplasty and therefore the way by which any potential anti-restenosis therapy may be measured are:

■ **Binary angiographic restenosis rates**, e.g. follow-up lesion diameter of < 50% of reference diameter. For coronary stenting this is generally in the region of 20–50% depending on the type of lesion.

■ **Clinical restenosis rate**; for coronary stenting this varies between 8 and 30%, depending on the lesion type.

Late loss, e.g. the loss of acute gain (in mm) at the lesion site at 6-month quantitative angiographic follow-up. For balloon angioplasty this value is generally around 0.7 mm. Clearly the lower this number the more effective the anti-restenosis treatment.

Late loss index, e.g. the late loss at the lesion site divided by the acute gain. This is accepted as the most sensitive measure of the effectiveness of any technique and generally measures 0.4–0.6 mm for balloon angioplasty. Once more the lower this value the more effective the anti-restenosis treatment.

BASIC CONCEPTS OF INTRA-VASCULAR RADIATION THERAPY

Due to the high integral dose seen with external beam irradiation and the difficulty in localising the dose precisely to the treatment volume (given the moving nature of the beating heart), external radiation treatment is currently not practical. The current systems therefore utilises 'brachytherapy' which refers to radiation therapy with a radioactive source placed in or near to the target cell (in this case intra-coronary brachytherapy). The radiation may be delivered via a stent, removable solid source or fluid/gas filled balloon (all placed at the site of the coronary lesion following standard intervention).

Broadly speaking two types of radiation source are currently being used for intra-coronary brachytherapy, that is those which deliver either beta or gamma radiation. Beta particles are high-speed electrons that are emitted from the nucleus of an unstable atom. They are high energy but have a low penetration so that the dose fall-off distant to the source is rapid. Gamma rays are high-energy photons again emitted from the nucleus of an unstable atom. The penetration of gamma rays in much higher than beta, meaning that the dose fall-off is much lower. The potential advantages and disadvantages of both types of source are discussed later.

The unit of dose of radiation therapy is the Gray (Gy) and refers to the mean energy imparted by ionising radiation to matter in a given volume divided by the mass of matter in that volume.

The mechanism of action of both beta and gamma radiation is identical. Radiation disrupts DNA by strand and cross-link breakage. This leads to cell death the next time the cell divides. The target cell for brachytherapy treatment is not entirely clear although the most likely candidate appears to be the myofibroblasts in the adventitial layer which migrate into the intima and transform to smooth muscle cells.[12] Most brachytherapy systems therefore aim to administer the target dose to the adventitial layer of the coronary artery. The dose of radiation appears crucial, too low a dose being ineffective or even stimulatory to neointimal growth and too high a dose being potentially associated with aneurysm formation due to thinning and weakening of the vessel wall. The potential for long-term fibrotic complications has not yet been seen in the human. The therapeutic window for dosing of radiation therapy is not yet clear, but may well be relatively narrow.

ANIMAL DATA

The principal of using brachytherapy post angioplasty to reduce restenosis has been proven in the animal model. This is true for both beta and gamma radiation and also in a number of different animal models.[13,14] There remain a number of outstanding issues however. The minimal dose required to show a favourable response is not yet established. There is some data to suggest that too low a dose may actually stimulate intimal hyperplasia. The minimal dose would appear to be in the region of 8 Gy to the adventitia. However it should be remembered that there is a major difference in the pathology of the balloon overstretch animal injury model (this is the mechanism used to create the lesion in the coronary artery of the animal model) and the human atherosclerotic artery. It is likely that doses that have been proven effective in the animal model could prove ineffective in the human because of the disease process is less predictable and often markedly eccentric.[15] There has also been some criticism of the animal models for the short-term follow-up and the young age of the animals (this may have some influence on radiation sensitivity). Despite these concerns following these encouraging results in the animal model human studies were commenced.

INITIAL CLINICAL HUMAN TRIALS

The encouraging results in the animal model led to the first human clinical trials. Condado performed the first intra-coronary brachytherapy cases in the world and reported an encouraging late loss index of 0.19 at 6 months. More recently the 2–3-year follow-up data have been reported with an encouragingly low binary angiographic restenosis rate of 28% (Ref. 16, data presented at Cardiovascular Radiation Therapy III, Washington February 17–19 1999). Despite the use of relatively high doses of radiation and one new pseudoaneurysm at early follow-up no progression of aneurysm formation or late adverse effects have been seen in this group of patients.

The SCRIPPS (the Scripps Coronary Radiation to Inhibit Proliferation Post Stenting Trial) trial was a landmark study which reported favourable results for the use of intra-coronary gamma brachytherapy in the human.[17] The trial was a double blind randomised placebo controlled trial comparing gamma radiation (iridium[192] embedded within an intra-coronary guidewire) vs placebo in a group of patients with coronary restenosis. Two-thirds of the patients presented with in-stent restenosis, a particularly high-risk group for repeat restenosis following further interventional therapies. The results are displayed below and indicate a major advantage of Ir[192] vs placebo (Fig. 16.1). Six months angiographic restenosis was dramatically reduced by Ir[192] from 53.6% to 16.7% (Fig. 16.1a). In addition there was a 63% reduction in late loss to 0.38 and an 80% reduction in late loss index to 0.12 (Fig. 16.1b). At 2-year follow-up these results were maintained and led to a marked clinical benefit with a

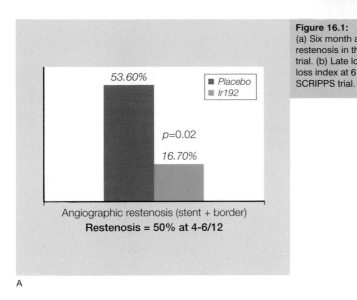

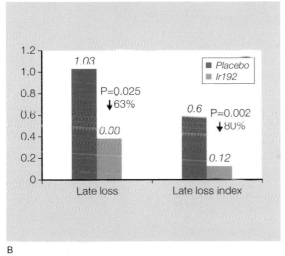

Figure 16.1:
(a) Six month angiographic restenosis in the SCRIPPS trial. (b) Late loss and late loss index at 6 months in the SCRIPPS trial.

target lesion revascularisation rate (TLR) of 15.4% in the Ir[192] group and 44.8% in the placebo group.

The SCRIPPS trial and Condado data[16] proved a major impetus to further clinical trials and to the development of multiple different brachytherapy systems by interventional cardiology companies.

INTRA-CORONARY BRACHYTHERAPY SYSTEMS

The various brachytherapy systems in development differ not only in the type of radiation which is delivered (beta or gamma) but also the mechanism by which it is delivered.

Solid vs liquid vs gas

The most common systems in development consist of a solid source which is deployed at the target site in order to deliver the radiation and subsequently removed after the necessary 'dwell time'. This source may be:

1. A 'wire' type system with the radiation source embedded in the distal portion.
2. A 'train' of several miniature cylindrical sealed sources which is flushed in and out of a blind-ending delivery catheter.

The alternative approach is to use balloon technology to deliver the radiation. A number of companies have developed this type of system. Balloon based systems have the advantage that the system is 'self-centering' (e.g. the balloon filled radiation system by its very nature centres the source of radiation within the lumen of the artery) and this technology is familiar to all interventionists. The disadvantages of this type of system is the potential for radiation 'spillage' if there is balloon rupture. Systems using both liquid (renium[188], renium[186]) and gas (xenon) filled balloons are in development.

Stents

Another attractive way to deliver radiation therapy is to use 'stent technology'. This has the advantage that the technique is similar to that which is used on a day-to-day basis in current standard practice. This technology has been used in the radioactive P^{32} stent. With this system the stent itself delivers the radioactivity (beta). The dose rate delivered using this platform is different to other systems, i.e. there is low dose radiation delivered for a prolonged period. The relevence of this to subsequent disappointing results with this technology is unclear. The stent delivery system is protected by a lucite shield which prevents excess radiation exposure to the operator.

SUBSEQUENT HUMAN CLINICAL TRIALS

The use of the above technologies and the enthusiasm of industry and interventionists following the publication of the SCRIPPS trial has led to a number of clinical trails in the human setting which are in the process of reporting either final or intermediate results.

THE 'IRIS' TRIALS USING THE P^{32} RADIOACTIVE STENT

The results of clinical trials thus far with the P^{32} stent have been disappointing.[18] The initial IRIS registry in the USA showed that the stent could be delivered with no early complications but with an angiographic restenosis rate of 39%. Subsequent dose-ranging studies performed in Europe have been equally disappointing. The principal difficulty with this device appears to be the so called 'edge effect' which may be difficult to combat using stent-based radiation technology. The 'edge effect' is a problem related to radiation dose. This occurs when the source length does not completely cover the 'injured segment' of coronary artery. This results in a previously injured area receiving a low dose of radiation and has led to the so-called 'Candy Wrapper' lesion being seen at follow-up. As the name suggests this is a lesion with no late loss at the actual site of the lesion but severe restenosis at the proximal and distal margins. Although this phenomenon may be theoretically more of a problem with beta radiation (because of the rapid fall-off in dose) it is also seen with gamma sources. The problem may be particularly difficult to solve with the radioactive beta stent as there is almost inevitably a segment of artery beyond the stented segment which is 'injured' by the deployment balloon. An extension of this is so-called 'geographic miss'. This term indicates that the source was not placed wholly within the injured segment at the initial procedure. The overall solution to both the edge effect and geographic miss is principally two-fold:

1. Operators must learn the importance of positioning of the source within the injured segment and ensure there is good overlap into non-injured segments.
2. The above will be facilitated by the industry developing source of much greater length.

The results of the European dose-ranging studies using the P³² stent are shown in Figure 16.2. Within stent restenosis of higher activity stents (3–6 µC) was found to be low (3.5%) but restenosis at the edges of the stents is high (39.3%) (Fig. 16.2). Subsequent development of this stent could revolve around differing radioactivity along the length of the stent and refining of the deployment technique.

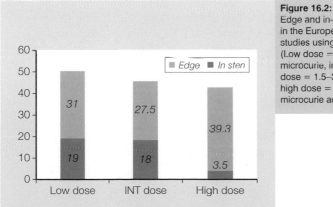

Figure 16.2:
Edge and in-stent restenosis in the European Dose ranging studies using the P³² stent. (Low dose = 0.75–1.5 microcurie, intermediate (INT) dose = 1.5–3.0 microcurie, high dose = 3.0–6.0 microcurie activity stents.)

THE 'WRIST' TRIALS

The 'Washington Radiation for In-Stent restenosis Trials' ('WRIST' trials) appear to be another landmark series of trials. The final results of the first of these trials was recently presented but has not yet been published (see Appendix A). The WRIST trial was a double-blind randomised trial of gamma radiation (Ir^{192}) vs placebo for the treatment of in-stent restenosis following standard treatment for this condition. In 90% of cases this meant the patient had already had debulking (by laser or rotablator) or repeat stenting before being randomised. The 6-month outcomes were dramatically in favour of the Ir^{192} arm with a 67% reduction in angiographic restenosis, 79% reduction in target lesion revascularisation, 61% reduction in target vessel revascularisation and 63% reduction in major adverse cardiac events (reported at American College of Cardiology [ACC] 1999).

Subsequent trials from the same institution will test a similar strategy for in-stent restenosis in saphenous vein grafts (SVG) (SVG WRIST), long lesions (long WRIST) and beta radiation for in-stent restenosis (beta WRIST).

THE 'BERT' (BETA ENERGY RESTENOSIS TRIAL) TRIALS

The 'BERT' studies have investigated the use of beta radiation (strontium^{90} delivered via the Novoste Beta-Cath system) to reduce restenosis following coronary angioplasty.[19] The Novoste device is non-centered but being a 5 F device (the strontium is delivered via a blind-ending 5 F catheter) it tends to 'self-centre' in the artery. The original trial was essentially a registry of the use of beta radiation to prevent restenosis following balloon angioplasty with no primary intention to deploy a stent. Bail-out stenting was required in 13% of cases. Three different doses of radiation were used during the study, i.e. 12 Gy, 14 Gy and 16 Gy. There was no control group. The results of the BERT study are shown in the Table 16.1. For the group as a whole the angiographic restenosis rate was 17% with an encouraging late loss index of 0.09. In addition the in-stent restenosis rates in the bail-out stent group were low and there was a suggestion of a dose effect with better results being achieved with higher radiation doses.

TABLE 16.1 – SIX-MONTH ANGIOGRAPHIC DATA FROM THE 'BERT' TRIAL. THE PATIENTS RECEIVING THE HIGHER RADIATION DOSES (14 AND 16 GY) ARE SHOWN IN THE RIGHT-HAND COLUMN.

	ALL	14 AND 16 GY
Patients (*n*)	78	52
Angiographic restenosis	17%	15%
Late loss index	9%	4%
Bail-out stenting	13%	9%
In-stent restenosis	8%	0%

THE 'PREVENT' TRIAL

This trial was performed using beta radiation delivered via a P^{32} source embedded in the end of a standard guidewire (Guidant Corporation). It was predominantly a phase 1 safety study. However radiation was compared with placebo therapy in a 2:1 randomisation fashion. Seventy-two lesions were included in the study (22 with in-stent restenosis). Of the 72 lesions treated 44 received a stent during the procedure. The 6-month angiographic and clinical data has been reported on 48 radiation patients and 15 control patients. These results are displayed in Table 16.2. Once more the P^{32} patients had an impressively low 'lesion' angiographic restenosis rate and late loss index but the 'edge effect' was clearly demonstrated by a vessel restenosis rate of 25%. Clinically this led to a target lesion revascularisation rate of only 4% but a target vessel revascularisation rate of 24%. These 'edge effects' with this device may be solved by:

- identification of the optimal dose;
- greater attention in ensuring that there are clear margins at the lesion site which receive radiation outside the injury site.

THE 'SCHNEIDER/SAUVERWEIN' TRIALS

The Schneider radiation system consists of a yttrium source embedded in a guidewire which delivers beta radiation via a computerised afterloader. The afterloader allows all functions such as dwell times to be automatically controlled. The initial animal data with this device was encouraging but the human phase 1 trial had a high restenosis rate (angiographic restenosis 40% with TLR 27%). The explanation for these results is likely to be that a relatively low dose of radiation was delivered. In this study 18 Gy was delivered to the endoluminal surface of the vessel. This equates to a dose of 5.4 Gy at 1 mm and 2.7 Gy at 2 mm. It appears that these doses are too low and ineffective at limiting neointimal proliferation.

These initial results have led to the current multicentre dose-ranging study. This trial will investigate the use of four different doses of radiation (9, 12, 15 and 18 Gy at 1 mm from the endoluminal surface) on

TABLE 16.2 – SIX-MONTH RESULTS OF THE 'PREVENT' TRIAL IN 63 PATIENTS WITH AVAILABLE DATA		
	P^{32} (n = 48)	CONTROL (n = 15)
Treatment site angiographic restenosis rate	6%	33%
Treatment site and adjacent site restenosis rate	25%	44%
Late loss index	0.05	0.51
Death	2%	0%
Myocardial infarction	11%	6%
Target lesion revascularisation	4%	18%
Target vessel revascularisation	24%	29%

angiographic restenosis rates in a group of patients undergoing balloon angioplasty without planned stent insertion.

ONGOING ISSUES

Dosimetry and type of radiation (beta vs gamma)

It appears clear that there will be a therapeutic window in which radiation therapy is effective. Too low a dose appears at best ineffective and may indeed be pro-proliferative. Too high a dose may potentially lead to coronary aneurysm formation in the future due to a weakening of the vascular wall. The therapeutic dose is likely to be around 10–18 Gy at 1 mm from the endoluminal surface. Dosimetry is undoubtedly more difficult with the beta sources because of the low penetration of the energy. Uniform dosimetry to the adventitia may prove difficult with beta sources (even with centring devices) resulting in both high and low doses to the adventitia even within the same lesion. This may be especially true in eccentric and calcified lesions.

However, beta radiation, because of its low penetration into tissues has the advantage of less radiation exposure to the catheter laboratory and hospital staff along with a lower total body radiation dose to the patient. The use of centring catheters to deliver a homogeneous dose to the target area is probably more important with the use of beta radiation.

The use of gamma radiation has some practical difficulties because of the need for more extensive radiation protection measures and increased total body dose to the patient. The dwell times of gamma sources are also much longer than beta sources (15–20 minutes vs 3–6 minutes). During the dwell time of gamma sources interventional staff also have to leave the cardiac catheter laboratory to limit radiation exposure. This is not necessary with beta radiation. However, the higher tissue penetration of gamma radiation has the advantage of easier dosing with centring of the delivery device being less important. It is also important to note that most of the initial positive trials using radiation to reduce restenosis are based on trials using gamma radiation.

Further trials on the efficacy of beta radiation will be necessary before this controversy is resolved.

Licensing

In order to perform intra-coronary brachytherapy within the UK currently three factors must be put in place:

1. Ethical Committee approval. Currently all procedures will be performed in either clinical trials or national/international registries.
2. Administration of Radioactive Substances Advisory Committee (ARSAC) licence approval. The licence allows the therapeutic delivery of radiation and is usually held by a radiation oncologist. It is unlikely,

given the training requirements, that this licence will be held by an interventional cardiologist in the foreseeable future.

3. Medical Device Agency approval of the delivery device.

In order to fulfill these requirements a 'team' consisting of an interventional cardiologist, clinical oncologist and medical physics representative needs to be set up. This 'team' approach will be a new one to most interventionalists!

Anxieties for the future

The longest follow-up of any patient who has undergone intra-coronary brachytherapy is approaching 4 years. There are clear worries about potential long-term complications of this procedure. These include:

■ Late fibrosis leading to 'delayed' restenosis.

■ Late 'thinning' of the vessel wall leading to aneurysm formation.

■ 'New' tumour formation either at a local or distant site.

These potential complications have thus far not been seen but in the field of radiation oncology they may be expected between 10–20 years following the index procedure.

CONCLUSIONS

Intra-coronary brachytherapy may prove to be the greatest breakthrough for interventional cardiology since the coronary stent. It is currently unclear where this procedure will fit into the interventional amourmentarium. Whether it will be used as a primary procedure, with or without a coronary stent, or whether it will be reserved for the treatment of in-stent restenosis remains to be seen. It is unlikely that intra-coronary brachytherapy will be delivered twice to the same site and this may play an important part of this decision making progress. Clearly the long-term follow-up of the pioneering work of Condado and Teirstein will be pivotal in the general acceptance of this form of treatment to the interventional community.

REFERENCES

1. Bergelson BA, Fishman RF, Tommaso CL *et al.* Abrupt vessel closure: changing importance, management, and consequences. Am Heart J 1997;134(3):362–81.

2. Fischman DL, Leon MB, Schatz RA *et al.* A randomised comparison of coronary-stent placement in the treatment of coronary artery disease. Stent Restenosis Study Investigators. N Eng J Med 1994;331:496–501.

3. Serruys PW, de Jaegere P, Kiemeneij F *et al.* A comparison of balloon-expandable stent implantation with balloon angioplasty in patients with coronary artery disease. BENESTENT Study Group. N Engl J Med 1994;331:449–95.

4. Williams IL, Thomas MR, de Belder A, Wainwright RJ, Jewitt DE. In-patient outcome and clinical restenosis in Benestent and non-Benestent lesions. Heart 1997;May (Suppl. 1):77–P46.

5. Zampieri P, Colombo A, Almagor Y, Maiello L, Finci L. Results of coronary stenting of ostial lesions. Am J Cardiol 1994;73:901–903.

6. Moussa I, Di Mario C, Moses J et al. Comparison of angiographic and clinical outcome of coronary stenting of chronic total occlusions versus sub-total occlusions. Am J Cardiol 1998;81:1–6.

7. Baim DS, Levine MJ, Leon MB, Levine S, Ellis SG, Schatz RA. Management of restenosis within the Palmaz–Schatz coronary stent (The US Multicenter Experience). Am J Cardiol 1993;71:364–6.

8. Schmog A, Kastrati A, Dietz R et al. Emergency coronary stenting for dissection during percutaneous transluminal coronary angioplasty: angiographic follow-up after stenting and repeat angioplasty of the stented segment. J Am Coll Cardiol 1994;23:1053–60.

9. Van den Brenk HAS, Minty CC. Radiation in the management of keloids and hypertrophic scar. Br J Surg 1959/60;47:595–605.

10. Mintz GS, Popma JJ, Pichard AD et al. Arterial remodelling after coronary angioplasty: a serial intravascular ultrasound study. Circulation 1996;94:35–43.

11. Hoffman R, Mintz GS, Popma JJ et al. Chronic arterial responses to stent implantation: a serial intravascular ultrasound analysis of Palmaz–Schatz stents in native coronary arteries. J Am Coll Cardiol 1996;28:1134–9.

12. Scott NA, Cipolla GD, Ross CE et al. Identification of a potential role for the adventitia in vascular lesion formation after balloon overstretch injury of porcine coronary arteries. Circulation 1996;93:2178–87.

13. Waksman R, Robinson KA, Crocker IR et al. Endovascular low-dose irradiation inhibits neointima formation after coronary artery balloon injury in swine. A possible role for radiation therapy in restenosis prevention. Circulation 1995;91:1533–9.

14. Verin V, Popowski Y, Urban P et al. Intra-arterial beta irradiation prevents neointimal hyperplasia in a hypercholesterolemic rabbit restenosis model. Circulation 1995;92:2284–90.

15. Verin V, Urban P, Popowski Y et al. Feasability of intra-coronary beta-irradiation to reduce restenosis after balloon angioplasty: A clinical pilot study. Circulation 1997;95:1138–44.

16. Condado JA, Waksman R, Gurdiel O et al. Long-term angiographic and clinical outcome after percutaneous transluminal coronary angioplasty and intra-coronary radiation therapy in humans. Circulation 1997;96(3):727–32.

17. Teirstein PS, Massullo V, Jani S et al. Catheter-based radiotherapy to inhibit restenosis after coronary stenting. N Engl J Med 1997;336:1697–1703.

18. Hehrlein C, Kubler W. Advantages and limitations of radioactive stents. Sem Intervent Cardiol 1997;2(2):109–113.

19. King SB 3rd, Williams DO, Chougule P et al. Endovascular beta-radiation to reduce restenosis after coronary balloon angioplasty: results of the beta energy restenosis trial (BERT). Circulation 1998;97(20):2025–30.

Section Three

Non-coronary Intervention

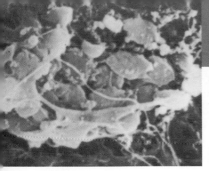

17

Percutaneous mitral balloon valvuloplasty

BERNARD D. PRENDERGAST AND
ROGER J.C. HALL

KEY POINTS

■ Approximately 300 mitral valvuloplasty procedures are carried out annually in the UK.

■ The procedure requires experience in trans-septal puncture.

■ It is ideal in non-calcified and non-regurgitant valves.

■ Expert echocardiographic assessment is required pre- and post-procedure.

■ Results similar to surgery in the long-term.

■ There is very large experience of the procedure in countries with high incidence of rheumatic fever.

■ The presence of left atrial thrombus is currently a contraindication.

INTRODUCTION

Despite the decline of rheumatic fever, mitral stenosis remains a common and important problem. The incidence of rheumatic heart disease in immigrants and ethnic minority groups is not inconsiderable and acute rheumatic fever is still a common problem in the developing world. In the West, rheumatic heart disease in the elderly represents a medico-historical remnant of widespread streptococcal infection earlier this century. Although degenerative valve disease now predominates in this age group, rheumatic mitral stenosis is by no means unusual. Older patients with mitral stenosis tend to fall into two categories: those who have restenosis after a previously successful surgical mitral valvotomy, and those with more slowly progressive rheumatic disease which has only become symptomatic in later life, these latter subjects illustrating selective survival in that the more seriously afflicted died at a young age.

Since the first publication on the implementation of the technique of percutaneous balloon mitral valvuloplasty by Inoue in 1984, numerous reports have confirmed its safety and efficacy. The technique has now replaced closed surgical commissurotomy for the treatment of mitral stenosis in young patients with pliable valves and indications for the technique in developed countries have now been extended to include older patients with more severe disease.

PATHOPHYSIOLOGY

The frequency of mitral stenosis parallels the incidence of acute rheumatic fever: the current prevalence, though clearly decreasing, is unknown. Rheumatic mitral valve disease is characterised by fusion of one or both commissures. The valve leaflets may be thickened, fibrous and calcified, causing reduced mobility, and the chordae tendinae may shorten and thicken, before fusing to form secondary subvalvular stenosis.

The normal mitral valve orifice is 4 cm^2, but in severe mitral stenosis this may be reduced to less than 1 cm.^{2} Pulmonary hypertension and increased pulmonary vascular resistance are frequent associated findings. These abnormalities usually become haemodynamically significant in the fourth and fifth decades, although initial presentation at the age of 70 or above is not uncommon. In mild–moderate disease the cardiac output may remain normal but is unable to increase with exercise, leading to exertional dyspnoea. With more severe degrees of stenosis, cardiac output becomes subnormal, even at rest. Symptoms may also be precipitated during tachycardia, when the abbreviation of diastole is associated with impaired left ventricular filling, and by the onset of atrial fibrillation when cardiac output may fall by 20–25% due to the loss of atrial transport and there is usually an associated sudden increase in heart rate.

The mechanism of balloon mitral valvuloplasty is splitting of the fused commissures and the procedure is only likely to work when there is significant fusion. The results of valvuloplasty are inversely related to the degree of leaflet thickening, calcification and mobility, and, in particular, the extent of subvalvular disease. In general, marked thickening and calcification of the subvalvular apparatus makes the valve less amenable to valvuloplasty.

PATIENT SELECTION

Patient selection is fundamental in predicting the immediate outcome of balloon mitral valvuloplasty. The procedure may have its most significant impact in the developing world where mitral stenosis is common, particularly in young patients, and cardiac surgical resources are sparse. In Western populations, patients with mitral stenosis may have moderately mobile and pliable valves, but generally are far older and have much more valvular thickening and calcification. Despite the lack of scientific evidence in this group of patients, a consensus regarding the place of balloon valvuloplasty is emerging which is consistent with common sense and a knowledge of the pathology of mitral stenosis. In practice, the choice of percutaneous balloon valvuloplasty will depend on the following factors: the patient's clinical condition, anatomical aspects and the experience of the practitioners concerned.

Clinical considerations

Clinical evaluation focuses on functional disability and the risks of the procedure in comparison with mitral valve replacement. Traditionally, surgical treatment of mitral stenosis has been withheld until symptoms become quite severe because of the very definite risk and inconvenience of surgery. In such markedly symptomatic patients the indication for balloon valvuloplasty is clear. However, now that the mitral valve can be dilated with excellent symptomatic results, a risk <1% and only a few days in hospital, it is also reasonable to consider the procedure in mildly symptomatic patients in the hope that early intervention may postpone the onset of atrial fibrillation and pulmonary vascular disease and allow the patient normal or near normal exercise tolerance. Truly asymptomatic patients are not usually candidates for mitral valvuloplasty, except in the following circumstances: a need for major non-cardiac surgery, to allow pregnancy, and possibly in patients with an increased risk of embolism (e.g. heavy left atrial spontaneous echo contrast) or with recurrent atrial arrhythmias.

Balloon valvuloplasty is the only interventional alternative when mitral valve replacement is contraindicated. It may also be preferable to surgery, at least as a first attempt, in patients with mitral stenosis who have undergone previous surgical mitral commissurotomy or aortic valve replacement. Although a good immediate outcome is frequently achieved, overall event-free survival is inferior in patients undergoing balloon valvuloplasty following previous valve surgery compared with those in whom balloon valvuloplasty is the primary procedure. However, the immediate outcome and long-term follow-up results are excellent in carefully selected patients with suitable valves and valvuloplasty is a valuable treatment option in this group.

The procedure may also be preferable to valve replacement in patients with impaired left ventricular function since the subvalvular apparatus is spared and the insult of cardiopulmonary bypass is avoided. In cases of co-existent mitral stenosis and moderate aortic valve disease, balloon valvuloplasty can be performed as an interim measure, and may postpone the need for eventual double valve replacement. In Western populations, many patients with mitral stenosis have concomitant non-cardiac disease which may increase the risk of surgery and balloon mitral valvuloplasty represents an attractive therapeutic option in this setting. This situation is particularly common in elderly patients, where balloon dilatation usually results in a moderate but significant improvement in valve function, associated with a clinically useful symptomatic result, although subsequent functional deterioration is frequent. The procedural mortality is 3% in the elderly, which is considerably less than the risks of mitral valve replacement in this group. Furthermore, in centres with greater experience, complication rates may be even lower.

Data from about 100 pregnant patients indicate that balloon valvuloplasty is a safe and efficacious treatment to improve the mother's haemodynamic status; it is also well tolerated by the foetus. The risks of exposing the foetus to radiation may be minimised by adequate lead screening of the abdomen and case reports describing a successful outcome using transoesophageal echocardiographic guidance alone, i.e. dispensing with radiation, have recently appeared. It must be borne in mind, however, that the procedure always carries a risk of complications, albeit small, so that it should be limited to pregnant women who remain symptomatic despite appropriate medical treatment.

Anatomical aspects

The evaluation of candidates for the procedure requires a precise assessment of valve morphology and function for advance planning of balloon dilatation and subsequent follow-up. Subsequent to clinical examination, two-dimensional echocardiography is currently the best and most widely used non-invasive technique for assessing the suitability of the mitral valve for balloon dilatation, allowing evaluation of the anatomical characteristics of the mitral valve and subvalvular apparatus, and the size of the valve annulus (Table 17.1).

In rheumatic mitral stenosis the valve leaflets are characteristically thickened (and often calcified) at echocardiography with evidence of commissural fusion. The degree of commissural fusion is usually best assessed using transthoracic echocardiography in the parasternal short axis view. Cusp mobility is reduced and bowing of the leaflets occurs in diastole. Associated features such as left atrial enlargement and/or thrombus, pulmonary hypertension and mitral regurgitation may also be apparent. Transthoracic imaging is satisfactory in most patients, but the valve is better defined by transoesophageal imaging. The aims of echocardiographic assessment prior to balloon valvuloplasty are to identify features predictive of a poor outcome, such as extensive valvular calcification, marked thickening and scarring of the subvalvular apparatus and the presence of associated mitral regurgitation. In addition, it is important to exclude the presence of left atrial thrombus, which increases the risk of systemic thromboembolism during or following the procedure. Since transoesophageal echocardiography allows more accurate assessment of the degree of leaflet involvement and subvalvular disease and is better at visualising left atrial and appendage thrombus, it is now considered mandatory in all patients prior to balloon valvuloplasty. The presence of thrombus within the left atrium (either floating or localised) or on the inter-atrial septum is a contraindication to balloon valvuloplasty. A number of small series have reported that the procedure is feasible in patients with thrombus localised to the left atrial appendage, but this remains controversial. Unless there is a need for urgent intervention or

TABLE 17.1 – ECHOCARDIOGRAPHIC ASSESSMENT PRIOR TO BALLOON MITRAL VALVULOPLASTY
■ Degree of mitral stenosis
■ Commissural fusion
■ Valvular calcification
■ Subvalvular involvement
■ Associated mitral regurgitation
■ Left atrial thrombus
■ Atrial septal anatomy

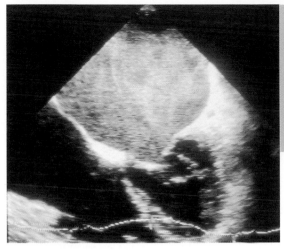

Figure 17.1:
Transoesophageal echocardiogram (horizontal plane, four chamber view) taken from a patient with severe rheumatic mitral stenosis. Note calcification of the anterior leaflet and spontaneous echo contrast within a grossly dilated left atrium, indicative of stagnant blood flow.

anticoagulation is contraindicated for other reasons, the patient can be treated with oral anticoagulants for 2 months, after which a follow-up transoesophageal echocardiographic examination usually shows disappearance of the thrombus. Spontaneous echo contrast, an echocardiographic marker of blood stasis within the left atrium, is a frequent finding in mitral stenosis and does not prohibit balloon valvuloplasty (Figures 17.1 & 17.2).

The valve area can be calculated using planimetry of the valve orifice in early diastole. This method is subject to error, however, and a more accurate assessment is obtained by measuring the velocity of flow across the valve using continuous wave doppler. By this means, a pressure half-time (the time interval for the velocity to fall from its peak value to the peak value divided by the square root of 2, normal <100 ms) can be derived and the valve area calculated as follows:

$$\text{Mitral valve area (cm}^2) = \frac{220}{\text{pressure half-time (ms)}}$$

Generally speaking, it is not advisable to define an arbitrary threshold valve area above which balloon valvuloplasty should not be performed, since overall assessment should also take account of functional disability and the presence of pulmonary hypertension. In practice, however, it is unusual to undertake the procedure in patients with a valve area greater than 1.5 cm^2 (or 1 cm^2/m^2 body surface area if the patient is unusually large).

Coexistent mitral regurgitation can be quantified using doppler techniques: moderate regurgitation contraindicates balloon valvuloplasty whereas mild regurgitation is acceptable. In cases where mitral stenosis is combined with severe aortic stenosis, the need for surgery is obvious. Tricuspid regurgitation is usually present to some degree and measurement of the velocity of the jet allows estimation of the pulmonary artery pressure. Preliminary reports in relatively small numbers of patients have

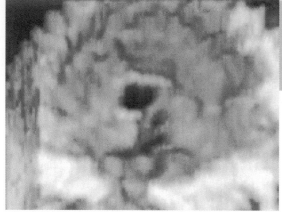

Figure 17.2:
Three-dimensional echocardiographic reconstruction of a severely stenosed mitral valve viewed from the ventricular aspect in late diastole.

suggested that balloon valvuloplasty can be performed safely and effectively in patients with severe pulmonary hypertension.

Clinician experience

In addition to these patient-related parameters, the experience of the medical team is important in reaching a management decision. Several series have confirmed that major complications are significantly fewer in centres undertaking a relatively large caseload. Inevitably, complications are more frequent when the operator has only a small throughput, since the procedure is technically demanding. In general terms, balloon valvuloplasty should only be performed by groups who are experienced in trans-septal catheterisation and who carry out an adequate number of procedures to maintain the technical skills required. These considerations are highly relevant in Western countries where mitral stenosis is relatively infrequent. Specialist experience is of particular importance in cases with minimal symptoms, cardiothoracic deformity or during pregnancy.

PATIENT PREPARATION

Patient preparation is essentially similar to that for routine left/right heart catheterisation. Informed consent should be obtained and the patient made aware of the small risks of systemic thromboembolism and severe mitral regurgitation requiring urgent surgery. Where appropriate, anticoagulant medication should be terminated 48 hours prior to the procedure, and then recommenced the day following valvuloplasty (assuming there are no vascular complications). All other medication is continued. A recent transthoracic and transoesophageal echocardiogram should be available to confirm valve suitability and exclude the presence of left atrial thrombus (see above). In practice, these are often performed during the 24 hours prior to the procedure.

On the day of valvuloplasty, the patient is fasted for 4–6 hours before the procedure and both groins are prepared for vascular access. A light sedative (e.g. diazepam 5 mg) may be helpful in anxious patients. Vascular sheaths are removed 3–4 hours following valvuloplasty when the anticoagulant effects of heparin have elapsed. Alternatively, the effects of heparin may be reversed with a small dose of protamine and sheaths removed immediately.

Generally, the patient can be discharged the day after a successful procedure providing there have been no complications. A further echocardiogram is performed before discharge (a transthoracic study is usually sufficient) to exclude significant mitral regurgitation or residual left-to-right shunt and to provide a baseline assessment of residual stenosis, which assists future follow-up.

TECHNIQUE

Two techniques – the Inoue and the double balloon techniques – are currently used to perform mitral valvuloplasty. The former has now gained widespread general acceptance, even though the equipment required is approximately twice as expensive, since it is simpler to perform and complications are less frequent. Both involve trans-septal catheterisation of the left atrium. Routine right heart catheterisation is undertaken via the femoral vein and right atrial angiography with late filling and filming of the left atrium is performed to guide trans-septal puncture. A retrograde pigtail catheter may also be positioned in the ascending aorta to delineate the position of the aortic valve and posterior aortic sinus, thereby reducing the risk of inadvertent aortic puncture. Trans-septal puncture is performed using a Brockenbrough needle and satisfactory left atrial positioning is confirmed by direct measurement of left atrial pressure and oxygen saturation. If satisfactory, the trans-septal catheter (either a Mullins or Brockenbrough catheter) is advanced into the left atrium, heparin (7500–10 000 IU) is administered, and mitral valve area is derived by measurement of the trans-valve pressure gradient and cardiac output.

The Inoue, single balloon technique makes use of a double loop guidewire, a 14 F dilator and the Inoue balloon catheter (Fig. 17.3). The size of Inoue balloon is selected according to the patients size (usually

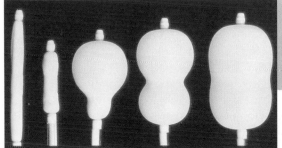

Figure 17.3:
The Inoue balloon at various stages of inflation. Note the initial selective inflation of the distal balloon which allows optimal positioning across the stenosed mitral valve.

TABLE 17.2 – INOUE BALLOON SELECTION	
HEIGHT (CM)	**BALLOON SIZE (DIAMETER IN CM)**
<150	24
>150	26
>165	28
>180	30

height or body surface area – Table 17.2) and the balloon prepared by successive inflation and deflation with contrast to extrude excess air. Balloon diameter at peak inflation is then verified using graduated calipers. The double loop guidewire is inserted into the left atrium through the trans-septal catheter, which is then removed. The 14 F dilator is introduced over this guidewire and advanced to dilate both the femoral vein and the atrial septal puncture site. It is then removed and the Inoue balloon catheter is inserted over the guidewire and placed in the left atrium. Following partial inflation of the distal balloon to assist flotation, the balloon catheter is then manipulated across the mitral valve. In cases where gross left atrial dilatation or puncture unduly low in the inter-atrial septum make this difficult, the catheter may be looped within the left atrium with the assistance of the guidewire – the so-called 'Kawasaki manoeuvre', thereby allowing more direct access to the valve orifice. Once across the valve, the distal balloon is then inflated, moved back and forth inside the left ventricle to ensure that it is mobile and not entangled between the mitral valve chordae, and then pulled back against the mitral valve until resistance is felt and immediately fully inflated. It is then deflated at once (maximal occlusion time 5 seconds) and the catheter allowed to retreat into the left atrium. The degree of success may then be estimated, either by measurement of the pressure gradient or immediate echocardiographic assessment, and serial inflations using stepwise increases in balloon diameter undertaken until a satisfactory result is obtained (see below). Before terminating the procedure, a left ventricular angiogram is usually performed to determine whether any mitral regurgitation has been induced (Figures 17.4 & 17.5).

The double balloon technique requires a Brockenbrough needle, a Mullins catheter and sheath, and a dilator. Trans-septal puncture is performed as described above, the Mullins sheath advanced over the dilator into the left atrium and heparin given. A 7 F floating balloon catheter is passed through the sheath antegradely across the mitral valve and valve area determined. Once the left ventricle has been catheterised, the sheath is advanced over the floating balloon catheter, which is subsequently withdrawn. One or two precured long exchange guidewires are then positioned at the left ventricular apex, or alternatively they are manipulated across the aortic valve into the ascending aorta. The sheath is removed and the dilating balloon catheters are advanced over the wires and positioned across the stenotic mitral valve. Occasionally, pre-dilatation of the atrial septum using a 6 mm balloon may be necessary. A variety of

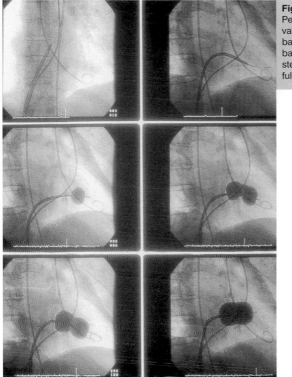

Figure 17.4:
Percutaneous balloon mitral valvuloplasty using the Inoue balloon. Note 'waisting' of the balloon as it straddles the stenosed mitral valve prior to full inflation.

dilating balloon combinations may be used: a 20 mm and 15 mm balloon, two 20 mm balloons, a Trefoil 3 × 10 mm and a 19 mm balloon or a Trefoil 3 × 12 mm and a 19 mm balloon. After 1–2 inflations (each no longer than 20 seconds to avoid prolonged hypotension and syncope), the balloon dilating catheters are removed, leaving the two wires in place, and the floating balloon catheter and Mullins sheath are replaced to allow calculation of mitral valve area. If a satisfactory result has been obtained, the floating balloon, Mullins sheath and wires are removed and mitral regurgitation assessed by left ventriculography.

There is controversy as to which of these antegrade techniques provides superior immediate and long-term results. Compared with the Inoue balloon, the double balloon technique usually results in a larger mitral valve area and a lesser degree of mitral regurgitation after valvuloplasty, particularly in patients with anatomically favourable valves. However, these differences in immediate outcome are poorly sustained, with no significant differences in survival, adverse clinical events or restenosis at long-term clinical follow-up. As indicated, the Inoue technique is now generally accepted at most major centres since it is easier to perform and has a lower risk of complications, particularly left ventricular perforation.

A third, rarely used approach is the retrograde trans-arterial technique. A long guidewire is introduced via the femoral vein and advanced trans-

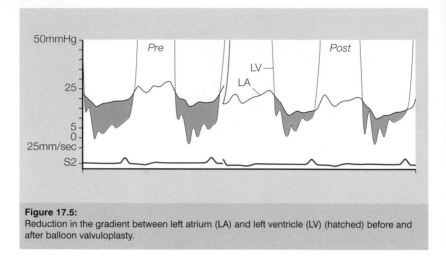

Figure 17.5:
Reduction in the gradient between left atrium (LA) and left ventricle (LV) (hatched) before and after balloon valvuloplasty.

septally through a Brockenbrough catheter into the left ventricle. The wire is snared using a retrieval catheter introduced from the femoral artery and exteriorised. The balloon dilating catheter is inserted from the femoral artery and positioned retrogradely across the mitral valve before dilatation as described above. A similar retrograde technique, which avoids the need for trans-septal puncture and creation of a left-to-right atrial shunt (with the inherent risk of a residual atrial septal defect), has also been described recently. However, although these techniques reduce the hazards associated with trans-septal catheterisation, the risks of significant arterial damage are increased.

OUTCOME

Initial results
Technical failure rates range from 1–17% and usually occur in the early stage of the operator's experience. Successful balloon mitral valvuloplasty converts severe mitral stenosis to a mild-moderate narrowing, usually providing an increase in valve area of over 100%, which results in an immediate decrease in left atrial pressure, pulmonary arterial pressure and pulmonary vascular resistance. These physiological changes are associated with a parallel improvement in the patient's clinical state, often by two or more New York Heart Association classes. These results are well maintained and encouraging 5 and 7-year follow-up results have been reported recently.

After the procedure, the most accurate evaluation of valve area is provided by echocardiography. There is a small loss in initial gain during the first 24 hours, and assessment should therefore ideally be performed 1–2 days after valvuloplasty, when planimetry, the pressure half-time or the continuity equation can be used to calculate valve area. Two definitions of an optimal initial result are in current use: a final valve area

> 1.5 cm^2 and an increase in valve area of at least 25%, or a final valve area > 1.5 cm^2 without significant mitral regurgitation.

Predictors of outcome

Initial reports stressed the predictive value of echocardiographic anatomical assessment using echo scores to predict immediate outcome. Of these, the best known is that originally developed by Wilkins *et al.* at the Massachusetts General Hospital. Leaflet rigidity, leaflet thickening, valvular calcification, and subvalvular disease are each scored on a scale from 0 to 4 yielding a maximum total echocardiographic score of 16. A higher score would represent a heavily calcified, thickened and immobile valve with extensive thickening and calcification of the subvalvular apparatus. Among the four components of the score, valve leaflet thickening and subvalvular disease provide the best correlates for the increase in mitral valve area produced by balloon valvuloplasty. Patients with lower echocardiographic scores have a higher likelihood of a good outcome with minimal complications and a haemodynamic and clinical improvement that persists at long-term follow-up. Furthermore, in long-term follow-up studies, patients with echocardiographic scores <8 display a higher rate of survival and freedom from combined events (death, mitral valve replacement, repeat valvuloplasty and symptoms in New York Heart Association class III or IV). Conversely, patients with higher scores have a relatively poor outcome. In particular, rigid thickened valves, extensive subvalvular fibrosis and valve calcification herald a suboptimal result.

However, these echocardiographic scores do not predict the outcome of balloon mitral valvuloplasty with complete reliability. Limitations of echo classification include the difficulties of reproducibility, underestimation of lesion severity, and the fact that the use of scores takes no account of localised changes in specific portions of the valve apparatus, particularly in the commissural area. Reflecting these limitations, recent publications have been less enthusiastic and found a poor correlation between echo scores and the initial increase in valve area. Furthermore, anatomical prediction of the development of severe mitral regurgitation following the procedure is even less reliable. It is now generally accepted that other factors influence immediate outcome, including the age, sex and size of the patient, the presence of mitral valve calcification, pre-existent mitral regurgitation, atrial fibrillation, left atrial dilatation or pulmonary hypertension, a small initial valve area, balloon size and a history of previous surgical commissurotomy. These parameters should therefore also be taken into consideration (Table 17.3)

Outcome following mitral balloon valvuloplasty in elderly patients is generally inferior compared with the younger population, particularly since other adverse factors such as valve calcification and atrial fibrillation are frequently present. Nevertheless, the procedure has an established useful role in carefully selected patients. Independent predictors of success in the elderly include a lower echocardiographic score, lower New York

TABLE 17.3 – FACTORS PREDICTING OUTCOME AFTER BALLOON MITRAL VALVULOPLASTY

- Age and sex
- Body size
- Valve anatomy
- Mitral valve calcification
- Pre-existent mitral regurgitation
- Previous surgical commissurotomy
- Small initial valve area
- Left atrial size
- Sinus rhythm
- Pulmonary arterial pressure
- Balloon size

Heart Association functional class and a larger mitral valve area prior to valvuloplasty. A low echocardiographic score, particularly the absence of valve calcification, is the strongest predictor of event-free survival.

Patients with heavily calcified valves, either on fluoroscopy or echocardiography, have a worse immediate outcome, as reflected in a smaller increase in valve area after balloon valvuloplasty and inferior long-term, event-free survival. These outcomes correlate closely with the degree of calcification. Similar findings have also been reported in long-term follow-up studies after surgical commissurotomy. Further studies are needed to refine the indications for balloon valvuloplasty in this frequently encountered, heterogeneous group of patients. Current strategy recommends surgery in patients with massive or bicommissural calcification, whereas balloon valvuloplasty can be attempted as an initial therapeutic approach in patients with mild or unicommissural calcification, particularly when other clinical factors are favourable. Traumatic mitral regurgitation requiring surgery is a more frequent complication of balloon valvuloplasty in this group. Patients with valve calcification who undergo uncomplicated balloon dilatation require careful appraisal and follow up – those with poor early results or subsequent clinical deterioration should be considered for surgery.

Many patients in atrial fibrillation have other factors associated with an inferior result, i.e. advanced age, unsuitable valve anatomy and a history of previous surgical commissurotomy. Nevertheless, it seems that atrial fibrillation predicts a poor outcome after balloon valvuloplasty, i.e. a smaller initial increase in mitral valve area after valvuloplasty and inferior event-free survival.

Restenosis

The incidence of restenosis following successful balloon valvuloplasty, (defined as a loss greater than 50% of the initial gain, with a valve area <1.5cm^2), is usually low (approximately 20% over 4 years in one recent series). Repeat balloon valvuloplasty has been successfully performed for restenosis in a small number of patients and may represent an attractive treatment option in cases of symptomatic restenosis occurring several years following the initial procedure, providing, of course, that valve anatomy remains suitable.

COMPLICATIONS

Reported mortality of balloon valvuloplasty averages 0.5% in experienced hands. Although this is considerably less than the risk associated with mitral valve replacement, a fairer comparison would be with closed mitral commissurotomy, which has a very similar risk. The main causes of death are left ventricular perforation or the poor initial condition of the patient. Important complications of balloon valvuloplasty are cardiac perforation leading to tamponade, embolic stroke due to displacement of thrombus from the left atrium, severe damage to the valve leading to severe regurgitation, and residual atrial septal defect (Table 17.4).

The rate of haemopericardium varies from 0.5–7%, and usually results from trans-septal catheterisation or, more rarely, from apex perforation, either by the guidewires or the balloon itself. This complication has become relatively infrequent since the widespread use of the Inoue balloon.

Embolism is encountered in 0.5–5% of cases but is seldom the cause of permanent incapacity. It may be due to fibrino-thrombotic material (despite the absence of detectable thrombus prior to the procedure), gas, or, on rare occasions, calcium. The risk of thromboembolism can be minimised by anticoagulation for several weeks before the procedure, and scanning of the left atrium using transoesophageal echocardiography before the dilatation.

Mild mitral regurgitation is relatively common and usually seems to occur via the commissures that have been split open by the balloon dilatation. Severe mitral regurgitation results from a tear in a valve cusp and is unusual, with rates ranging from 2–19%. Effective balloon dilating area normalised for body surface area (EBDA/BSA) and valve calcification are the only established predictors of increased mitral regurgitation following balloon valvuloplasty. More recently, an echocardiographic score evaluating uneven distribution of thickness in the anterior and posterior leaflets, the degree of commissural disease, and subvalvular disease has been proposed, consistent with the longstanding clinical impression that mitral regurgitation occurs most often in patients with unfavourable anatomy, especially in those with extensive subvalvular

TABLE 17.4 – COMPLICATIONS FOLLOWING BALLOON MITRAL VALVULOPLASTY

- Cardiac perforation
- Systemic embolism
- Mitral regurgitation
- Residual atrial septal defect
- Vascular damage
- Arrhythmias

disease. Moderate–severe regurgitation may be well tolerated initially, but surgery is often necessary, usually on a scheduled basis. Valve replacement is needed in most cases because of the severity of the underlying valve disease, but conservative surgery, combining suture of the valve tear and commissurotomy may be possible in cases with less severe valve deformity if appropriate surgical expertise is available. Promising results using this approach have been recently reported by Acar in Paris (Fig. 17.6).

The frequency of residual atrial septal defect varies from 10–20%, as assessed by oximetry, and from 60–90% by colour flow doppler. The associated shunts are nearly always small and without clinical consequence. Some data suggest that the incidence of significant left-to-right atrial shunting is higher in patients with anatomically unsuitable valves. The vast majority (45–80%) close spontaneously. Persistence is related to size (>0.5 cm diameter), unsatisfactory relief of valve obstruction meaning that left atrial pressure remains high, or to the development of restenosis.

Other complications, including arrhythmias and vascular damage, are rare.

Urgent surgery (i.e. within 24 hours) is rarely needed (<1%) for complications of mitral balloon valvuloplasty. It may occasionally be required for massive haemopericardium or less frequently for severe mitral regurgitation which is poorly tolerated. Overall, the procedure is of low risk when performed by experienced operators on properly selected patients.

COMPARISONS WITH SURGICAL COMMISSUROTOMY

Balloon valvuloplasty may achieve an increase in mitral valve area comparable with that obtained using the established surgical techniques of open and closed mitral commissurotomy. Furthermore, the technique overcomes the need for thoracotomy, general anaesthesia and cardiopulmonary bypass, and requires a short hospital stay and brief

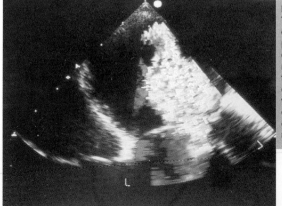

Figure 17.6: Transoesophageal echocardiogram (horizontal plane, four chamber view) demonstrating severe mitral regurgitation secondary to a tear in the anterior leaflet complicating balloon valvuloplasty. This patient developed acute pulmonary oedema and required urgent mitral valve replacement.

convalescence. Most patients return to normal activities within a day or two of the procedure. Such advantages are meaningless, however, unless the dilatation procedure and conventional surgery have comparable safety and efficacy.

Interpretation of long-term follow-up studies of patients undergoing balloon mitral valvuloplasty and their comparison with surgical series are confounded by heterogeneity in the patient populations studied. In patients with optimal mitral valve morphology, surgical commissurotomy has favourable long-term haemodynamic and symptomatic results. However, as observed following balloon valvuloplasty, elderly patients and those with calcified valves or atrial fibrillation do less well.

Several recent randomised studies from developing countries have compared the techniques of balloon valvuloplasty and surgical commissurotomy. The two methods appear to be comparable in safety and give similar immediate and mid-term clinical and haemodynamic improvement. However, a valid comparison remains difficult since (i) these series are few and concern relatively small numbers of patients; (ii) the duration of follow-up after balloon valvuloplasty is still insufficient, given that deteriorating valve function following surgical commissurotomy is most commonly seen after a period of 8–10 years; and (iii) the patients in these series were nearly always young with favourable mitral valve morphology.

Although long-term follow-up studies will continue to define the precise role of balloon valvuloplasty, these initial randomised controlled trials comparing the technique with surgical commissurotomy are encouraging and support the percutaneous approach for the treatment of patients with rheumatic mitral stenosis who have suitable valve anatomy. Given its practical advantages, balloon valvuloplasty should be considered in all patients with mitral stenosis who are symptomatic despite medical treatment.

CONCLUSIONS

Balloon valvuloplasty is now firmly established as the procedure of choice for the treatment of patients with rheumatic mitral stenosis whose valves are anatomically suitable for balloon dilatation, and in patients where surgery is contraindicated or represents too high a risk. The best results are obtained when the valve shows definite commissural fusion, is pliable, has little or no disease of the subvalvular apparatus and is not heavily calcified. Despite these ideal criteria, good palliation may also be obtained by dilating quite heavily calcified valves in patients who are unfit for surgery. Good results have also been reported in the elderly. The procedure results in a significant decrease in the mitral gradient and an increase in mitral valve area in the majority of patients with minimal mortality and morbidity. These haemodynamic changes are usually associated with a marked immediate clinical improvement which persists at medium and long-term follow-up. Although immediate and long-term results are comparable with established surgical procedures, it is important to consider percutaneous and surgical approaches as complementary techniques in the management of patients with mitral stenosis, each applicable at the appropriate stage of the disease.

FURTHER READING

Inoue K, Okawi T, Nakamura T et al. Clinical application of transvenous mitral commissurotomy by a new balloon catheter. J Thorac Cardiovasc Surg 1984;87:394–402.

Iung B, Cormier B, Ducimetière P et al. Immediate results of percutaneous mitral commissurotomy. A predictive model on a series of 1514 patients. Circulation 1996a;94:2124–30.

Iung B, Cormier B, Ducimetière P et al. Functional results 5 years after successful percutaneous mitral commissurotomy in a series of 528 patients and analysis of predictive factors. J Am Coll Cardiol 1996b;27:407–14.

Iung B, Cormier B, Elias J et al. Usefulness of percutaneous balloon commissurotomy for mitral stenosis during pregnancy. Am J Cardiol 1994;73:398–400.

Jang IK, Block PC, Newell JB et al. Percutaneous mitral balloon valvotomy for recurrent mitral stenosis after surgical commissurotomy. Am J Cardiol 1995;75:601–5.

Lau KW, Hung JS, Ding ZP et al. Controversies in balloon mitral valvuloplasty: the when (timing for intervention), what (choice of valve), and how (choice of technique). Cathet Cardiovasc Diagn 1995;35:91–100.

Palacios IF. Farewell to surgical mitral commissurotomy for many patients. Circulation 1998;97:223–6.

Palacios IF, Tuczu ME, Weyman AE et al. Clinical follow-up of patients undergoing percutaneous mitral balloon valvotomy. Circulation 1995;91:671–6.

The National Heart, Lung and Blood Institute Balloon Valvuloplasty Registry Participants. Multicenter experience with balloon mitral commissurotomy: NHLBI balloon valvuloplasty registry report on immediate and 30-day follow-up results. Circulation 1992;85:448–61.

Tuzcu EM, Block PC, Griffin B et al. Percutaneous mitral balloon valvotomy in patients with calcific mitral stenosis: immediate and long-term outcome. J Am Coll Cardiol 1994;23:1604–9.

Tuzcu EM, Block PC, Griffin BP et al. Immediate and long-term outcome of percutaneous mitral valvotomy in patients 65 years and older. Circulation 1992;85:963–71.

Wilkins GT, Weyman AE, Abascal VM et al. Percutaneous balloon dilatation of the mitral valve: an analysis of echocardiographic variables related to outcome and the mechanism of dilatation. Br Heart J 1988;60:299–308.

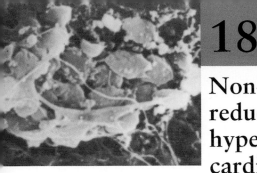

18

Non-surgical septal reduction in hypertrophic cardiomyopathy

ROD STABLES AND ULRICH SIGWART

KEY POINTS

- Non-surgical septal reduction (NSSR) is a promising new therapy for the treatment of classical hypertrophic obstructive cardiomyopathy (HOCM).

- Patients should have symptoms related to a significant left ventricular outflow tract (LVOT) gradient that have proven resistant to conventional medical therapy.

- The procedure involves the selective injection of absolute alcohol into the hypertrophied basal septum via the epicardial coronary vessels.

- This results in localised infarction with septal thinning and other changes that tend to reduce the LVOT gradient.

- The procedure is well tolerated with low mortality. The principal complication is the development of heart block which demands pacemaker implantation in around 20% of patients.

- Haemodynamic and functional improvement can take some time to become evident and may continue to improve for several months after the procedure.

- Emerging medium term follow-up data suggest that the benefits are sustained with no late morbidity.

- The long-term outcome of the procedure is not known and its value has never been compared with other therapeutic options in randomised controlled trials.

INTRODUCTION

Hypertrophic cardiomyopathy (HCM) is a genetic disease characterised by hypertrophy of the left ventricle (LV), with markedly variable haemodynamic consequences and clinical manifestations.

In a subset of patients, the site and extent of cardiac hypertrophy results in obstruction to left ventricular outflow tract (LVOT). This may be present at rest but, in others, significant obstruction occurs only under conditions that tend to reduce ventricular pre-load (dehydration, sudden adoption of the upright posture and the Valsalva manoeuvre) or increase ventricular after-load, particularly exercise.

In the classic form of hypertrophic obstructive cardiomyopathy (HOCM), patients manifest asymmetric septal hypertrophy (ASH), systolic anterior motion (SAM) of the anterior leaflet of the mitral valve and, in most cases, mitral regurgitation (Fig. 18.1). The inward movement of the hypertrophied septum during systole further narrows the LV outflow tract resulting in high LVOT blood velocities that pull the mitral valve leaflet toward the interventricular septum (Venturi effect). The SAM

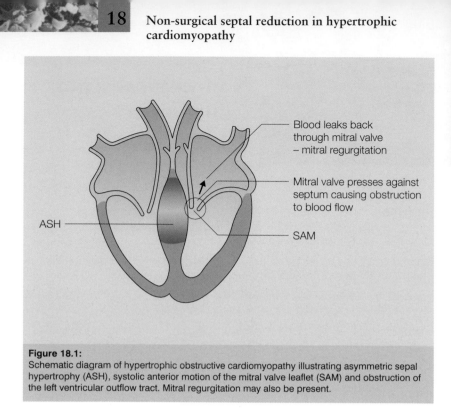

Blood leaks back through mitral valve – mitral regurgitation

Mitral valve presses against septum causing obstruction to blood flow

ASH

SAM

Figure 18.1:
Schematic diagram of hypertrophic obstructive cardiomyopathy illustrating asymmetric sepal hypertrophy (ASH), systolic anterior motion of the mitral valve leaflet (SAM) and obstruction of the left ventricular outflow tract. Mitral regurgitation may also be present.

of the mitral valve with valve–septal contact is, in many patients, the most important determinant of the severity of LV outflow obstruction and the cause of the mitral regurgitation.

A number of variants of obstructive HCM have been characterised.

■ Mid cavity obstructive hypertrophic cardiomyopathy – due to the systolic apposition of hypertrophied papillary muscle and LV wall at the level of the mid-LV, producing two distinct LV chambers.

■ Complex obstructive HCM – consists of obstruction at the level of both the papillary muscle (mid-LV cavity) and the aortic valve leaflets.

■ Obstructive HCM in the elderly – associated with calcification of the mitral valve annulus and anterior displacement of the mitral valve.

Although patients with these variants may manifest high LVOT gradients and limiting symptoms, current experience with the non-surgical septal reduction is restricted to the classical form of HOCM.

TREATMENT OPTIONS IN CLASSICAL HOCM

Many patients with HOCM eventually develop one or more of the following symptoms: dyspnoea, chest pain, syncope, palpitations, and fatigue. Symptoms are variable and not exclusively related to left ventricular outflow tract obstruction – with which there is a poor correlation. Other mechanisms include:

■ Impaired myocardial function in the absence of obstruction.

■ Arrhythmia or conduction delay.

■ Impaired filling due to diastolic dysfunction.

Drug therapy with beta blockers or other negative inotropes can be effective, but a number of patients are intolerant of these agents or remain symptomatic despite treatment. Right ventricular contraction immediately following atrial systole reduces LV outflow tract gradients without adversely affecting systemic arterial pressure. This observation provided the rationale for the evaluation of dual chamber (DDD) pacing for the treatment of HOCM. Randomised controlled trials (RCT) have demonstrated only very limited haemodynamic and clinical improvement with DDD pacing and the inability to predict response in an individual patient means that this is rarely used as routine therapy.[1]

Patients with resistant symptoms have traditionally been considered as candidates for cardiac surgery. Left ventricular myectomy, performed in the septal area and sometimes combined with mitral valve replacement, eliminates or improves symptoms in most patients and significantly reduces LV outflow tract pressure gradients. The long-term efficacy of this procedure has been demonstrated in a number of reports though there is an associated procedural mortality of around 5% and considerable morbidity including complete heart block, ventricular septal defect formation and cerebrovascular accident.[2,3]

NON-SURGICAL SEPTAL REDUCTION

Percutaneous methods of septal reduction have been developed as an alternative to open surgical therapy. A number of terms have been used to describe these procedures including 'percutaneous transluminal septal myocardial ablation (PTSMA)', 'the Sigwart procedure', 'alcohol septal ablation' and 'transcoronary ablation of septal hypertrophy' (TASH).[4–6] We prefer the more generic description 'non-surgical septal reduction' (NSSR) that encompasses the variety of techniques that can be employed in this setting.

Initial observations in this field had demonstrated that transient occlusion of a septal artery with an angioplasty balloon resulted in a reduction in the LVOT gradient. In 1994 Ulrich Sigwart extended this approach, introducing a small volume of absolute ethanol by selective injection into a septal vessel to create an area of localised myocardial infarction in the area of the left ventricular outflow tract.[7] This technique has been adopted by a number of groups worldwide and several hundred procedures have now been performed. As with all new interventions there has been a process of rapid evolution in patient selection and operative technique. This chapter describes our current approach and identifies aspects that are the subject of ongoing evaluation.

PATIENT SELECTION AND INITIAL INVESTIGATION

Subjects should exhibit symptoms despite medical therapy or have proven intolerant of drug agents. Patients with previous surgical myectomy or DDD pacemaker implantation can be treated.

Echocardiography confirms the anatomical diagnosis. Magnetic resonance imaging provides comprehensive diagnostic information in almost all patients and may be an alternative when echocardiography is suboptimal. The patient should manifest classical HOCM with SAM as described in the introduction. Although we have performed a small number of procedures in patients with the mid-cavity obliteration variation of HOCM, experience in this clinical setting is limited.

Doppler examination can be used to measure the LVOT gradient at rest and under conditions of exercise or pharmacological stress. A resting gradient of > 50 mmHg or a stress gradient of > 100 mmHg are commonly used thresholds for intervention though highly symptomatic patients with less significant findings may benefit from the procedure. Exercise testing is safe in HOCM and for research purposes we document exercise capacity with measurement of maximal oxygen uptake.

Diagnostic cardiac catheterisation provides important information. Left ventriculography can demonstrate LV outflow obstruction, SAM, and mitral regurgitation. Coronary angiography is performed to exclude co-existing significant coronary disease and to identify the probable anatomy of blood supply to the septum

We measure the LV outflow tract pressure gradient with simultaneous recordings from a Brockenbrough catheter in the left ventricle (placed via a trans-septal approach) and a coronary angioplasty guide catheter in the ascending aorta. Other units use bilateral femoral artery puncture for retrograde cannulation of the LV cavity and aorta with separate catheters. It is best to employ an end-hole catheter in the LV since the level of obstruction can be very localised. The pressure gradient may also be measured with a double lumen catheter or by withdrawing an end-hole catheter slowly from the apex of the LV to the ascending aorta (Fig. 18.2). These methods do not allow continuous examination of changes in the gradient over the course of the procedure.

Manoeuvres designed to detect provoked obstruction are indicated when the gradient at baseline is less than 30–50 mmHg. The stimulation of ventricular premature beats may reveal a gradient in the post extra-systolic cycles. Ectopics can be induced with manipulation of the ventricular catheter or using a single paced beat from a temporary wire. The most reliable method of gradient provocation is to use a slow infusion of isoprenolol at an initial rate of 1 μg/min. The rate is then increased until the heart rate reaches 100–110 beats per minute or the LV outflow pressure gradient reaches diagnostic values. Operators should note that there is often a delayed heart rate response with a lag time of up to a minute and close control of the infusion is essential.

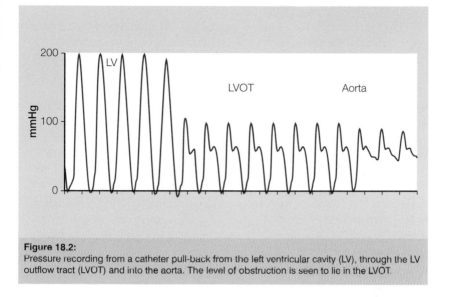

Figure 18.2:
Pressure recording from a catheter pull-back from the left ventricular cavity (LV), through the LV outflow tract (LVOT) and into the aorta. The level of obstruction is seen to lie in the LVOT.

A significant systolic pressure gradient often develops between the ascending aorta and femoral artery during isoprenolol infusion, particularly in young patients. This may give rise to an exaggerated estimation of the provoked LV outflow obstruction if pressures are recorded from the femoral sheath.

PERFORMANCE OF THE NON-SURGICAL SEPTAL REDUCTION PROCEDURE

Preparation

The procedure is performed under local anaesthetic with light pre-medication (e.g. temezapam 10–20 mg). An intravenous cannula should be placed in a peripheral vein. The right groin is prepared in the usual manner and venous and arterial sheathes placed. The first venous sheath is used to introduce a temporary pacing electrode to the apex of the right ventricle. This is essential, as heart block (usually transient) is very common following alcohol injection. In our unit a second venous sheath is used for the trans-septal puncture (TSP) equipment. An alternative strategy is to perform an arterial puncture (perhaps at the left groin) and use this to position an end-hole catheter at the apex of the LV.

The third and final sheath is placed in the femoral artery and is used to introduce the left coronary guide catheter. This can be selected from routine stock and sized for optimal access to the left coronary system. We favour the Judkins left short tip, but patient anatomy and local preference will influence the choice. After the TSP has been performed, systemic anti-coagulation is induced with a bolus of heparin (7.5–10 thousand units as dictated by body weight) and diagnostic evaluation of the LVOT gradient performed (see above).

Identification of the target vessel

Angiographic images are acquired to identify the anatomy of blood supply to the septum. The vessel pattern is variable and can be confusing. Multiple angiographic projections may be required to distinguish septal and diagonal vessels (Fig. 18.3). The ideal target vessel is a proximal septal of diameter 1.0–2.0 mm. If more than one potential target is identified then additional techniques (described below) are required to identify the most suitable vessel. These methods, using intra-coronary echo contrast agents, are also of value in the very rare circumstances when the blood supply to the proximal septum is derived from the circumflex or an intermediate coronary trunk.[8]

An angioplasty guidewire is introduced into the selected septal vessel. A flexible, low trauma wire is the first choice though some times a stiffer shaft (intermediate or standard) may be needed to ensure balloon access to a septal arising at an acute angle from the main left anterior descending (LAD) vessel. An over the wire (OTW) angioplasty balloon catheter is advanced over the wire and positioned in the proximal part of the septal vessel. Any semi-compliant, OTW balloon system is acceptable, but it is best if the balloon is of short length (maximum 10 mm). Longer devices mean that the alcohol is be delivered into a more distal portion of the target vessel, limiting its myocardial distribution, particularly if the balloon tip lies distal to a branch in the septal vessel. If the septal has an early bifurcation, each distal branch can be approached as if it were an individual vessel.

The balloon diameter should be sized to ensure complete occlusion of the septal at low or nominal inflation pressure. A two-marker balloon

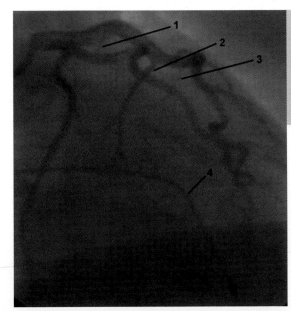

Figure 18.3:
Selective coronary injection of the left coronary system in a right anterior angiographic projection. Potential target septal vessels are identified (1, 2, 3). A temporary pacing wire has been placed in the apex of the right ventricle (4).

allows more precise positioning. The entire length of the balloon must be within the septal to eliminate the possibility of LAD barotrauma or the balloon 'melon-pipping' back into the LAD vessel (Fig. 18.4). Sometimes balloon occlusion of the vessel reduces the resting gradient. This is a very favourable sign that an appropriate target septal vessel has been identified but the positive and negative predictive value of this observation is limited and does not obviate the desirability of a contrast echo study (see below).

With the balloon inflated, two injections of radiographic contrast are performed. In the first of these a standard, selective left coronary injection through the guide catheter demonstrates that the target septal vessel is sealed to the antegrade flow of dye and hence, by presumption, any subsequent retrograde leak of alcohol. In the second injection, contrast is introduced through the central lumen of the OTW balloon into the target vessel (Fig. 18.5). This is to ensure that there is no major collateralistion

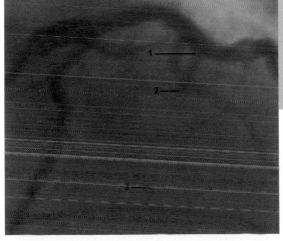

Figure 18.4:
An over the wire angioplasty balloon is inflated in the proximal portion of the septal vessel. The margins of the balloon are illustrated (1, 2). An angioplasty guidewire marks the course of the septal vessel (3).

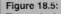

Figure 18.5:
The angioplasty balloon is inflated in the proximal portion of the septal vessel. An injection of radiographic contrast has been made through the central lumen of the over the wire balloon. The contrast distribution in the septal vessel and its branches is clearly seen (2).

that takes dye (and hence in due course alcohol) to the LAD or other major epicardial vessel. The ideal image seen at this stage is a septal myocardial blush.

Additional anatomical confirmation is provided with a myocardial echo contrast study. Trans-thoracic images in the para-sternal long axis or apical four chamber views are used with recording for immediate play-back analysis. An echo contrast agent is injected through the central lumen of the OTW balloon. (Suitable agents include Levovist™ manufactured by Schering or Optison, though the latter has a very short dwell time in the myocardium) The region of myocardial distribution is then visible as a bright area on the echo images. The ideal target region is the hypertrophied muscle at the point where the SAM of the mitral valve touches the septum. If the septal vessel selected is too distal then contrast illuminates the septal muscle in mid cavity or near the apex. Contrast appearance in the left or right ventricular free walls identifies that the target vessel is a diagonal branch rather than a septal.

Alcohol injection

After final angiographic confirmation of balloon positioning and septal occlusion a small volume of absolute alcohol is injected through the OTW system. The dose depends on the size of the septal and the extent of the myocardial run-off. There has been a trend towards the use of reduced alcohol doses and typical injection volumes now lie in the range 0.5–1.5 ml. We favour the use of a single bolus injection rather than a slow infusion. We believe that this will promote dispersion in the perfusion bed without the risk of selective distribution caused by small vessel thrombus and occlusion in the early phase of the injection. The alcohol should be followed by 1–2 ml of saline to clear the dead space of the OTW balloon.

The patient will get immediate pain and should be warned to expect this symptom. If required, diamorphine can be administered before the injection, but we do not do this as a routine as the pain eases after 30–45 seconds and is rarely severe. ST segment change and ventricular ectopic activity are routine. Transient heart block is common but the heart rate is supported by the temporary pacemaker, which is set to initiate capture if the native rate falls below 40 beats per minute.

The balloon is kept inflated for 5–7 minutes after alcohol injection. After this time the guidewire can be re-introduced into the distal septal though this is not essential. Deflation of the balloon and withdrawal into the guide catheter should be performed in a rapid and positive fashion to limit the possibility of any residual alcohol entering the LAD circulation.

It is possible to repeat this process with a second, third or even fourth septal vessel. Multiple vessel injection was our norm in the early series and may still be indicated in cases when the septal territory is supplied by a leash of small vessels or two proximal septal perforators. Other groups have adopted a policy of single vessel injection with the option to perform a subsequent staged procedure on a second vessel if the patient does not demonstrate a good clinical response at medium term follow-up.

Repeat diagnostic evaluation

A coronary angiogram usually reveals occlusion of the target septal with a no re-flow appearance. A repeat resting or stress gradient study can be performed, often with gratifying results though, as discussed below, myocardial remodelling and hence the full benefits of the intervention may take many months to become apparent.

EFFICACY AND COMPLICATIONS

Like all new surgical and interventional procedures NSSR has undergone a period of rapid evolution and refinement. Coincident with this a number of operators and centres have gained their initial experience with the technique. As a result it may be expected that the results from the earliest cases may be less good than in current practice. Certainly the use of myocardial contrast echocardiography has allowed more precise targeting of the alcohol injection and the trend towards the delivery of smaller alcohol volumes into fewer septal vessels has reduced the immediate procedure-related complications, particularly complete heart block.

Follow-up data has been published describing the short term results in around 200 patients and medium-term data in less than 100 cases. The longest reported follow-up period is to a mean of 30 months in 25 patients.[9] All outcome data were recently reviewed by Knight[4] who observed that the mortality rate was low (2%) both at the initial procedure and in subsequent follow-up. It must be remembered that early cases were often performed in patients with significant co-morbidity and involved more aggressive dose regimes. The current procedural mortality rate is probably well below this value.

The main complication of the procedure is the induction of permanent atrioventricular conduction block necessitating permanent pacemaker implantation. The presence of trifasicular or complete heart block persisting at 48 hours post procedure is an indication for implantation of a dual chamber pacing device. To date this has occurred in around 20% of cases though with better myocardial targeting we expect that this may fall to a value of 10%.

Some observers have been concerned that the induction of septal infarction may result in a range of adverse effects.[10] To date there have been no reports of late ventricular arrhythmia or induced ventricular septal defect. Another concern relates to the impact of the procedure on ventricular function, both systolic and diastolic. The natural history of HOCM can involve progression to a phase of poor ventricular function and this may be hastened or exacerbated by the infarction of healthy muscle. Fortunately follow-up studies have not demonstrated any trend to increasing ventricular cavity dimensions or reduced systolic performance, **241** though the current observation period is too short and involves too few patients to draw any firm conclusions in this respect.

There is little doubt that NSSR is effective in the reduction of LVOT obstruction. Echocardiographic studies have observed that the procedure results in thinning of the basal septum with reduced SAM and mitral regurgitation. Left atrial size may also be reduced. Serial follow-up has revealed that the magnitude of the gradient continues to fall as the myocardium remodels with scar formation. The benefits of the procedure may take up to 3 months to become apparent and may continue to develop over the first post-operative year. In the German series with 2–3 year follow-up, the stress LVOT gradient was reduced from a pre-procedure mean of 147 mmHg to a mean of 12 mmHg at final assessment. All patients experienced a greater than 50% reduction in gradient and there was complete elimination in over 70% of subjects.[9]

The technique also results in an improvement in left ventricular diastolic function with improved relaxation and compliance.[11] In addition there is consistent alteration of septal activation with secondary incoordination of contraction – similar to that seen with dual chamber pacing.[12] These factors could play a significant role in gradient reduction and subjective functional improvement.

The assessment of symptomatic benefit is complicated by the potential for a placebo effect. Nevertheless, follow-up reports suggest a substantial and sustained improvement of greater than one New York Heart Association functional class. Objective tests of functional capacity have also shown increases of around 40% in exercise performance at medium term follow-up.

FUTURE DIRECTIONS FOR NSSR THERAPY IN HOCM

Developments in technique, principally the use of myocardial contrast echocardiography have refined the procedure and hold the prospect of reduced complication rates. Questions concerning the selection of a single or multiple target vessels, the total alcohol dose and its rate of administration may be subject to further evaluation. We suspect that there will be an increase in the use of single vessel procedures with the option of repeat intervention if medium term maturation of the infarct area fails to bring the desired clinical benefit.

The elegance, simplicity and apparent efficacy of this procedure has led to its rapid dissemination in the cardiology community. Maron has observed that the number of NSSR procedure performed over the last few years is ten times that predicted by the historic activity of the best surgical units offering the surgical myectomy procedure.[6] NSSR is a promising therapeutic option for the management of a selected group of patients with symptomatic HOCM, resistant to medical therapy. The procedure may be best performed in specialist centres with a developed interest in the management of HOCM. All cases should be documented for inclusion in collaborative registries and other research ventures. Its long-term efficacy is yet to be evaluated and its value, compared to intensive medical therapy or traditional surgery has not been assessed in prospective randomised trials. Such studies are now indicated, but may be difficult to complete given the very disparate nature of the treatments under consideration.

REFERENCES

1. Nishimura RA, Trusty JM, Hayes DL *et al.* Dual-chamber pacing for hypertrophic cardiomyopathy: a randomized, double-blind, crossover trial. J Am Coll Cardiol 1997;29:435–41.

2. Brunner-La Schonbeck MH, Rocca HP, Vogt PR *et al.* Long-term follow-up in hypertrophic obstructive cardiomyopathy after septal myectomy. Ann Thorac Surg 1998;65:1207–14.

3. Robbins RC, Stinson EB. Long-term results of left ventricular myotomy and myectomy for obstructive hypertrophic cardiomyopathy. J Thorac Cardiovasc Surg 1996;111:586–94.

4. Knight CJ. Five years of percutaneous transluminal septal myocardial ablation. Heart 2000;83:255–6.

5. Gietzen FH, Leuner CJ, Raute-Kreinsen U *et al.* Acute and long-term results after transcoronary ablation of septal hypertrophy (TASH). Catheter interventional treatment for hypertrophic obstructive cardiomyopathy. Europ Heart J 1999;20.1342 54.

6. Maron BJ. Role of alcohol septal ablation in treatment of obstructive hypertrophic cardiomyopathy. Lancet 2000;355:425–6.

7. Sigwart U. Non-surgical myocardial reduction for hypertrophic obstructive cardiomyopathy. Lancet 1995;346:211–14.

8. Faber L, Seggewiss H, Gleichmann U. Percutaneous transluminal septal myocardial ablation in hypertrophic obstructive cardiomyopathy: results with respect to intra-procedural myocardial contrast echocardiography. Circulation 1998;98:2415–21.

9. Faber L, Meissner A, Ziemessen P *et al.* Percutaneous transluminal septal myocardial ablation in hypertrophic obstructive cardiomyopathy: long-term follow up of the first series of 25 patients. Heart 2000;83:326–31.

10. Oakley CM. Non-surgical ablation of the ventricular septum for the treatment of hypertrophic cardiomyopathy. Br Heart J 1995;74:479–80.

11. Nagueh SF, Lakkis NM, Middleton KJ *et al.* Changes in left ventricular diastolic function 6 months after nonsurgical septal reduction therapy for hypertrophic obstructive cardiomyopathy. Circulation 1999;99:344–7.

12. Henein MY, O'Sullivan CA, Ramzy IS, Sigwart U, Gibson DG. Electromechanical left ventricular behavior after nonsurgical septal reduction in patients with hypertrophic obstructive cardiomyopathy. J Am Coll Cardiol 1999;34:1117–22.

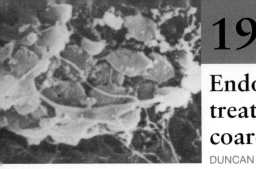

19

Endovascular treatment of aortic coarctation

DUNCAN F. ETTLES AND ANTHONY NICHOLSON

KEY POINTS

■ Localised juxtaductal coarctation often presents later in life.

■ It is commoner in males; associations include bicuspid aortic valve and ventricular septal defect.

■ Non-invasive investigation confirms diagnosis and severity.

■ Balloon angioplasty provides good long-term results with low morbidity.

■ Use of primary stenting is under evaluation.

INTRODUCTION

A spectrum of anatomical lesions exist which result in varying degrees of obstruction of the aortic arch. These abnormalities range from a localised narrowing of the aortic lumen to diffuse narrowing or even interruption of a longer segment of the aortic arch. Coarctation of the aorta is a rare condition and is often classified either according to anatomical site or age of presentation. Distinction between adult (juxtaductal) and infantile (preductal) types is often made, but can be misleading as presentation depends on the haemodynamic effects of the lesion and co-existing abnormalities. Localised juxtaductal coarctation is a discrete shelf-like narrowing of the aortic lumen related to the aortic wall opposite to the site of insertion of the ductus arteriosus and this is the commonest type seen in clinical practice. It has a male to female preponderance of around 5:1 and is associated with Turner's syndrome. Additional abnormalities occur in the majority of patients and include bicuspid aortic valve, ventricular septal defect and intra-cerebral aneurysms. The less common preductal form of coarctation affects a variable portion of the aortic arch and usually occurs in conjunction with a patent ductus arteriosus. The associated abnormalities commonly include more complex cardiac anomalies such as transposition of the great vessels and hypoplastic left heart. Management of this type of coarctation is generally much more complex because of these factors.

The remainder of this chapter will consider the approach to treatment of juxtaductal aortic coarctation.

PRESENTATION

Clinical features

The manner of presentation of juxtaductal coarctation depends on the severity of aortic obstruction. With severe coarctation in infancy, there may be left ventricular failure with systemic hypoperfusion and left to right shunting. When there is less severe aortic obstruction, compensatory left ventricular hypertrophy and collateral circulation develop and in these cases presentation is more likely in later life.

In the adult patient symptoms include claudication, cold extremities and headache, but detection of hypertension resistant to standard therapy at routine examination may be the only clue. On examination there is radiofemoral delay, reduced lower limb blood pressure and a systolic murmur. Untreated, the major risks to the patient are those of the cerebral and cardiac effects of hypertension. In addition there are increased risks of bacterial endocarditis and thoracic aortic dissection

Non-invasive investigation

The chest radiograph may show dilatation of the ascending aorta and the '3' sign in the left mediastinum which reflects pre- and post-stenotic aortic dilatation. Collateral circulation via the intercostal vessels gives rise to rib notching which develops between 4 and 12 years of age and is seen on the inferior rib surfaces. Co-exisiting features of cardiac decompensation are rarely present. The ECG confirms left ventricular hypertrophy.

Cross-sectional echocardiography can visualise the coarctation site in most patients using the suprasternal approach and continuous wave Doppler provides accurate measurements of the severity of stenosis. In addition, echocardiography is used to detect any additional cardiac abnormalities prior to invasive investigation and treatment.

Magnetic resonance imaging (MRI) is able to provide additional multiplanar views of the site of coarctation as well as the heart and mediastinum. In addition the technique can identify collateral vessels and show any undue tortuosity or kinking which would influence endovascular treatment. MRI has an important role in post-treatment follow-up.

Invasive investigation

With modern imaging methods such as MRI and duplex ultrasound it is possible in most cases to confirm the diagnosis and the severity of coarctation prior to the definitive procedure. Cardiac catheterisation may still be necessary where non-invasive imaging is inconclusive, and in centres where some modalities are unavailable.

Cardiac catheterisation and aortography may be performed solely as a diagnostic procedure or in combination with coarctation angioplasty or stenting. The left anterior oblique and lateral projections best demonstrate the site of coarctation. Angiography can usually be performed using a femoral approach, but a brachial or combined approach may be needed if severe aortic narrowing precludes easy catheter manipulation into the ascending aorta from below.

MANAGEMENT OF JUXTADUCTAL COARCTATION

Surgical treatment for aortic coarctation was introduced in the 1940s and remained the only method of treatment for the next 50 years. Surgical treatment involves the use of autologous or synthetic patch grafting or alternatively, excision of the coarctation site with end to end anastomosis. Results from early surgical series were relatively poor, but more recent work has shown effective and sustained reduction in blood pressure with low complication rates[1-4] (Table 19.1).

Over the last decade, experience has grown in the use of balloon angioplasty in coarctation and more recently evaluation of stent placement has also been reported. Considerable experience of balloon angioplasty exists in the literature and there is a wealth of available short-term and follow-up data. Long-term follow-up data are more limited. In one of the largest published series there were 43 patients with no mortality, 7% aneurysm formation rate and a 7% restenosis rate. A total of 73% of patients had normalisation of blood pressure following angioplasty.[5] The summated experience from four series describing a total of 136 patients demonstrates significant sustained reduction in blood pressure in 60–90% of cases.[5-8] The observed complications in these four studies are shown in Table 19.2.

In the management of uncomplicated juxtaductal coarctation, angioplasty offers several important advantages over surgical treatment, not least of which is the avoidance of general anaesthesia and thoracotomy. Comparing the surgical and angioplasty complication rates it is clear that mortality is lower with angioplasty and that paraplegia, one of the most disastrous complications of surgical treatment, is not reported following angioplasty. Rates of aneurysm formation at the treated site are comparable for the two modalities, but the residual stenosis rate is higher with angioplasty.

TECHNIQUE OF COARCTATION ANGIOPLASTY

The procedure is performed in the angiography suite either under general anaesthesia or neuroleptanalgesia depending on the patient. Although

TABLE 19.1 – SURGICAL COMPLICATION RATES

Mortality	2.6–3.1%
Paraplegia	0.5–1%
Aneurism	5.4%
Residual stenosis	3%

TABLE 19.2 – BALLOON ANGIOPLASTY COMPLICATION RATES

Mortality	0.7%
Aneurism	3–10%
Residual stenosis	7–26%
Aortic dissection	0–10%
Femoral arterial complications	2–7%

immediate complications are rare, cardiothoracic surgical back-up should be available on site. Following sterile preparation, the common femoral artery is punctured and a 7 F haemostatic sheath placed. In some cases the femoral pulse is impalpable and may be located prior to puncture using a hand-held Doppler probe. A shaped catheter, such as a right coronary catheter, is advanced to the level of the coarctation and using a steerable wire the obstruction is gently probed until the stenosis is crossed. The use of a hydrophilic guidewire may be necessary in some cases, but great care is needed with such wires as they are more likely to result in intimal dissection. The wire and catheter are then advanced into the ascending aorta and the steerable wire is removed and replaced by a 260 cm long stiff guidewire. The shaped catheter is then withdrawn and replaced by a 5 F marker pigtail catheter and 5000 units of heparin is given. At all times from now until completion of the procedure either the catheter or wire are always positioned across the coarctation. Simultaneous pressures are measured in the ascending aorta and at femoral level via the sheath (Fig. 19.1).

Angiography is performed in a left anterior oblique projection and using the marker catheter for calibration the diameter of the aorta immediately below the left subclavian artery is measured. A balloon catheter 2 mm less than this diameter is selected for the dilatation. With the long stiff wire in place an appropriately sized sheath is inserted into the femoral artery (usually 11 or 12 F). The large balloon catheter (commonly 18–24 mm) is advanced over the stiff wire into the coarctation site and inflated using

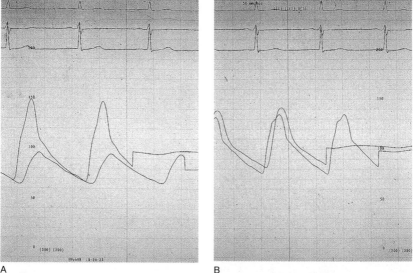

A   B

Figure 19.1:
(a) Simultaneous pressure recordings from ascending aorta and right femoral artery prior to balloon angioplasty. (b) Following PTA the gradient has been abolished.

dilute contrast. An indentation will confirm its position in the coarctation and it can then be fully inflated until the waist is abolished. The balloon is then deflated and withdrawn through the sheath. The pigtail catheter is reinserted and repeat pressure recordings made. If a gradient of 10 mmHg or less is obtained completion angiography is performed to confirm a good anatomical result and to confirm that there is no evidence of intimal tear or extravasation (Fig. 19.2). If a satisfactory result is demonstrated, the pigtail is withdrawn over the guidewire and both are removed. Removal of the sheath is followed by manual compression of at least 30 minutes to

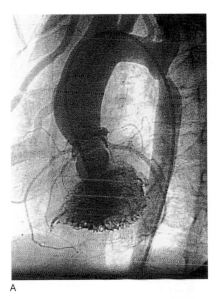

A

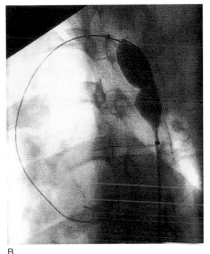

B

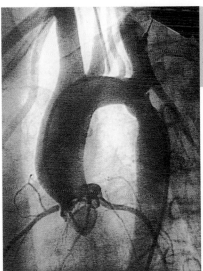

C

Figure 19.2:
(a) Pre-treatment angiogram demonstrating severe juxtaductal coarctation. (b) The balloon is inflated until the waist is abolished. (c) Post-treatment angiogram demonstrates a satisfactory result.

obtain haemostasis. It is usually only necessary to perform a single balloon inflation to obtain a satisfactory result. However, if there is a significant persisting gradient, then repeated balloon dilatation or use of a slightly larger balloon (1–2 mm) may be required.

Aftercare and follow-up

Because of the size of the introducer sheath used (11 or 12 F) the patient should be maintained on bed rest for 24 hours, lying flat for the first 6 hours. Blood pressure and ECG should be continuously monitored during this period. The patient is then mobilised and prior to discharge has Doppler echocardiographic and MRI studies as baseline for follow-up. These investigations are repeated at 1 month, 6 months and 1 year. Annual clinical follow-up is undertaken thereafter. Ambulant blood pressure monitoring is performed if the patient was taking antihypertensive medication prior to the procedure.

RESULTS AND COMPLICATIONS

High technical success with minimal complications can be expected in the treatment of native and post-operative coarctation using balloon angioplasty. Follow-up of children with native coarctation treated by balloon angioplasty shows an appreciable rate of recoarctation, which has been reported at between 39%[9] and 46%[10] in infants, the recoarctation rate being lower in older children. A lower restenosis rate of 18% is seen after angioplasty of recoarctation following previous surgical repair.[10] Recoarctation is especially common if there is associated hypoplasia of the transverse aortic arch.[11] In the authors' experience, small residual pressure gradients (less than 20 mmHg) can be detected across the coarctation site several years after treatment, but sustained reduction in systolic pressure and reduction in the need for antihypertensive drugs can be expected in all patients.

Immediate complications at the angioplasty site are extremely rare, but potentially include aortic rupture, dissection and disruption of large collateral vessels. Careful measurement of the aorta and balloon sizing are essential to minimise these risks. The risk of stroke or transient ischaemic episodes must be borne in mind during the procedure and the authors recommend early systemic heparinisation. Potential iliofemoral arterial complications such as stenosis, thrombosis and pseudoaneurysm formation relate to use of the large calibre sheaths which are required. Their reported incidence is 14%, but in the majority of cases such complications do not require surgery and can be managed by endovascular means.[9] Aneurysm formation at the site of angioplasty is reported in approximately 5% of cases at follow-up.[9] The long-term significance of aneurysms at the coarctation site is debatable. Experience with follow-up of 14 patients for a mean of 7.3 years suggests that small aneurysms at the dilatation site are likely to resolve with time and that later formation of such aneurysms does not occur.[12]

STENTING IN COARCTATION

The currently available data suggest that balloon angioplasty is safe and effective in both native and post-operative coarctation with good medium to long-term outcomes. Whether primary stenting offers a more effective strategy has yet to established. The potential use of stents in children for treatment of coarctation would necessitate a device that could be expanded sequentially with negligible damage to the overlying neointima. There is evidence from animal studies that stents can be sequentially distended without adverse consequences and this has been performed in a preliminary clinical study where a previously deployed stent was dilated to 3 mm above its initial size with good clinical and objective follow-up outcomes.[13] In the adult patient with coarctation, the use of stents seems an attractive option, but one which clearly requires fuller evaluation. Long-term stability and structural integrity of implanted stents remains an important concern particularly in this group of young and otherwise fit patients.

CONCLUSION

Balloon angioplasty is an established, safe and effective treatment for thoracic aortic coarctation in both children and adults. Various technical considerations must be made in patient selection. Further evaluation of the place of stenting in coarctation repair is required.

REFERENCES

1. Bobby JJ, Emami JM, Farmer RDT, Newman CGII. Operative survival and 40 year follow up of surgical repair of aortic coarctation. Br Heart J 1991;65:271–6.

2. Kirklin JW, Barratt-Boyes BG (eds). Cardiac surgery, Chapter 34, Part IV. Harlow: Churchill Livingstone, 1986.

3. Sabiston DC, Spencer FC (eds). Surgery of the chest, Chapter 33. Philadelphia: WB Saunders, 1990.

4. Knyshov GV, Sitar LL, Glagola MD, Atamanyuk MY. Aortic aneurysm at the site of repair of coarctation of the aorta: a review of 48 patients. Ann Thorac Surg 1996;61:935–9.

5. Fawzy ME, Sivanandam V, Galal O et al. One to ten year follow-up of balloon angioplasty of native coarctation of the aorta in adolescents and adults. J Am Coll Cardiol 1997;30(6):1542–6.

6. Schrader R, Bussmann WD, Jacobi V, Kadel C. Long-term effects of balloon coarctation angioplasty on arterial blood pressure in adolescent and adult patients. Cathet Cardiovasc Diag 1995;36:220–25.

7. Tyagi S, Arora R, Kaul UA, Sethi KK, Gambhir DS, Khalilullah M. Balloon angioplasty of native coarctation of the aorta in adolescents and young adults. Am Heart J 1992;123(3):674–80.

8. Biswas PK, Mitra K, De S *et al*. Follow-up results of balloon angioplasty for native coarctation of aorta. Ind Heart J 1996;48:673–6.

9. Rao PS, Galal O, Smith PA, Wilson AD. Five to nine year follow-up of balloon angioplasty of native aortic coarctation in infants and children. J Am Coll Cardiol 1996;27(2):462–70.

10. Ino T, Nishimoto K, Kato H *et al*. Balloon angioplasty for aortic coarctation – report of a questionnaire survey by the Japanese Pediatric Interventional Cardiology Committee. Jap Circ J 1997;61:375–83.

11. Yetman AT, Nykanen D, McCrindle BW *et al*. Balloon angioplasty of recurrent coarctation: a 12 year review. J Am Coll Cardiol 1997;30(3):811–6.

12. Dyet JF, Paddon AJ, Ettles DF, Nicholson AA. Long-term follow-up of balloon angioplasty for native adult aortic coarctation. Cardiovasc Interv Rad 1998;21(Suppl. 1):S145.

13. Ebeid MR, Prieto LR, Latson LA. Use of balloon expandable stents for coarctation of the aorta: initial results and intermediate term follow-up. J Am Coll Cardiol 1997;30:1847–52.

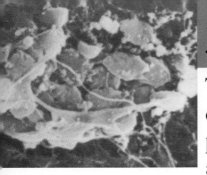

20

Transcatheter occlusion of the patent arterial duct and atrial septal defect

ERIC ROSENTHAL

KEY POINTS

- Transcatheter occlusion of the patent arterial duct is now the method of choice in all except small infants and neonates.

- Atrial septal defect closure is possible in about 60% of secundum defects.

- The patent foramen ovale can be closed to prevent paradoxical embolism but the indications are unclear.

- These procedures may be technically demanding and require a range of closure devices to be available. It is essential to have retrieval equipment in the event of device embolisation.

- Patients are usually discharged the following day.

Surgical ligation of a patent arterial duct was first performed successfully by Gross in 1939 and patch closure of an atrial septal defect by Gibbons in 1953 using cardiopulmonary bypass. With the advent of percutaneous transcatheter occlusion, surgery and its associated risks and complications can be avoided and the hospital stay considerably reduced (most patients being discharged the following day).

OCCLUSION OF THE PATENT ARTERIAL DUCT (PDA)

Transcatheter occlusion of a patent arterial duct was first reported by Porstmann in 1966 using a compressed Ivalon plug.[1] The Ivalon plug was chosen according to the angiographic size of the arterial duct and the device was passed up a large bore femoral arterial sheath into the duct. The 10–14 F sheaths precluded use in small children (who have the highest incidence of a patent arterial duct) and the technique was not used widely. The Rashkind double umbrella device, introduced in 1984, gained wide acceptance and use in many European centres and rapidly became the method of choice for duct closure.[2,3] This device is now no longer used but the occluding and implanting principles remain in use for transcatheter occlusion of both patent arterial ducts and atrial septal defects.

Rashkind double umbrella

The Rashkind occluding device consisted of two thin discs of polyurethane foam (12 or 17 mm in diameter) fixed onto a folding double umbrella-like frame with a narrow central connecting body. After initial aortic angiography to define the anatomy and size of the duct, a long 8 F or 11 F sheath was passed from a femoral vein across the duct into the descending aorta. The device was advanced through the sheath so that only the distal umbrella opened in the aorta. The sheath and device were then withdrawn into the duct until the distal umbrella was impacted into the aortic ampulla. The sheath alone was withdrawn further to expose the proximal umbrella which opened in the pulmonary artery to straddle the duct. Aortic angiography was used to confirm device position prior to release. The device was then detached from the delivery wire. Embolisation to the pulmonary artery or distal aorta was uncommon, and virtually all devices could be retrieved with intravascular snaring tools.

A residual leak was commonly present immediately after the procedure, but in most patients the duct occluded by 6 months as the device was covered by endothelium. In those not occluded by 6 months, there was a further incidence of closure over the next few years. Implantation of a second device was undertaken if a large leak persisted.[4] After implantation of one or two devices the occlusion rate was over 90%, a figure similar to that obtained with surgical closure.[5]

The Rashkind device could not be used in very large ducts (greater than 8 mm) as stability could not be guaranteed. In very small infants (weighing less than 8 kg) the 11 F sheath was too big for the femoral and iliac veins, though a modified loading technique allowed passage of the 17-mm device through an 8 F sheath. In these infants, there was a risk of left pulmonary artery obstruction by the device.

Coil occlusion

These drawbacks and the occlusion rate of only 90% led to introduction of further devices. Various types of coil including the standard Gianturco stainless steel spring coil were found effective in small ducts.[6,7] A transarterial or less commonly transvenous approach using 4 F sheaths was used to deploy 1 or 2 loops of the coil distal to the duct and then the catheter was withdrawn to deploy the remainder (Fig. 20.1). Embolised coils were retrieved with snaring catheters. The development of controlled release PDA coils (3–8 mm in diameter) reduced the incidence of embolisation and multiple coils could be placed in moderate size ducts (initial coil diameter usually twice the minimum duct diameter) with occlusion rates approaching 99%.[8] Recanalisation occurred infrequently during the first year after implantation.[9] Another major advantage to coils was the substantial reduction in cost (approximately 1/20th the cost of an umbrella).

Cardioseal and Amplatzer

For larger ducts the Cardioseal device – a modification of the Rashkind-occluder for atrial septal defect occlusion with device diameters of 17 to 33 mm – and the Amplatzer device – a modification of that designed for atrial septal defect occlusion (see later) – came into use. Like the Rashkind umbrella they are deployed from a venous approach: extruding first the distal 'disc' and then withdrawing the sheath to deploy the remainder of the device.[10]

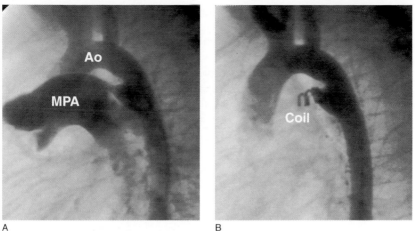

Figure 20.1:
Implantation of a single 5 mm PDA controlled release coil in a moderate arterial duct. (a) Before implantation. Ao: aorta; MPA: main pulmonary artery. (b) After implantation demonstrates complete occlusion.

Advantages over surgical ligation

■ Avoidance of thoracotomy and hence avoidance of:
  – Scar
  – Bleeding
  – Risk of recurrent laryngeal nerve palsy
■ Shorter hospital stay

Disadvantages of transcatheter occlusion

■ Not possible (yet) in premature neonates and infants.
■ Left pulmonary artery obstruction in small children with large devices.
■ Femoral vessel haemorrhage or occlusion.
■ Device embolisation is usually managed successfully by transcatheter retrieval.

Indications for duct occlusion

It is commonly accepted that all patent arterial ducts of 'haemodynamic' importance require closure to prevent eventual deterioration in function of the left ventricle. By definition this would include ducts causing volume overload to the left ventricle as judged either clinically, radiographically or by echocardiography. The second group in whom there is little argument for recommending closure is the patient with an audible continuous murmur but no clinical or other evidence of a large shunt. The rationale for closure in these patients is that there is a continuing risk of bacterial endocarditis with dental procedures (and less commonly after no apparent invasive event) which can be eliminated by successful closure of the duct. Once the duct has been demonstrated to be occluded for 6 months then antibiotic prophylaxis can be dispensed with.

Controversies

Silent patent arterial duct

A third group of patients with a patent arterial duct generates the most discussion. These are the patients in whom the duct is 'silent' and was detected at incidental echocardiography. The increased use of echocardiography with colour flow mapping enables even the smallest of ducts to be detected – indeed some are so small that at catheterisation it is not even possible to cross with a 0.014–0.018 inch guidewire. Many of these patients undergo echocardiography for evaluation of a soft systolic murmur which is clinically innocent. The discovery of a tiny patent arterial duct then raises issues of endocarditis prohylaxis and closure of the duct. Opinion is divided between those who close all ducts (is it always 'silent'?, endocarditis has been reported on a 'silent' duct in one case,[11] unexplained endocarditis may have had a 'silent' duct as the substrate) and those who only close ducts that are clinically detectable ('silent' duct endocarditis is vanishingly rare, the incidence of patent ducts is low in adults so many of these detected in childhood close spontaneously, the risk of the procedure outweighs any theoretical risk of endocarditis). There are yet others who do not recommend closure for 'silent' ducts but who still recommend antibiotic prophylaxis. The ease of closure of small ducts with a single coil has swayed many towards eliminating the duct and any of these concerns.

Residual leak after device closure

While in the era of duct ligation it was assumed that ligated ducts were all closed, it is now apparent, using colour flow doppler, that there is a significant patency rate.[5] In these the surgical constriction serves as a perfect point for coil deposition and occlusion. It is notable however that post duct ligation endocarditis does not seem to have been a well recognised problem. Patency after device implantation is perhaps more worrying as there may be device material that is not fully endothelialised at the site of turbulence. These leaks are usually only detectable using colour flow doppler and as with post-ligation duct leaks, the significance is uncertain. While device endocarditis has been reported rarely as a result of the procedure it does not seem to occur as a late event.[12] Prophylaxis against endocarditis is however, usually advised until complete closure. There is therefore a tendency to complete duct occlusion at a second procedure if the duct remains patent after a year or two.[4]

OCCLUSION OF SECUNDUM ATRIAL SEPTAL DEFECTS

Transcatheter atrial septal defect occlusion was first attempted in 1976 by King and Mills,[13] but reliable occlusion devices have only recently become available. The first device to be used with some success was the Clamshell double umbrella modelled on the Rashkind duct occluder.[14] Encouraging early results were reported but subsequently it became apparent that the supporting struts underwent fatigue, and fractures and displacements were seen in some patients. The device was withdrawn pending modification.

Occlusion devices

A range of devices made of different materials with different shapes and release mechanisms is now available.[15-19] The ASDOS device consists of two polyurethane patches mounted on nitinol umbrellas which are screwed together from each side of the atrial septum. The device is retrievable and repositionable but needs to be advanced over a long arteriovenous guidewire circuit (femoral vein, atrial septal defect, femoral artery) and is complicated to implant. The Sideris device incorporates a button mechanism to sandwich two opposing polyurethane foam sheets mounted on Teflon coated wire frames around the defect but has a tendency to unbutton spontaneously and embolise. It has undergone numerous modifications since its introduction. The Angelwings device is comprised of two Dacron squares on a nitinol frame which are joined together in a central ring that acts as a partial self centring mechanism. The sharp corners have resulted in atrial and aortic perforation and the device is being modified. These two devices are difficult to retrieve after partial deployment or embolisation. The modified Clamshell device with fatigue resistant arms (called Cardioseal) has performed better than the original Clamshell but lacks a self-centring mechanism. The Amplatzer device consisting of a double disc joined in the middle by a short 'stent' the size of the defect, is made of nitinol mesh with Dacron patches inside it to promote thrombosis and occlusion. Its popularity is due to it being able to close defects up to 38 mm in diameter and the 'self-centring' mechanism of the stent in the defect between the two discs. This completely occludes the defect and the adjacent discs only have diameters up to 14 mm larger than the stent. It is available in a much larger range of sizes than the other devices (4–38 mm in increments of 2 mm). It can easily be retrieved prior to release and repositioned. The other devices with a narrow central junction between the left and right atrial discs do not centre as readily and diameters of twice the defect size are required to prevent the device from embolising. This limits the size of defect closable with these devices to around 20–25 mm and they have a higher incidence of residual shunting. More recently the Cardioseal device has been modified with nitinol strands joining the two umbrellas (Starflex) as a 'self-centring' mechanism. All these devices have also been used in occluding the atrial fenestration created during the fenestrated Fontan operation. Small muscular ventricular septal defects (congenital or post-myocardial infarction) have also been closed by these devices.

Implantation technique

The method of implantation is similar with all the devices. Transoesophageal echocardiography is invaluable for determining suitability of the defect, presence of additional fenestrations, normal pulmonary venous drainage and correct positioning away from the atrioventricular valves and pulmonary and systemic veins prior to release. The need for a rim of atrial septum onto which the device will rest and grip excludes sinus venosus and primum defects and secundum defects with deficient margins (aortic margin deficiency excepted as devices can grip around the aortic root).

The defect is crossed from a femoral vein and a stiff guidewire placed in a left pulmonary vein. Over this wire a sizing balloon catheter is advanced and inflated to occlude the defect. The size of the balloon that is just able to close the defect without excessive force is called the 'stretch' diameter of the defect and is used to select the correct device size (Fig. 20.2a). Accurate sizing is imperative to reduce the likelihood of device embolisation. An 8–12 F long sheath is advanced over the guidewire into the left atrium and meticulously de-aired. The chosen device is advanced and the distal (left atrial) umbrella or disc is extruded into the left atrium. The sheath and device are withdrawn simultaneously to the atrial septum and using fluoroscopy and transoesophageal echocardiography, the sheath is withdrawn further to deploy the proximal right atrial disc (Fig. 20.2b). The Amplatzer and ASDOS devices are completely retrievable and repositionable at this stage and the Cardioseal and Starflex devices can be retrieved (though not repositioned). Once the device appears to be correctly sited and stable it is released. If the device is correctly sized, embolisation is uncommon. When it does occur, transcatheter retrieval is not as easy as with the Rashkind ductal umbrella and surgical retrieval and atrial septal defect closure are often required. [20]

A small leak is common across the device in the first few days and months until it is fully endothelialised. While the presence of fenestrated

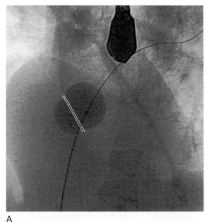
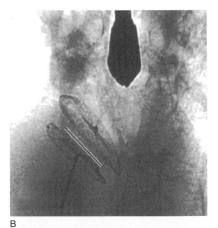

A   B

Figure 20.2:
(a) Balloon sizing of an atrial septal defect. The waist in the balloon represents the 'stretch' diameter' of the defect. (b) Deployment of an Amplatzer atrial septal defect occluder. The diameter of the central 'stent' of the device matches that of the measured stretch diameter in (a).

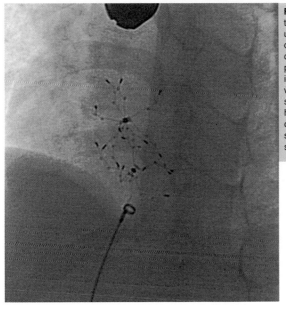

Figure 20.3: Implantation of two Cardioseal double umbrella atrial septal defect devices into two atrial septal defects at the same procedure. Note that the inferior device is seen side on while the superior device is seen en face (each device has eight radio-opaque arms) demonstrating that the atrial septum does not lie in a single plane.

defects was originally a contraindication to device closure, it is possible to implant either a larger device to cover over any fenestrations or two devices if the defects are not in proximity to each other (Fig. 20.3). An atrial septal aneurism can be sandwiched between the proximal and distal discs. Aspirin is given for 6 months after device implantation to prevent thromboembolism from the device during endothelialisation.

Advantages over surgical repair

■ Avoidance of sternotomy and cardiopulmonary bypass and hence avoidance of:
  – Scar
  – Bleeding
  – Risk of cerebral events
  – Post-pericardiotomy syndrome, which has risk of:
    Effusion
    Arrhythmias
  – Mortality (1% in adults, lower in children)
■ Shorter hospital stay.

Disadvantages

■ Not suitable for all defects (~ 60%) including:
  – Stretch diameter >38 mm
  – Deficient rim (<4 mm) – although deficiency towards the aorta is no longer a contraindication
■ Risk of cerebral events (air or clot in the sheath)
■ Femoral vessel haemorrhage or occlusion
■ Device embolisation may require surgical removal (and atrial septal defect repair) if transcatheter retrieval is not possible

■ Mitral regurgitation

■ Arrhythmias from atrial irritation in first few weeks

■ Atrial or aortic perforation (late) with some devices

■ Residual shunt.

Indications
The indications for atrial septal defect closure vary but in childhood is recommended for right ventricular volume overload (clinical, radiographic or echocardiographic). In addition a pulmonary to systemic flow ratio (usually by a radionuclide first pass scan, but also by echocardiography or even cardiac catheterisation) of greater than 2:1 is commonly accepted. There are those who accept a flow ratio of 1.5:1 as an indication. In adults who are asymptomatic there are some who conclude that atrial septal defect closure is not of any benefit although longer follow-up has shown improvements in exercise capacity and survival.[21,22] Patients with small atrial septal defects or a patent foramen ovale and paradoxical cerebral embolism should also have their defects closed. Similarly, divers who have experienced systemic complications from decompression sickness should have closure of the foramen ovale or atrial septal defect.

Controversies
Atrial septal defect device closure
Device closure for atrial septal defects is still in its infancy and long-term results are not available. The range of available devices and the moderate applicability (~60%) also indicate that the ideal device is yet to be developed. Nevertheless in suitable patients it seems to be a highly effective method of closing atrial septal defects and in these patients has advantages over surgical closure.

Patent foramen ovale
The greatest controversy is in patients who are discovered to have a small atrial septal defect or patent foramen ovale with or without an atrial septal aneurysm during work-up of a presumed embolic cerebral event. The incidence of a patent foramen ovale is increased in those patients without another cause for the embolic event compared with patients with a recognised cause for the event.[23] While thrombi have occasionally been seen to cross such a defect, it is difficult to prove that the cerebral event is due to a paradoxical embolus in any particular patient. Thus even after successful closure, there may still be an ongoing risk for recurrent cerebral events if the presumed alerting embolus was not paradoxical – 3.4% per annum in one study.[24] Thus simply continuing anticoagulation without foramen ovale closure is an option. Furthermore, if these patients did have recurrent venous thrombi and paradoxical embolism, there may still be a continuing need for anticoagulation after closure of the foramen to prevent pulmonary embolism. A cerebral event occurring during

pregnancy (with the increased thrombotic tendency) is a more convincing reason to close a patent foramen ovale to prevent a recurrence in a future pregnancy.

CONCLUSIONS

Transcatheter occlusion of the patent arterial duct is now the method of choice with a high success rate, low complication rate and applicability to all except small infants and neonates. Atrial septal defect closure is being increasingly used but an ideal device does not yet exist and only about 60% of defects are currently suitable for transcatheter closure. While foramen ovale closure is invariably possible the indications remain uncertain.

REFERENCES

1. Porstmann W, Wierny L, Warneke H. Closure of the persistent ductus arteriosus without thoracotomy. Ger Med Mon 1967;12:259–61.

2. Rashkind WJ, Mullins CE, Hellenbrand WE, Tait MA. Non-surgical closure of patent ductus arteriosus: clinical application of the Rashkind PDA occluder system. Circulation 1987;75:583–92.

3. Tynan M. Transcatheter occlusion of persistent arterial duct. Report of the European Registry. Lancet 1992;340:1062 6.

4. Huggon IC, Tabatabaei AH, Qureshi SA et al. The use of a second transcatheter Rashkind arterial duct occluder for persisting flow following implantation of a first device: indications and results. Br Heart J 1993;69.544 50.

5. Sorenson KE, Kristensen B, Hansen OK. Frequency of occurrence of residual ductal flow after surgical ligation by color-flow mapping. Am J Cardiol 1991;67:653–4.

6. Lloyd TR, Fedderly R, Mendelsohn AM et al. Transcatheter occlusion of patent ductus arteriosus with Gianturco coils. Circulation 1993;88:1412–20.

7. Rosenthal E, Qureshi SA, Reidy J, Baker EJ, Tynan M. Evolving use of embolisation coils for occlusion of the arterial duct. Heart 1996;76:525–30.

8. Celiker A, Qureshi SA, Bilgic A et al. Transcatheter closure of patent arterial duct using controlled-release coils. Europ Heart J 1997;18:450–4.

9. Daniels CJ, Cassidy SC, Teske DW, Wheller JJ, Allen HD. Reopening after successful coil occlusion for patent ductus arteriosus. JACC 1999;31:444–50.

10. Masura J, Walsh KP, Thanopoulous B et al. Catheter closure of moderate- to large-sized patent ductus arteriosus using the new Amplatzer duct occluder: immediate and short-term results. JACC 1998;31:878–82.

11. Balzer DT, Spray TL, McMullin D, Cottingham W, Canter CE. Endarteritis associated with a clinically silent patent ductus arteriosus. Am Heart J 1993;125:1192–3.

12. Latson LA, McManus BM, Doer C, Kilzer K, Cheatham JP Endocarditis risk of the USCI PDA umbrella for transcatheter closure of patent ductus arteriosus. Circulation 1994;90:2525–8.

13. King TD, Mills NL. Secundum atrial septal defects: non-operative closure during cardiac catheterisation. JAMA 1976;235:2506–9.

14. Lock JE, Rome JJ, Davis R et al. Transcatheter closure of atrial septal defects. Circulation 1989;79:1091–9.

15. Hausdorf G, Schneider M, Franzbach B et al. Transcatheter closure of secundum atrial septal defects with the atrial septal defect occlusion system (ASDOS): initial experience in children. Heart 1996;75:83–8.

16. Sideris EB, Leung M, Yoon JH et al. Occlusion of large atrial septal defects with a centering buttoned device: early clinical experience. Am Heart J 1996;131:356–9.

17. Rickers C, Hamm C, Stern H et al. Percutaneous closure of secundum atrial septal defect with a new self centring device ('angel wings'). Heart 1998;80:517–21.

18. Kaulitz R, Paul T, Hausdorf G. Extending the limits of transcatheter closure of atrial septal defects with the double umbrella device (CardioSEAL) Heart 1998;80:54–9.

19. Chan KC, Godman MJ, Walsh K, Wilson N, Redington A, Gibbs JL. Transcatheter closure of atrial septal defect and interatrial communications with a new self expanding nitinol double disc device (Amplatzer septal occluder): multicentre UK experience. Heart 1999;82:300–306.

20. Bohm J, Bittigau K, Köhler F, Baumann G, Konertz W. Surgical removal of atrial septal occlusion system-devices. Eur J Card Thorac Surg 1997;12:869–72.

21. Ward C. Secundum atrial septal defect: routine surgical treatment is not of proven benefit. Br Heart J 1994;71:219–23.

22. Konstantinides S, Geibel A, Olschewski M et al. A comparison of surgical and medical therapy for atrial septal defect in adults. N Engl J Med 1995;333:469–73.

23. Lechat P, Mas JL, Lascault G et al. Prevalence of a patent foramen ovale in patients with stroke. N Engl J Med. 1988;318:1148–52.

24. Lock JE. Patent foramen ovale is indicted, but the case hasn't gone to trial. Circulation 2000;101:838.

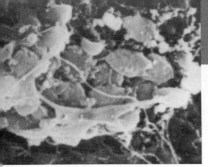

21

Percutaneous balloon pericardiotomy

JOHN L. CAPLIN

KEY POINTS

- PBP is effective in recurrent (usually malignant) pericardial effusion.

- It is performed in a cardiac catheterisation laboratory by an experienced operator.

- Cardiac and pulmonary injury are avoided by fluoroscopic guidance.

- Pleural effusion are common but usually transient.

- PBP is useful in critically ill patients with advanced malignancy.

INTRODUCTION

Most recurrent pericardial effusions are due to malignant disease, but it is unusual, which is perhaps surprising as cardiac metastases are relatively common. Patients with recurrent effusions often spend a long time in hospital for treatment of their underlying condition, and effective pericardial drainage, in addition to relieving symptoms, can reduce hospital stays in a group of patients who particularly value the quality of life and the remaining time spent at home. Sclerosant therapies have been shown to be ineffective in the management of recurrent malignant pericardial effusions, and the choices facing the physician managing these patients include open pericardiectomy, surgical subxiphisternal pericardial window, and video assisted thoracoscopic surgery to create a pericardial window. The development of percutaneous balloon pericardiotomy (PBP) has allowed the interventional cardiologist to contribute to the management of these patients.[1] The procedure has been shown to be a safe and effective procedure with a low recurrence rate.

PATIENT SELECTION

Patients with recurrent pericardial effusions irrespective of the aetiology may be considered. In patients with definite malignant effusions who have not had previous pericardiocentesis, a decision can be made to perform PBP if the effusion is felt likely to recur. Echocardiography is the most important pre-procedure investigation. There must be at least 1 cm of fluid inferior to the heart when viewed subxiphisternally. In addition if the effusion is loculated then the procedure is unlikely to succeed. If the patient has clinical signs of tamponade, but the procedure cannot be carried out promptly, pericardiocentesis with the removal of a few hundred millilitres of fluid will relieve the symptoms and allow PBP to be performed electively. If pericardiocentesis is performed a sheath should be left in the pericardial space for future access.

PROCEDURE

It is recommended that the procedure be performed in a cardiac catheterisation laboratory with access to X-ray screening, haemodynamic monitoring and resuscitation equipment.[2] The patient is placed on the operating table with a back wedge to bring the patient's chest to about 30 degrees from horizontal. Subxiphisternal echocardiography is performed to confirm that there is adequate fluid inferior to the heart and the depth from the skin to the effusion is measured so that an adequate needle length can be selected. The balloon dilatation stretches both the pericardium and the diaphragm and is painful. I use intravenous sedation with a small dose of a short-acting benzodiazepine, and pain prevention with narcotic analgesia. Continuous electrocardiographic monitoring is required and saturation monitoring is suggested in view of the sedation. The subxiphisternal region is prepared and a small skin incision is made about 2 cm below the subxiphisternal notch. The pericardium is punctured in the normal manner, directing the needle towards the left shoulder. A 0.035 inch J-tipped guidewire is inserted through the needle and a 7-F angiographic sheath inserted into the into the percardial sac. I routinely inject 5–10 millilitres of contrast into the pericardial sac. This confirms the position of the sheath, that the effusion is not loculated, and that there is adequate pericardial fluid inferior to the heart for the procedure. A 0.038 inch soft-tipped stiff shaft Amplatz wire is then inserted into the pericardial space. The tip of the wire is positioned in the superior part of the pericardial sac if possible. A 20 mm diameter 3 cm long dilating balloon is prepared in the usual way by suction using a syringe containing contrast diluted to half-strength with saline. The track is then pre-dilated using a 10-F dilator and the balloon catheter is advanced over the guidewire. The aim is to centre the balloon across the parietal pericardium and diaphragm. The balloon catheter is then connected via a three-way tap to an indeflator. The balloon is initially filled by hand injection using half-strength contrast until a 'dog-bone' shape is noted (Fig. 21.1). The indeflator is then used to fill the balloon to a pressure of approximately 3 atmospheres. The aim is to abolish, if possible, the indentation caused by the diaphragm and pericardium (Fig. 21.2). It may be necessary to perform more then one inflation to open a hole. The balloon may not fill completely if the proximal part of the balloon is within the skin or superficial tissues. If this occurs gentle traction of the skin downwards is sometimes necessary. In my experience the main problem is that the balloon prolapses into the pericardial sac when the indeflator is used. In order to prevent this the balloon should be partially filled within the pericardial sac and then pulled back and fully inflated.

Once the dilatation is completed the balloon catheter is withdrawn over the wire and replaced with a 7 or 8-F pigtail catheter. It is my practice to drain off as much pericardial fluid as possible at this stage as this probably limits the size of any pleural effusions. The catheter is then

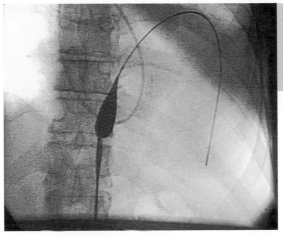

Figure 21.1:
The balloon catheter having been connected, the balloon is initially filled by hand injection using half-strength contrast until a 'dog-bone' shape is noted.

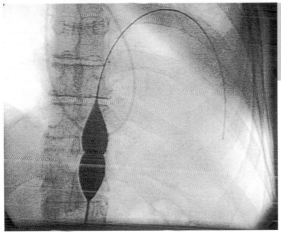

Figure 21.2:
The indeflator is used to fill the balloon to a pressure of ~3 atm. The aim is to abolish the indentation caused by the diaphragm and pericardium.

sewn in place and left on free drainage. There have been reports of the use double balloons, Inoue balloon catheters,[3] and the apical approach.

POST-PROCEDURE MANAGEMENT AND FOLLOW-UP

The patient should be monitored on the ward after return from the catheter laboratory. The volume of pericardial drainage should be noted every 6 hours. Once the volume is negligible (<75 millilitres in 24 hours), echocardiography should be performed, and provided the effusion is absent or very small the catheter should be withdrawn. If there is persistent fluid the pigtail catheter should be gently flushed with 5–10 millilitres of heparinised saline and manipulated around to enter the residual fluid. Once the catheter is removed the patient should be monitored for a further 24 hours, a departmental chest radiograph obtained and echocardiography performed. If there is no large pleural effusion and the pericardial sac is dry, the patient can be discharged home. I review the patient in clinic after 1 month with repeat chest radiograph and echocardiogram to check for complications or recurrent effusion.

Complications:

■ **Pleural effusions:** The development of left pleural effusions occurs in most successful PBP procedures. Most are small and temporary, but between 10 and 15% of patients develop effusions large enough to require pleural drainage.[4] The highest risk is in patients with a pre-existing effusion. In patients with borderline pulmonary function who would be severely compromised by a large pleural effusion, close monitoring of the size of any pleural effusion is important.

■ **Cardiac or pulmonary injury:** Pericardiocentesis is a potentially hazardous procedure. Before echocardiography was widely available there was significant morbidity and mortality due to myocardial or pulmonary injury. Echocardiography has substantially reduced these risks, but PBP should only be performed by operators experienced in pericardiocentesis.

■ **Balloon rupture:** Rupture of the balloon is not uncommon: not surprisingly it is related to the use of high pressure and large balloons and the presence of an inelastic pericardium. Generally there are no other complications and the catheter is removed over a guidewire. If dislodgement of the balloon or catheter fracture occur, then the fragments may be removed using a snare inserted through a second pericardial catheter.[5]

■ **Fever:** Pyrexia was noted frequently in initial reports, but sepsis is rare. Some authors recommend prophylactic antibiotics,[2] although this is not my practice.

RESULTS OF THE MULTICENTRE PBP REGISTRY

Data were collected from 130 patients in the years 1987–94.[4] The mean age was 59 years (range 25–78). There was an equal sex distribution. Malignant disease was present in 85%; the majority were from lung or breast primaries. Of the non-malignant aetiologies four of 20 were HIV related. Tamponade was present in 69%, and prior pericardiocentesis had been performed in 58%.

The overall success rate of the procedure, defined as an uncomplicated procedure without the need for surgical pericardial window, and no recurrent effusion over an average follow-up of 5 months, was 85%. Five patients required surgery for pericardial bleeding. Thirteen patients had recurrent effusion usually within 3 months, and 12 of these had surgery; however six of the surgical patients had further recurrences.

There were minor complications in 13% of patients with fever as the most frequent complication; however no patients had septicaemia. About one in six patients required thoracocentesis, and this was more common in patients with pre-existing pleural effusions. Survival in the majority of patients was consistent with the diagnosis of disseminated malignancy. The success rate in this registry was better than that reported for surgical procedures such as pericardiectomy, pleuropericardial window and subxiphisternal pericardiotomy, and much better than pericardiocentesis alone and sclersosant therapy.[6]

CONCLUSION

Percutaneous balloon pericardiotomy is a safe and effective treatment of pericardial effusions, especially when due to disseminated malignant disease. It can reduce the duration of hospitalisation, and is less invasive and more effective than surgical therapy. In experienced hands the risks of the procedure are low, and it should be available in cardiac units which serve specialist cancer centres.

REFERENCES

1. Palacios IF, Tuzcu EM, Ziskind AA *et al.* Percutaneous balloon pericardial window for patients with malignant pericardial effusion and tamponade. Cathet Cardiovas Diagn 1991;22:244–9.

2. Ziskind AA, Palacios IF. Percutaneous balloon pericardiotomy for patients with pericardial effusion and tamponade. In: Topol EJ (ed.) Textbook of interventional cardiology, 3rd edn. Philadelphia: WB Saunders, 1999, pp. 869–77.

3. Chow WH, Chow TC, Yip AS, Cheung KL. Inoue balloon pericardiotomy for patients with recurrent pericardial effusion. Angiology 1996;47:57–60.

4. Ziskind AA, Lemmon C, Rodriguez S *et al.* Final report of the percutaneous balloon pericardiotomy registry for the treatment of effusive pericardial disease. Circulation 1994;1–121.

5. Block PC, Wilson MA. Hemi balloon dislodgement during percutaneous balloon pericardial window procedure: removal using a second pericardial catheter. Cathet Cardiovasc Diagn 1993;29:289–91.

6. Vaitkus PT, Herrmann HC. LeWinter MM. Treatment of malignant pericardial effusion. JAMA 1994;272:59–64.

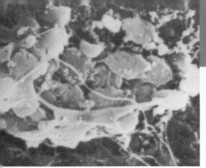

22

Intracardiac foreign body retrieval

EVER D. GRECH AND DAVID R. RAMSDALE

KEY POINTS

- With the widespread use of intravascular catheters for diagnostic use and therapeutic purposes, the iatrogenic embolisation of materials employed for catheterisation has increased and is probably more prevalent than previously recognised.

- Many intravascular foreign bodies can be successfully removed using a variety of devices such as loop-snares, retrieval baskets or grasping forceps.

- The requirement for pacemaker/ICD electrode extraction will continue to increase as device implantations escalate. Adequate training and experience in lead extraction techniques is necessary.

- Intra-coronary stent deployment failure is a problem that has received little attention in the medical literature and is associated with significant morbidity and mortality. It can be avoided by prudent interventional techniques. Retrieving detached stents may be difficult and should only be performed by experienced operators.

- Operators should have a wide selection of retrieval devices and equipment, and be familiar in their use.

INTRODUCTION

The volume and complexity of percutaneous diagnostic and therapeutic techniques involving the heart and circulation has increased worldwide. These procedures are carried out not only by the cardiologist, but also by radiologists, anaesthetists, surgeons and physicians. Procedures commonly involve insertion of temporary or permanent pacing electrodes and central venous lines or catheters. Moreover, subcutaneously implanted long-term intravenous cannulae, such as Hickman lines, have proved useful for treating various conditions. Catheter-based coronary diagnostic and interventional procedures have also become widely practised.

Unfortunately, hand-in-hand with this rise in vascular intervention has come an increase in the incidence of lost or embolised foreign bodies in the venous and arterial circulations. It is therefore necessary for practising interventional cardiologists to become familiar with retrieval equipment and the techniques for their percutaneous removal. This not only circumvents the need for major thoracic or open heart surgery, but may also avoid potentially life-threatening complications. For the adult cardiologist, the commonest sites for retrieval of lost components are the great veins and right heart including the pulmonary arteries, and the coronary arterial tree. This chapter reviews the various types of retained components and the different methods for their successful retrieval.

DEVICES

A variety of transcatheter devices for retrieval of components are available. These include the following:

Loop-snare retrieval systems

The loop-snare device is often the first choice in view of its safety and ease of use. Two examples of loop-snare systems are shown in Figure 22.1. The Welter retrieval loop catheter consists of a wire snare and is operated from a proximal handle. Its design permits orientation of the loop at right angles to its shaft, enabling access to free-floating foreign bodies. Other examples are the Curry loop snare (Fig. 22.1) and the Amplatz goose neck snare, which has a nitinol 90 degree snare-loop to shaft orientation and remains co-axial to the vessel lumen (Fig. 22.2).

Retrieval baskets

Examples of retrieval baskets include the Dotter retrieval catheter (Fig. 22.1, bottom), the minibasket and the Dormia stone catcher. These consist of an outer sheath enclosing movable parallel metal wires, which can be opened or closed by sliding a cone in and out of the coronary catheter. To deploy

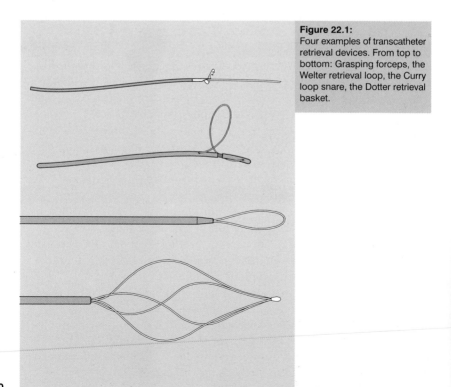

Figure 22.1:
Four examples of transcatheter retrieval devices. From top to bottom: Grasping forceps, the Welter retrieval loop, the Curry loop snare, the Dotter retrieval basket.

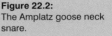

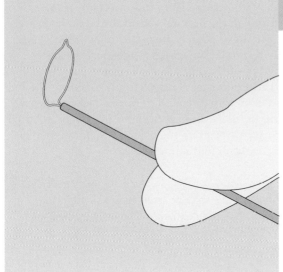

Figure 22.2:
The Amplatz goose neck snare.

these devices, the basket is placed beyond the fragment and then opened. It is then withdrawn, allowing entrapment of the foreign body, at which time the basket is pulled shut and removed as a single unit. Retrieval basket devices are particularly useful in retrieving objects in the great veins or intracardiac chambers. In the arterial circulation, they are only useful if the object extends into the aorta.

Bioptome/grasping forceps
Different types of jaw forceps are available and an example is the Cook retrieval grasping forceps (Fig. 22.1, top). The grasping jaws are operated from a proximal handle, and care is needed when used to retrieve foreign bodies in less resilient vascular areas.

Miscellaneous techniques
Handmade wire snares
A simple, handmade snare may be fashioned using single or twin guidewires. The snare is created by doubling over an exchange-length wire at its midsection and inserting it down a 4 F probing catheter. Alternatively, a snare may be created by looping the distal 5 cm of a standard-length wire, or tying together the flexible ends of two 0.014-inch wires. The probing catheter is then passed through the guide catheter and positioned just proximal to the retained fragment. The loop is front-loaded through the probing catheter and gently passed over the object. Ideally, the loop should have a moderate bend to help encompass the

fragment. Once the object is trapped, the wire ends are pulled firmly to secure the object against the catheter tip. The whole assembly is then withdrawn until it passes through the femoral sheath. If the snare device cannot be steered into a tortuous or acutely angled coronary artery, twin 0.014-inch guidewires may be used. The wires are advanced separately into the coronary artery and positioned beside the fragment. The proximal wire ends are inserted into a torquer and clamped firmly together. The torquer is then rotated in a clockwise direction to form a helix of the two wires. With the Y-connector partially open, the double helix is propagated distally into the coronary artery, ensnaring the object, which can then be withdrawn into the guiding catheter and removed.

Balloon catheters
Inflated or deflated balloon catheters may be used to physically drag fragments from the vessel into the guide catheter. The inflated-balloon technique has the potential for significant mechanical vascular injury and must be used cautiously.

Pigtail ventriculography catheter
A pigtail ventriculography catheter has been used to snare a catheter fragment in the venous system[1] and a broken guidewire in a coronary artery.[2] Again the potential for causing vessel wall damage demands caution when attempting this procedure.

SITES OF RETAINED COMPONENTS
Retained components can only be removed percutaneously if they are radio-opaque. High-resolution fluoroscopy is required, preferably digital with magnification options to enable accurate definition of the object. Full haemodynamic monitoring is essential. Systemic heparin (10 000–15 000 units) should be administered if not already given beforehand, to avoid thrombus formation on the retrieval device or the retained fragment.

Right heart
For retrieval of central venous or right heart objects, the preferred technique is to use the right femoral vein for access. Under local anaesthetic, an 8 F haemostatic sheath is inserted into the right femoral vein using a Seldinger technique. A long sheath is then advanced over a 0.035 mm diameter long guidewire into the appropriate part of the great veins or right heart chamber. On removing the guidewire, the retrieval device is inserted to grip or ensnare the free end of the foreign body. Once captured, the device is withdrawn into the long sheath and the long sheath, retrieval device and foreign body are removed intact from the vein. A second venous sheath may sometimes be useful for insertion of another catheter such as a pig-tail, Judkins or Cournand which can be used to help unfold loops of catheters in order to present a free end for the retrieval

device. Alternatively, a grasping forceps or snare device can be used. At the end of the procedure, haemostasis can be achieved by simple direct pressure when larger objects, knots or loops have been removed. Protamine sulphate can be given to reverse heparin anticoagulation.

Pacemaker electrodes

The transvenous extraction and/or repositioning of chronically implanted permanent pacemaker electrodes presents special difficulties due to scar-tissue adhesion at the lead tip, which may extend along the length of the lead. If a lead has failed, the usual practice is to cap it at the connector terminal so that it is sealed, leaving it buried under the patient's skin. However, removal is essential if the lead becomes infected, the patient develops septicaemia or there is a free-floating lead in the vascular system.

In some instances, removal of an adherent electrode can be achieved by continuous traction on the lead until it comes away from the myocardium. However, this is generally unsatisfactory because of the risk of myocardial avulsion. Until recently, the alternative and more complex option has been thoracotomy. However, a purpose-made lead extraction system enables removal to be performed reasonably safely without the need for surgery. The system uses a countertraction technique and hence lessens the risk of myocardial avulsion (Fig. 22.3a).

Lead extraction can be performed via the superior approach, when the lead is extracted through the implant vein (the subclavian, cephalic or jugular vein). Alternatively, the femoral approach is used if the lead is inaccessible or if the superior approach is difficult or unsuccessful.

Using the superior approach, surgical cutdown to the pacemaker generator is performed and it is removed. The terminal connector of the pacing lead is cut off cleanly using the clippers supplied. The two main tools used are the special locking stylet and the dilator sheath set. The locking stylet, which stiffens the lead, is passed down the lumen of the lead to its tip. It consists of a loop handle at the proximal end and an expandable wire coil at the distal end. The size of the locking stylet is selected beforehand using gauge pins. By rotating the loop handle anti-clockwise several times, the fine-wire filament unwinds inside the coil, wedging the stylet shaft tightly into the coil at the lead tip and locking it there. A system of two telescoping dilator sheaths is advanced over the protruding lead end and manipulated along its length via the subclavian vein and on into the heart, thus disrupting the scar tissue along the lead. If the lead has not been freed by the time the sheaths reach the myocardium, the outer sheath is advanced onto the myocardium (Fig. 22.3b). With firm traction on the lead via the locking stylet and countertraction on the sheath supporting the myocardial wall, the lead can be freed and pulled through the sheath (Figs 22.3c and d). If required, a new lead can now be inserted through the outer sheath. Lead removal using this system may not be possible if there is excessive scar tissue along the length of the lead or if the locking stylet will not pass through a damaged lead. It may therefore

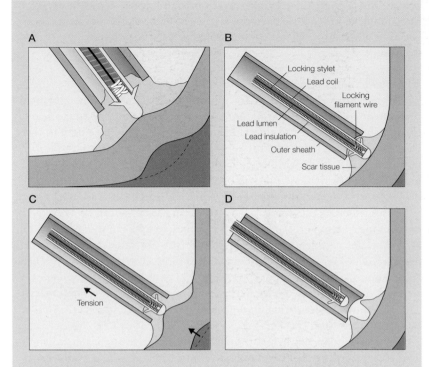

Figure 22.3:
(a) Pacing lead tension applied with countertraction within the sheath. (b) The stylet is locked inside the lead coil. If the lead has not been freed by the time the sheaths reach the heart, the outer sheath is advanced to the myocardium. (c) Firm traction is placed on the locking stylet, whilst the sheath provides countertraction, preventing invagination of the heart and confining the force within the circumference of the sheath. (d) When the lead tip is freed from the scar tissue, it is removed through the sheath. The outer sheath can even be used as an introducer for a new lead.

be necessary to use the femoral approach if the lead has retracted into the venous system and cannot be reached with the superior approach.

The femoral system comprises a long sheath with a tip-deflecting guidewire threaded through a Dotter retrieval basket. A long sheath system is inserted via the femoral vein using routine Seldinger technique and advanced up to the right atrium. A tip-deflecting wire is lassoed around the lead and is pulled down onto the Dotter basket. A longer sheath is then advanced over the lead in a similar manner to the superior approach, thus removing the lead from the scar tissue and myocardium. The femoral system with the lead attached is then removed from the body.

In the largest published series using the above technique, Byrd *et al.* performed 3540 lead extractions in 2338 patients over a period of 28 months. The indications for extraction were infection (27%), non-

functional or incompatible leads (25%), removal of Accufix or Encor
atrial J-leads following their re-call by Teletronics due to the risk of
potential fracture and protrusion of their J-retention wires (46%), or other
causes (2%). A superior approach was used for 84.4% of leads, a femoral
approach in 4.3% and a combined approach in 11.3%. Additional
devices, such as retrieval baskets, loop snares, coronary guiding catheters
and pigtail catheters were also used. A total of 93% of leads were
completely extracted (and 5% partially extracted) with a major
complication rate of 1.4%, which was statistically significantly higher in
women than in men (2.3% vs 0.8%, $p < 0.01$). Only one death was
reported (0.04%) and the minor complication rate was also low at 1.7%.
The overall complication risk increased significantly with the number of
leads removed and less operator experience. The authors concluded that
the indication for extraction should be balanced against the risk of
complication, and that experienced operators should be conscious of the
need to be fully equipped and prepared for every eventuality before
undertaking lead extraction.[3]

A newer technique using excimer laser has recently been introduced by
Spectranetics (Colorado Springs, CO, USA). Data from the randomised
PLEXES (**P**acemaker **L**ead **EX**traction with the **E**ximer laser **S**heath) trial
indicate that this system is more effective than standard non-laser
methods.[4] The Spector laser sheath (SLS) contains optical laser fibres,
which allow 308 nm ultraviolet light pulses from a xenon–chloride laser
to ablate tissue at the sheath tip allowing it to cut through adherent scar.
It is threaded over the pacemaker (or ICD) electrode and advanced
towards further fibrous binding sites until the tip of the electrode is
reached (Fig. 22.4a–c). This system is used in conjunction with the lead
locking device (LLD) which is comprised of a loop wire handle and a core
mandrel that has a stainless steel mesh fixation mechanism (Fig. 22.5).
This is inserted down the lumen of the electrode and the proximal end of
the mesh is attached to a proximal connector which is used to deploy and
lock the device in the electrode.

Left heart

There are only limited data concerning the incidence of retained
components within the left heart. However, two series that reviewed 500
and 5400 consecutive elective coronary angioplasty procedures, estimated
the risk of retained components to be 0.2%.[5,6] Within this system, the
most frequently reported retained fragments are angioplasty guidewires[7]
often within the coronary tree. Occlusion devices such as embolisation
coils, umbrella duct occluders and detachable balloons are becoming more
widely used and may also become misplaced.[8]

Intra-coronary stents

Failure of stent delivery or embolisation has been widely reported and
although it is not frequent, may occur in up to 8% of cases.[9] However,

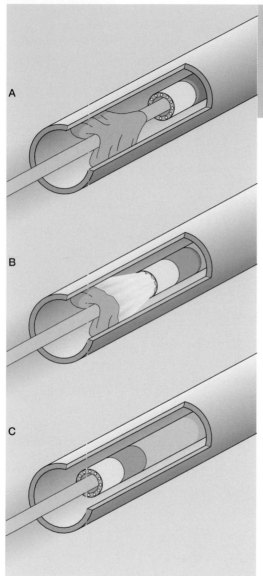

Figure 22.4:
(a) The laser sheath is advanced over the pacemaker/ICD electrode towards the binding site. (b) Controlled bursts of excimer laser energy photo-ablate fibrous tissue. (c) The laser sheath is advanced through the binding site to the next site until the lead is released.

delivery success rates have improved with more modern premounted, lower-profile, flexible, slotted-tube stents compared with the previous bare, hand-crimped, rigid Palmaz–Schatz stents. Displaced stents, which have not been fully deployed, can be retrieved using snares, baskets and grasping forceps. Meticulous attention to procedural and peri-procedural details is required if stent loss is to be prevented, although such events are usually unpredictable. Although systemic stent embolisation does not

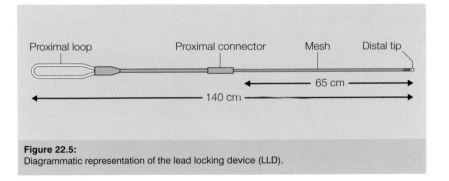

Figure 22.5:
Diagrammatic representation of the lead locking device (LLD).

usually result in clinical sequelae, undeployed stents in the coronary arteries should be removed immediately. However, there is surprisingly little literature describing retrieval methods of undeployed stents retained within the coronary tree. Using a technique where a second guidewire was twisted around the first, Veldhuijzen *et al.* were unsuccessful in removing an undeployed Palmaz–Schatz stent within a right coronary artery in one patient, although they were successful in retrieving an undeployed Wiktor stent, also within a right coronary artery, in another patient.[10] Foster-Smith *et al.* used a snare to retrieve an undeployed Wiktor stent and a forceps device to retrieve an deployed Wiktor stent from a vein graft, in the same patient.[11] In another patient, an undeployed Gianturco-Roubin stent was removed from the left main coronary artery by inflation of a balloon catheter to 5 atmospheres to trap the stent. It could not, however, be drawn into the guide catheter and was dislodged from the balloon catheter during the attempt. The stent was then retrieved using a multipurpose basket.[11] More recently, Columbo has described the use of the Amplatz goose neck snare (Fig. 22.2) to retrieve stents both within and outside the coronary tree, and the Cook grasping forceps (Fig. 22.1, top) outside the coronary tree.[12] The goose neck snare may be used in one of two ways (Fig. 22.6). In the proximal grab method, the balloon catheter is removed and the loop of the snare is placed over the proximal end of the guidewire. The snare is advanced until the distal end of the microcatheter is positioned just proximal to the stent. The loop is then opened and advanced around the proximal end of the stent. The loop is then closed to grab the stent and removed into the guide catheter. In the distal wire grab method, the balloon catheter is removed and a second guidewire is positioned adjacent to the stent and distal to the original guidewire. The snare is looped over the proximal end of the second guidewire and advanced until the distal end of the microcatheter is positioned distal to the stent and original guidewire. The loop is opened to snare the distal end of the original guidewire. The snare, both guidewires and the stent can then be withdrawn together into the guiding catheter.

277

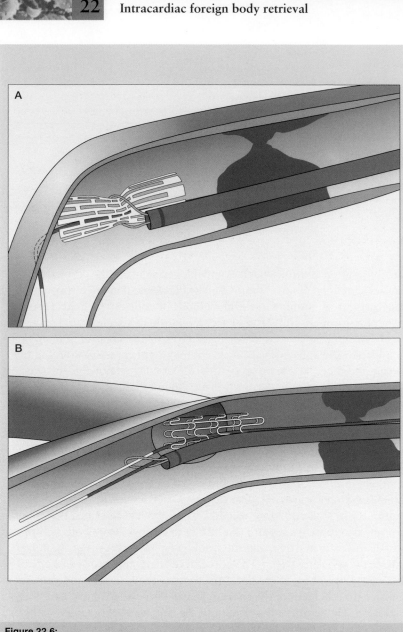

Figure 22.6:
Two methods of stent retrieval using the Amplatz 'Goose neck' microsnare. (a) The 'proximal grab' and (b) the 'distal wire grab' methods.

MANAGEMENT

The optimal management of intravascular fragment retention has been controversial and remains undefined. It is dependent on the site and situation in which the event occurs and must be tailored to the individual patient's needs and risks. Thus, the retrieval of an undeployed stent within a coronary artery may differ in technique and complexity from that of a pacemaker lead within a great vein.

Although retained components may be removed surgically or percutaneously, they may also be left *in situ*. There are instances when it may be appropriate and safe to leave a metallic fragment contained within a previously occluded coronary artery, when there is no clear indication for coronary artery bypass grafting. In their series, Hartzler *et al.* observed that the intra-coronary retention of equipment fragments were at times well tolerated.[6] However, it is worth noting that in this series only one wire fragment was left *in situ* in a patent coronary artery. Thus the benign clinical course characteristic of the patients in that series primarily reflected detached wire fragments in chronically occluded arteries. The potential for late perforation, dissection, infection, arrhythmia and proximal propagation of thrombus resulting in myocardial infarction must be considered as possible risks when this strategy is adopted. While there is some evidence that fragments may become endothelialised and remain benign, there is no long-term or pathological data to support this hypothesis.

In some cases, surgery will be required primarily because the initial procedure was unsuccessful and, in these circumstances, the retained fragment can be removed intra-operatively. If myocardial ischaemia is present or threatened, surgical removal of components should be considered early. In unstable patients, attempts at catheter extraction may cause unnecessary delay in mobilising an operating team.

Although transcatheter removal of retained components may be the optimal solution, it may itself result in serious complications. Thrombus deposition on protruding hardware with subsequent systemic embolisation must be considered, although adequate heparinisation should reduce this. Wires and retrieval devices may themselves break and become retained. In addition, fragments may slip free during removal and embolise to other locations.[6] The stiffer devices such as the Dotter retrieval basket should be handled carefully to avoid myocardial or venous perforation.

CONCLUSION

The morbidity and mortality associated with retained intravascular fragments are difficult to assess and it is likely that reported cases underestimate the true incidence and early deaths. It is often difficult to conclusively implicate retained fragments as the main cause of death, as this may be ascribed to other causes.

As the applications of conventional angioplasty and intra-coronary stenting expand, the probability of experiencing equipment failure will increase. Therefore, the option of percutaneous extraction of such components in place of invasive surgery will assume increasing importance. Where it can be executed successfully it should substantially diminish clinical risk. In order to achieve this, operators should have a wide selection of retrieval devices and equipment, and be familiar with their use.

REFERENCES

1. Auge JM, Orial A, Serra C, Crexells C. The use of pigtail catheters for retrieval of foreign bodies from the cardiovascular system. Cathet Cardiovasc Diagn 1984;10:625–8.

2. Krone RJ. Successful percutaneous removal of retained broken coronary angioplasty guidewire. Cathet Cardiovasc Diagn 1986;12:409–410.

3. Byrd CL, Wilkoff BL, Love CJ et al. Intravascular extraction of problematic or infected permanent pacemaker leads: 1994–1996. PACE 1999;22:1348–57.

4. Wilkoff BL, Byrd CL, Love CJ et al. Pacemaker lead extraction with the laser sheath: results of the pacing lead extraction with the excimer sheath (PLEXES) trial. J Am Coll Cardiol 1999;33(6):1671–6.

5. Steffanino G, Meier B, Finci L et al. Acute complications of elective coronary angioplasty: a review of 500 consecutive procedures. Br Heart J 1988;59:151–8.

6. Hartzler GO, Rutherford BD, McConahay DR. Retained percutaneous transluminal coronary angioplasty equipment components and their management. Am J Cardiol 1987;60:1260–64.

7. Keltai M, Bartek I, Biro V. Guidewire snap causing left main coronary occlusion during coronary angioplasty. Cathet Cardiovasc Diagn 1986;12:324–6.

8. Huggon IC, Qureshi SA, Reidy J, Dos Anjos R, Baker EJ, Tynan M. Percutaneous transcatheter retrieval of misplaced therapeutic embolisation devices. Br Heart J 1994;72:470–75.

9. Cantor WJ, Lazzam C, Cohen EA et al. Failed coronary stent deployment. Am Heart J 1998;136:1088–95.

10. Veldhuijzen FLMJ, Bonnier HJRM, Michels R, El Gamal MIH, van Gelder BM. Retrieval of undeployed stents from the right coronary artery: Report of two cases. Cathet Cardiovasc Diagn 1993;30:245–8.

11. Foster-Smith KW, Garratt KN, Higano ST, Holmes DR Jr. Retrieval techniques for managing flexible intra-coronary stent misplacement. Cathet Cardiovasc Diagn 1993;30:63–8.

12. Colombo A. Stent retrieval. In: Serruys P, Kutryk MJB (eds). Handbook of coronary stents. London: Martin Dunitz 1998:275–81.

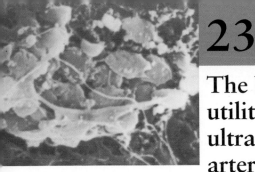

23

The basics and clinical utility of intravascular ultrasound in coronary artery disease

NEAL G. UREN

KEY POINTS

■ The appearance of the three-layered appearance by intravascular ultrasound occurs due to the acoustic impedance between adjacent structures.

■ The earliest accumulations of atherosclerotic plaque consist of crescentic intimal thickening of an intermediate echointensity.

■ With a greater accumulation of plaque, there is a greater complexity to the plaque which may be differentiated by broad ultrasound criteria relating to echoreflectivity.

■ Intravascular ultrasound provides accurate on-line quantitative information regarding lumen size and residual plaque load before and after interventional procedures.

■ Intravascular ultrasound has confirmed that with increasing plaque accumulation, there is a remodelling process whereby the vessel initially expands to accommodate the plaque load up to around 40% of vessel area.

■ During balloon angioplasty, localised calcium has a direct role in promoting dissection by increasing shear stress within the plaque at the junction between tissue types with differing elastic properties.

■ A strong argument for the use of IVUS in balloon angioplasty is that it may allow a 'stent like' result to be achieved by optimising the acute lumen gain from balloon dilatation alone.

■ In the MUSIC trial of additional IVUS guidance in optimal stent deployment, criteria for stent expansion were defined and even with only 80% of patients achieving these criteria, a 6-month angiographic restenosis rate of 8.3% was reported.

■ In the CRUISE study comparing IVUS and angiographic guidance of stenting, the former group demonstrated superior stent expansion and at 9-month follow-up, a 44% reduction in target vessel revascularisation was demonstrated.

■ In the OPTICUS trial comparing IVUS and angiographic guidance of stenting with angiographic follow-up, clinical and angiographic outcome was no different comparing both groups.

INTRODUCTION

The development of intravascular ultrasound (IVUS) has been a major development in the invasive imaging of coronary arteries. Clinical studies in intravascular ultrasound began in 1989 with the development of catheters initially in the 5–6 French gauge (F) range with the most recent catheter size miniaturised to 2.6 F.[1] Intravascular ultrasound has permitted not only a greater understanding of plaque morphology and its response to interventional procedures but has provided accurate on-line quantitative information regarding lumen size and residual plaque load, an important predictor of restenosis. The presence of disease not only at the site of focal stenosis but also in reference segments believed by angiography to be free of disease has modified interventional practice significantly. With continued improvement in image quality through increasing ultrasound frequency from 30 MHz through 40 MHz currently available and ultimately 50 MHz, the morphology of plaque and the off-line ability to characterise plaque will provide additional information in the management of atherosclerotic disease. It is likely that continued technical developments will enhance and define the role of intravascular ultrasound in coronary interventional practice.

BASIC INTERPRETATION

An appreciation of the coronary anatomy and its relationship to structures around it is important to the accurate interpretation of intravascular ultrasound images. These spatial relations are best appreciated at the time of slow catheter pull-back from distal to proximal vessel done using an automated pull-back device. Advances in image quality and improved tissue penetration has allowed the use of epivascular structures in addition to side branches as reference points for tomographic and axial orientation (Fig. 23.1).

There are three concentric layers in the epicardial coronary arterial wall demonstrable at histology and seen by intravascular ultrasound imaging. The intima is the innermost layer and consists of endothelial cells

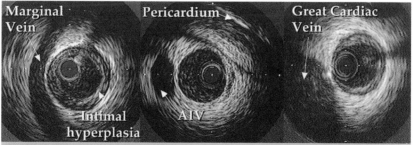

Figure 23.1:
The left panel is an image in the mid-right coronary artery. Marginal veins cross around the artery in a horseshoe pattern, often associated with and opposite to the branch points of the right ventricular marginal arteries. Recurrent atrial branches generally emerge on the opposite side of the artery to the marginal branches.

The middle panel is an image of the proximal left anterior descending artery (LAD). The anterior interventricular vein (AIV) lies to the left of the proximal artery in the majority of people (85%), with the first two diagonal branches on the same side. In one-third of people, the anterior interventricular vein branches into two after the second diagonal to lie either side of the LAD more distally. Pericardium may be seen as a bright reflection on the anterior side of the artery. Diagonal branches emerge on the same side as the AIV. Septal branches emerge from the LAD in a perpendicular fashion to myocardium, on the opposite side to pericardium.

The right image is of the proximal left circumflex artery. Distally, the CFX is accompanied by the posterior left ventricular vein whereas in its proximal section, it is crossed and shadowed superiorly by the great cardiac vein. Recurrent atrial branches emerge from the circumflex artery towards the great cardiac vein in the opposite direction to obtuse marginal branches.

and the subendothelial layer of smooth muscle cells and fibroblasts in a connective tissue matrix. The overall thickness of this layer can be just a few cells thick in childhood expanding to 150–200 μm in the adult. Beneath this, there is the internal elastic lamina which is intact in the normal state, consisting of fenestrated elastic fibres with a thickness less than 25 μm.

The media consists of multiple layers of smooth muscle cells arranged helically and circumferentially around the lumen of the artery, woven through a matrix of elastic fibers and collagen. The coronary arteries are less elastic than other similar sized arteries and thus resemble a transition towards more muscular peripheral arteries. The normal medial thickness ranges from 125–350 μm (mean 200 μm) although in the presence of plaque, the medial thickness may be considerably thinner, approximately 100 μm,[2] or completely involuted and replaced by plaque in severe disease. The external elastic lamina encircles the medial layer. It is composed of elastin but is thinner and more fenestrated than the internal lamina, and is not more than 20 μm in thickness.

The adventitia is essentially fibrous tissue, i.e. collagen (type III) and elastin, with the collagen orientated longitudinally in general, and to a lesser tissue density than media. It is a layer that is surrounded by the vaso vasorum, nerves and lymphatic vessels. The adventitia can extend from 300 to 500 μm in diameter beyond which it is considered perivascular stroma and epicardial fat.

The appearance of the three-layered appearance by intravascular ultrasound occurs due to the acoustic impedance between adjacent structures. For example, the lumen and intima are usually well-delineated due to the large acoustic impedance between fluid and tissue. The three-layered appearance of the vessel wall is dependent on the intima being of sufficient size to be identified with the resolution of the current generation of ultrasound transducers and in the presence of a sufficient acoustic interface between media and adventitia.[3] At a frequency of 30 MHz, the threshold of intimal thickening required to resolve a definite intimal layer is approximately 160 μm. Previous work has shown that there is a progressive increase in the thickness of the intimal layer with increasing age.[4] In an autopsy study done to evaluate the relationship between ultrasound images and tissue histology in 16 intact hearts from subjects ranging in age from 13 to 55 years with no history of coronary artery disease, segments with a three-layered appearance had a significantly greater intimal thickness (243 ± 105 μm) than non-layered segments (112 ± 55 μm) with a threshold between the two of 178 μm.[4] As this threshold is crossed in males over the age of 30 years, it is apparent that histologically normal arteries will only have a two-layered appearance in the rare patients younger than this undergoing ultrasound examination.

The media appears as a thin middle layer by intravascular ultrasound and is often referred to as the sonolucent zone as it is less echodense than the intima or adventitia due to a lesser collagen content. Intravascular ultrasound imaging was performed *in vitro* on six histologically normal and 104 minimally diseased arteries in patients aged 13 to 83 years to test the hypothesis that normal coronary arteries produce a three-layer image that corresponds to the histologic layers of intima, media and adventitia.[5] The results showed a very strong correlation between area of the echolucent ultrasound layer with the media and the inner echogenic layer with intimal area. In addition, a three-layered appearance was consistently seen when the internal elastic membrane was present with or without intimal hyperplasia. If the internal elastic membrane was absent, a three-layer appearance was still seen if the collagen content of the media was low. However, a two-layer appearance was observed when there was absence of the internal elastic membrane as well as a high collagen content of the media.[5] In addition, the relative composition of the intimal layer also determined the ability to discriminate the three vessel wall layers. Thus, over a given coronary artery segment, the three-layered appearance may alternate with a two-layered appearance due to the relative content of elastin and collagen. However, for the purposes of quantitation, the acoustic impedance between the combination of adventitia and external elastic lamina with the intima permits accurate measurement of plaque and vessel area. In the left main stem and at the proximal part of the right coronary artery, the three-layered appearance may be lost due to the increase in elastin content in transition from the highly elastic aortic root.

ATHEROSCLEROTIC DISEASE

Intravascular ultrasound is the current imaging technology of choice for studying the morphology of atherosclerotic plaque *in vivo* and continues to have an important diagnostic role (Table 23.1). Early studies used a large 8 F catheter to correlate ultrasound appearances with histological findings in arteries collected at the time of autopsy.[6] The arteries studied were a combination of elastic, transitional (musculo-elastic) and muscular types with respect to media/adventitia appearance. The results confirmed that a highly accurate measurement of luminal area was achieved comparing ultrasound to direct measurement of perfused isolated arteries. A distinct interface between media and adventitia was obtained only where there was a significant difference in the acoustic qualities of the two layers (namely, loose collagen in the adventitia of elastic arteries or where there was a minimal smooth muscle cell component in the adventitia of transitional/muscular arteries). The interface between plaque and media

TABLE 23.1 – DIAGNOSTIC ROLE OF IVUS

- Detection of angiographically silent disease
  - ostial lesions
  - syndrome X
  - transplant vasculopathy
- Assessment of an ambiguous angiographic appearance
- Estimation of functional stenosis severity

was only apparent where there was a dense internal elastic lamina or a significant amount of necrotic material in the plaque.

The earliest accumulations of atherosclerotic plaque consist of crescentic intimal thickening of an intermediate echointensity. A common site for initial and increased plaque accumulation occurs at branch points and bifurcations due to the shear stress effect of blood flow. Transplant vasculopathy is a good model for the early development of coronary artery disease as these patients undergo ultrasound studies at angiographic follow-up early after transplantation. In one study, intravascular ultrasound was used to study epicardial arteries in 25 recently transplanted hearts from young donors (mean age 28 years).[7] In this unique study group, all donors aged under 25 years had a homogeneous non-layered vessel wall. Another group of donors of mean age 32 years manifested a three-layered appearance. In five hearts, significant eccentric intimal thickening > 500 µm was shown in donors with risk factors for coronary disease, implying early coronary disease in the presence of angiographically normal arteries. Subsequent work by the same group in a larger group of transplant recipients over a period of long-term follow-up has shown that all 60 hearts had variable degree of concentric intimal thickening after 1 year, 42 of whom had normal coronary arteries at angiography.[8]

Occasionally, image interpretation can be obscured in abnormal vessels due to incorrect assumptions of the borders of the vessel layers traced manually. This can occur because the internal elastic lamina may not be a separate layer in the presence of plaque. Media may also appear unusually thick due to attenuation of the ultrasound beam passing through intimal plaque. By contrast, the media layer may also be thinner than expected due to the spread of the signal from an area of high reflectivity (plaque) to a low one (media). For these reasons, the outer border of the plaque is usually defined as at the media/adventitia border (the external elastic lamina) which is believed to be a fair assumption given the relative contribution of media to the plaque area. It is implicit in image interpretation that frames are selected with the best image quality and done so by an experienced operator.

With a greater accumulation of plaque, there is a greater complexity to the plaque which may be differentiated by broad ultrasound criteria. A fibrous plaque has an echodensity intermediate between less echodense media or lipid and more echodense calcification. Thus by comparing the brightness of the tissue in question to that of the adventitia, a relative grading of the plaque may be obtained. Such fibrous plaques with similar brightness to adventitia may then be described as hard or soft (with respect to the grey scale) depending on the presence or absence of shadowing behind the plaque (Fig. 23.2). Fatty plaques are significantly more echolucent and when large may be appreciated as lipid pools. However, because shadowing in relation to a fibrous plaque may be misinterpreted as a lipid collection, there is a tendency to broadly classify plaques containing lipid as fibrofatty in nature.

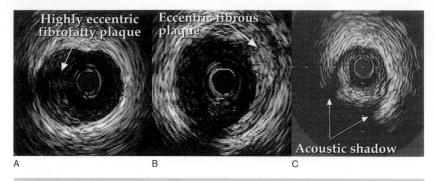

Figure 23.2:
These three panels demonstrate different plaque morphologies. (a) The left panel shows a concentric mild fatty plaque which is less echodense than adventitia. (b) The middle panel shows an extensive fibrofatty plaque with echodensity similar to adventitia. (c) The right panel is a more echodense eccentric plaque with an area of acoustic shadowing between 5 and 8 o'clock due to the presence of dense fibrous plaque.

Calcification is commonly seen by intravascular ultrasound as a bright echo with shadowing behind often associated with reverberation artifact in the area of the shadow due to oscillation of the ultrasound beam between calcium and transducer (Fig. 23.3). Calcium may be seen in relatively small plaque accumulations indicating the age of the plaque or the site of previous plaque rupture and repair. In one series of patients undergoing balloon angioplasty, 82% of arterial segments exhibited small areas of calcium which were visible in only 8% of angiograms at the lesion site or in 155 of more proximal segments by fluoroscopy.[9] In the

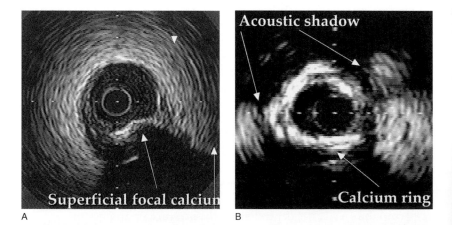

Figure 23.3:
These two images demonstrate the ultrasound fingerprint of (a) a superficial fibrocalcific plaque with an acoustic shadow immediately behind the calcific rim and an acoustic reverberation in this area at 5 o'clock, and (b) a dense cicatrix of calcium in all four quadrants of the image with extensive acoustic shadowing.

GUIDE (Guidance by Ultrasound Imaging for Decision Endpoints) trial (Phase I), 70% of target lesions had areas of calcium by ultrasound, compared to 40% of angiograms.[10] Calcification may be graded from absent (0) to severe (3+) by the extent of the arc subtended by a fibrocalcific matrix.[11] In general, at least 180 degrees of calcium is required to achieve a mass of calcium identifiable by angiography (74% identification by fluoroscopy) increasing to 86% of cases identified if more than two quadrants or calcium length ≥ 6 mm is present.[12]

By definition, plaque calcification results in shadowing of deeper structures, obscuring evaluation of underlying arterial wall components. Furthermore, shadowing may occur without any obvious calcification as the calcium may be out of plane and not visualised unless hit by the ultrasound beam in a perpendicular fashion. The calcium may be distributed in the plaque in several ways: as a deep deposit in an arc at the intima-media border, in a superficial rim at the luminal surface, or as a concretion within a fibrous plaque (Fig. 23.4). In one study of 110 patients, superficial calcium was present in 50%, deep calcium in 15% and both in 35%.[12] On occasion, the fibrous cap may be intensely echoreflective with shadowing extending to and around the periphery of the artery suggesting a more uniform distribution of calcium throughout the wall. Dense fibrotic plaques may be sufficiently underpenetrated by the ultrasound beam to cause significant shadowing, and such plaques are usually referred to as fibrocalcific.

The presence of thrombus is often more difficult to establish as it is frequently mistaken for soft plaque.[13] Thrombus often appears as a scintillating mass with a lobular edge and classically moves in an

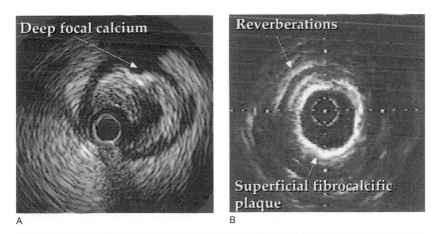

A   B

Figure 23.4:
These images demonstrate different distributions of calcium. (a) The left panel demonstrates an area of echodensity between 12 and 1 o'clock posterior to the intimal plaque indicative of deep wall calcium. (b) The right panel represents a superficial ring of calcium with reverberations readily visible (arrows).

undulating manner separate from the movement of the artery. Incomplete microchannels are sometimes identified but many intra-coronary thrombi may be very difficult to differentiate as they may be relatively small and not very separate from the arterial wall. Luminal blood is characterised by a continually mobile speckled pattern. In contrast to conventional echocardiography, the gain of the intravascular ultrasound console should be set to allow its identification separate from possible thrombus. Where the flow of blood is significantly impaired, the backscatter may be sufficiently intense to mimic thrombus or soft plaque. It may be differentiated from the latter by injection of saline converting the lumen briefly to greater echolucency. Advanced signal analysis of the radiofrequency pattern may help to provide a rational and objective criteria to differentiate thrombus from fibrofatty plaque.[14]

Intravascular ultrasound has confirmed the observations first made by Glagov *et al.* that with increasing plaque accumulation, there is a remodelling process whereby the vessel expands to accommodate the plaque load.[15] The extent of remodelling in a given artery may be highly variable with segments of positive remodelling, no change, and negative remodelling (shrinkage). Even in angiographically normal segments, the average plaque burden in the normal reference segment may comprise 40% of the total vessel cross-sectional area. The inability of angiography to detect this occult disease is due to the presence of positive arterial remodelling and the diffuse nature of disease throughout the entire vessel length in many patients. It has been suggested that discrete coronary artery lesions only become apparent angiographically when the accumulation of plaque above a threshold of 40% of vessel area for example overcomes the ability of the vessel to expand any further.[16–18]

CORONARY INTERVENTION

Intravascular ultrasound has provided an invaluable insight into the characteristics of atherosclerotic plaque with an accurate on-line means for measuring the dimensions of the index artery prior to and after intervention. Furthermore, the reduction in the diameter of ultrasound catheters (to less than 1 mm in diameter) has allowed an assessment to be made prior to intervention as well as describing vessel morphology after the procedure. Additionally, it may provide additional prognostic information regarding the likelihood of acute and subacute vessel closure and longer-term restenosis. In the context of stenting, an improved clinical outcome may be achieved with ultrasound guidance (Table 23.2).

Pre-intervention imaging

With the development of catheters as small as 2.6 F, intravascular ultrasound may be used to assess lesions prior to intervention and direct appropriate therapy. In general, there are two major determinants of device selection – plaque load or burden, and the extent and severity of calcification. With an extensive plaque load, a debulking strategy has

TABLE 23.2 – INTERVENTIONAL ROLE OF IVUS

PRE-INTERVENTION

- Accurate quantitation and balloon sizing
- Assessment of reference segment disease
- Device selection strategy with respect to plaque load and calcification

POST-INTERVENTION

- Recognition of dissection and thrombus
- Prognostic assessment
- Optimal stent deployment

become common in interventional practice. Directional coronary atherectomy has been used to debulk lesions although it is only generally successful when the lesion is free of superficial calcium. In the latter case, high speed rotational atherectomy may be used to ablate superficial calcium in lesions with a large plaque load, either as a stand alone procedure or in preparation for further treatment.[19]

In one study of pre-intervention imaging, 313 target lesions underwent intravascular ultrasound resulting in a change of therapy in 40% of cases.[20] This comprised 6% of patients who underwent therapy where none had been planned due to a significant disparity in the assessment of lesion severity between ultrasound and angiography; 7% had revascularisation deferred for the same reason, and a further 13% had a change in revascularisation strategy or selection including referral for bypass surgery in 1% due to demonstration of unsuspected significant unprotected left main involvement.[20]

Accurate balloon sizing is central to achieving the largest acute lumen gain after balloon angioplasty and with ultrasound, it is possible to demonstrate arterial remodelling and vessel expansion adjacent to diseased segments and balloon size accordingly. A strong argument for the use of intravascular ultrasound (IVUS) in balloon angioplasty is that it may allow a 'stent-like' result to be achieved by optimising the acute lumen gain from balloon dilatation alone. To investigate the safety of such an approach in selected cases, the CLOUT (Clinical Outcomes with Ultrasound Trial) pilot trial has been reported.[21] This is a multicentre investigation of the use of IVUS in balloon 'over-sizing' to achieve an improved acute outcome. The authors hypothesised that adaptive remodelling at the lesion site and in adjacent segments would accommodate this approach. Angiographically guided balloon angioplasty was performed in 104 lesions in 102 patients (types B1 and B2 lesions). IVUS was then performed to measure the proximal and distal reference segments, and if remodelling was present, a larger balloon size was calculated from whichever of the proximal or distal reference segments was smallest from the formula: balloon size = (mean lumen diameter + mean vessel diameter)/2. Quarter size balloons were then used to achieve this with increased balloon sizes ranging from 0.25 to 1.25 mm. The mean   **289** reference segment plaque area was 51 ± 15%. A total of 73% of patients had balloon up-sizing, increasing the balloon:artery ratio from 1.12 ± 0.15 to 1.30 ± 0.17. As a result, minimum lumen diameter increased from 1.95 ± 0.49 to 2.21 ± 0.47 mm (percent diameter stenosis decreased from 28 ± 15% to 18 ± 14%). Despite this more aggressive balloon sizing strategy, the angiographic dissection rate was unchanged (37% vs 40%) with no increase in major complication rate (1.9%). Whether or not this more aggressive approach impacts on clinical outcome is awaited.

One study performed to see whether IVUS guidance of balloon angioplasty leads to better outcome is the SIPS (Strategy of IVUS-guided PTCA and Stenting) trial.[22] Patients enrolled in the study were randomised to either IVUS-guidance using the ORACLE FOCUS™ balloon – a combined balloon catheter and ultrasound transducer – or angiographic guidance of standard practice of balloon dilatation. The aim of the study was to achieve > 65% reference minimal lumen area. A total of 355 lesions in 269 patients were enrolled with a 50% stent rate in both arms of the study. IVUS-guided angioplasty resulted in an increased MLD with a reduction in percent diameter stenosis (Table 23.3). A similar acute gain was also seen in patients receiving stents with IVUS-guidance, perhaps reflecting smaller vessels in the IVUS-guided stent group. Procedural success was higher in the IVUS-guided group. No significant difference in duration, contrast use, maximum inflation pressure or equipment used was seen although there was a trend towards a lower number of balloon catheters used in the IVUS-guided arm, 1.22 ± 0.94 vs 1.39 ± 1.03. With respect to acute outcome, there were no deaths and no difference in myocardial infarction (MI), but there was an increase in target vessel revascularisation in the standard angioplasty group, 4.6% vs 0.8%, resulting in a major adverse cardiac event rate (MACE) of 6.1% vs 0.8% ($p < 0.05$), compared with the IVUS-guided group. Of interest, those undergoing IVUS-guided percutaneous transluminal coronary angioplasty (PTCA) had the lowest target segment revascularisation over the follow-up period of almost 2 years. This reflected the fact that stenting was conditional and many patients received a stent because of a complication

TABLE 23.3 – THE SIPS TRIAL			
	ANGIO-GUIDED	IVUS-GUIDED	*p* VALUE
Follow-up (days)	594 ± 280	623 ± 294	–
Acute gain (mm)			
– All	2.36 ± 0.6	2.54 ± 0.6	0.02
– PTCA	1.94 ± 0.5	2.16 ± 0.5	<0.0001
– Stent	2.75 ± 0.5	2.88 ± 0.5	NS
Acute success	87.7%	94.5%	0.03
TLR (total)	29%	18%	NS
TLR in vessels <3 mm	28%	15%	0.04

TLR: target lesion revascularisation.

at the time of intervention. Furthermore, with IVUS-guidance, larger balloons were used due to the recognition of remodelling in diseased segments, accounting for stenting in smaller vessels in this group. Once stented, no difference was seen with respect to major events however. The long-term clinical results of this trial are awaited.

Post-intervention imaging

One of the common indications for an intravascular ultrasound study is to assess the appearance of a coronary artery following an interventional procedure. This is performed for several reasons – to examine the resulting morphologic appearance from the intervention, to judge success, to complement angiographic assessment, to quantitate lumen enlargement and plaque reduction, and to consider whether or not to proceed to further intervention including stent implantation. Once stenting is undertaken, ultrasound may used to guide optimal expansion which has been investigated in several trials completed or nearing completion.

Balloon angioplasty

Initial *in vitro* validation studies were done to correlate the appearance of diseased arteries at ultrasound post-balloon dilatation with histology.[23] The consistent finding following balloon dilatation was tearing of the plaque with separation of the ends of the tear and an increase in lumen cross-sectional area, with some stretching of the less diseased wall. In this study, the lumen area by ultrasound and at section were similar ($R = 0.88$).[23] Dissection of the plaque (separation of intima from media) was a common finding which appeared as an increase in the sonolucent area corresponding to media. One feature described was the presence of arterial flaps with protrusion of plaque into the lumen, less frequently seen *in vivo* due to blood flow.

The presence of calcium in a coronary lesion determines the response of the artery to balloon dilatation. In one study of patients after balloon angioplasty of peripheral and coronary vessels, intralesional calcium and the relative size of dissection for each lesion was determined.[24] A total of 76% of patients had significant dissection/plaque fracture after angioplasty. In 71% of these patients, significant localised calcium deposits were identified within the plaque, and the vast majority of dissections (87%) were adjacent to the calcific portion of the wall. Comparing the relative size of dissections with respect to the neoluminal area, dissections in calcified areas were larger than those in lesions without calcium, 28% vs 11%, respectively. It was concluded that localised calcium had a direct role in promoting dissection by increasing shear stress within the plaque at the junction between tissue types with differing elastic properties.[25] Given these findings, it may be that deep calcium deposits protect against deep medial injury despite a large plaque fracture by deflecting the pressure axially. Further characterisation of lesion morphology with newer ultrasound catheters is required to address these issues in a clinical context.

An important use for intravascular ultrasound in interventional procedures is that it can accurately measure lumen and vessel area both at the lesion site and at the reference segment allowing the operator to size angioplasty balloons more exactly. In a key study of 223 coronary vessels treated by a Palmaz–Schatz stent, directional atherectomy or laser balloon angioplasty, 83% of patients underwent follow-up angiography 6 months after treatment.[25] The traditional dichotomous definition of restenosis (≥ 50% diameter stenosis) was used along with a cumulative graphical method. Although the restenosis rates were 19%, 31% and 50% for stents, directional atherectomy, and laser balloon angioplasty respectively, the late lumen loss was equivalent across the groups. This indicated that the major procedural determinant on restenosis was the acute lumen gain (2.6, 2.2, and 2.0 mm in the three groups) leading to the 'Bigger is Better' hypothesis.[25]

Stent deployment

The MUSIC (Multicentre Ultrasound guidance of Stents In Coronaries) trial was designed to examine the additional value of IVUS in determining optimal stent deployment with aspirin alone in vessels >3.0 mm (Fig. 23.5). Using the initial criteria of complete apposition (symmetry >0.7) and complete expansion (minimum stent area [MSA] >90% average of proximal/distal segments or MSA >100% of lowest reference segment or MSA >90% proximal segment, and subsequently revised to 80%, 90%, 80% respectively if MSA >9 mm²), a subacute thrombosis rate of 1.3% was reported at follow-up of mean 198 days.[26] The need for bypass surgery was 0.6% and repeat angioplasty was 4.5%. Of interest, even using the revised IVUS criteria, only 80% of patients achieved this.

A 6-month angiographic restenosis rate of 8.3% was reported (9.3% if the stent thrombosis cases were included) which is a remarkable result suggesting a major clinical benefit form IVUS-guided stent deployment and this data largely led to the design of the OPTICUS trial.

In OPTICUS (OPTimal Intra-Coronary Ultrasound in Stenting), a multicentre, *randomised* trial of 550 patients with angiographic follow-up has been recently reported.[27] The primary endpoints were defined as binary restenosis and angiographic MLD at 6 months follow-up. The secondary endpoints were 6- and 12-month clinical follow-up and the economics of ultrasound-guided stenting. Again, patients were randomised to angiography- or IVUS-guided stent deployment of either Palmaz–Schatz or NIR stents (thus giving OPTICUS the angiography arm for comparison that MUSIC didn't have). Lesions were more challenging that described in the Benestent or Stress trials with 62% AHA/ACC type B2 and 15% type C lesions. The MUSIC expansion criteria were achieved in 64% of patients. Initial reports from the study have confirmed a reduction in the need for repeat in-hospital angioplasty although at follow-up despite an

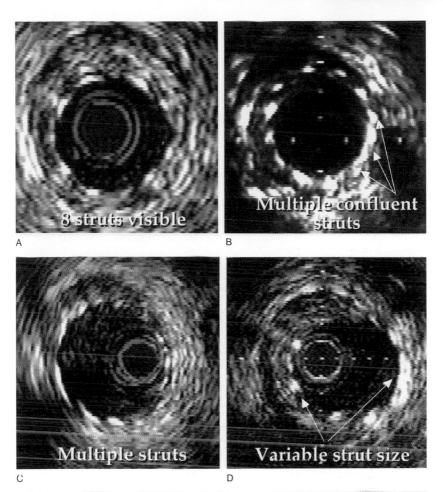

Figure 23.5:
A series of fully deployed intra-coronary stents. (a) The MicroStent™, which has a basic design of continuous wire segments in a zig-zag design with eight axial struts connected by eight radiused crowns. On ultrasound imaging, this stent is identifiable by the presence of eight equally spaced struts/frame when fully expanded. (b) The Wallstent, which is a self-expanding mesh design and made of a cobalt-based alloy with a platinum core. The ultrasound appeareance is characterised by a multiple struts closely apposed around the lumen interface. (c) The MultiLink™ Stent, a slotted tube stent with multiple visible struts by ultrasound. (d) The Crossflex stent, which is a coil design with the stainless steel wire describing a sinusoidal pattern giving an appearance of unequal arcs by ultrasound.

improved minimal luminal diameter (MLD) post-stent (and an impressive increase in angiography-guided post-stent MLD), clinical and angiographic outcome was no different comparing both groups.[27]

To evaluate objectively whether ultrasound-guided stent deployment results in an additional clinical benefit over angiography alone, the CRUISE (Can Routine Ultrasound Influence Stent Expansion?) substudy of STARS (STent Anti-thrombotic Regimen Study) has now been reported.[28] Patients undergoing ultrasound-guided stent deployment in nine centres were compared with seven centres in which stenting was guided by angiography alone followed by blinded IVUS assessment (IVUS-documentary). A total of 499 patients were followed up from an initial 525 patients with larger balloon sizing (3.88 ± 0.51 vs 3.69 ± 0.59 mm, $p < 0.001$) and greater dilatation pressure (18.0 ± 2.6 vs 16.6 ± 3.0 atmospheres, $p < 0.001$) used in the IVUS-guided and IVUS-documentary groups, respectively. A total of 36% of patients in the IVUS-guided group had a change in deployment strategy based on the ultrasound images. This was associated with superior stent expansion (MSA) in the IVUS-guided group, 7.78 ± 1.72 mm^2 vs 7.06 ± 2.13 mm^2 ($p < 0.001$). At 9-month follow-up, a 44% reduction in the clinical end-point of target vessel revascularisation (TVR) was demonstrated (8.5% vs 15.3%, $p < 0.05$) (Table 23.4).[28] This was an encouraging clinical outcome although the apparent benefits of IVUS guidance could have been accentuated by other differences in treatment between the different centres, given the operators' individual discretion regarding optimisation of final stent deployment. Also, a clinical restenosis rate (TVR) rather than angiographic restenosis rate was selected as a primary endpoint in CRUISE and yet a significantly greater number of multivessel disease patients were in the IVUS-documentary group (44%) compared with the IVUS-guided group (27%), although this was not an independent predictor of TVR by multivariate analysis.[28]

The AVID (Angiography Versus Intravascular ultrasounD) trial is a multicentre comparison of IVUS-guided stenting with angiography-guided stenting, similar in concept to the CRUISE study. The initial results were reported in 1999.[29] A total of 759 patients undergoing elective single or multiple stent placement in native vessels >2.5 mm or saphenous vein grafts in 24 centres were included. Patients were randomised after optimal angiography-guided stent deployment (<10% residual stenosis). In the angiography-guided group, documentary IVUS was performed (with un-blinding only if significant dissection was noted [2.6%]). In the IVUS-guided group, larger balloons or additional stents were required in 43% of cases to achieve the criteria of full stent apposition and MSA >90% of the distal reference area. As a result, the final MSA was greater in the

TABLE 23.4 – THE CRUISE TRIAL			
	ANGIO-GUIDED	IVUS-GUIDED	p VALUE
Number of patients	229	270	–
Death	2	0	NS
MI	14	19	NS
TVR	35 (15.3%)	23 (8.5%)	0.02

MI: myocardial infarction.
TVR: target vessel revascularisation

IVUS-guided group (7.54 ± 2.86 mm^2 vs 6.94 ± 2.46 mm^2, $p < 0.01$). After 12 months follow-up, the primary clinical endpoint of target lesion revascularisation (TLR) was 8.4% in the IVUS-guided group versus 12.4% in the angiography-guided group ($p = 0.08$). When protocol violations such as the inclusion of vessels smaller than 2.5 mm were excluded, the difference achieved statistical significance, 4.9% vs 10.8% ($p = 0.02$). The benefit of IVUS-guidance was particularly evident in three subgroups – saphenous vein grafts (TLR 5.7% versus 20.4%, $p = 0.05$), vessels with a diameter stenosis greater than 70% (TLR 3.5% vs 14.9%, $p = 0.003$), and vessels with a distal reference diameter less than 3.25 mm (TLR 7.9% vs 14.6%, $p = 0.04$).

Although the availability of recent generation balloon expandable stents has diminished the practice of high pressure (>14 atmospheres) dilatation, the OSTI (Optimal StenT Implantation) trial was completed in North America. This trial was designed to study the relationship between balloon pressure and stent deployment by IVUS. To date, 89 Palmaz–Schatz stents have been implanted in 79 lesions in 76 patients, post-dilating at 12, 15 and 18 atmospheres.[30] Palmaz–Schatz stent dimensions increase with increasing post-dilatation pressure which was described by IVUS but not quantitative angiography. Of interest, routinely used criteria for stent expansion, e.g. MUSIC criteria (37% at 12 bar, 61% at 15 bar, 74% at 18 bar) may still not be met despite 18 atmospheres pressure and a balloon: artery ration > 1.1 (Table 23.5). In the second OSTI study, focal balloons achieved maximal stent expansion within 0.2 mm of the external elastic lamina resulting in a clinical restenosis rate (target lesion revascularisation) of 8.3%.[31]

High-speed rotational atherectomy

Rotational atherectomy uses a rotating diamond-coated burr to abrade atherosclerotic plaque at speeds as high as 180 000 rpm. The technique works through the method of differential cutting whereby the burr selectively abrades harder tissue and is deflected away from normal vessel

TABLE 23.5 – THE OSTI TRIAL				
	12 atm	**15 atm**	**18 atm**	**p VALUE**
Balloon diameter (mm)	3.30	3.38	3.48	0.0001
Balloon: artery ratio	1.06	1.08	1.13	0.0001
MLD by QCA (mm)	2.78	2.84	2.86	NS
MLD by IVUS (mm)	2.72	2.91	3.04	0.0001
% Diameter stenosis (QCA)	10.6%	9.1%	8.5%	NS
% Diameter stenosis (IVUS)	6.2%	-0.4%	-4.7%	0.0001
Lumen area by IVUS (mm^2)	7.1	8.0	8.6	0.0001

MLD: minimal luminal diameter.
QCA: quantitative coronary angiography.

wall thus removing superficial calcium and dense fibrous plaque through micro-embolisation, pushing softer plaque away from the cutting path of the device. The appearance of vessels undergoing rotational atherectomy as a debulking strategy has been described.[32] In this study, 28 patients (22 calcified plaques, a third of which were circumferential) underwent ultrasound imaging after the procedure (with 71% having adjunct balloon angioplasty). Following rotablation, a distinct, circular intima-lumen interface was achieved with the lumen size 20% larger than the largest burr used. Deviations from a circular geometry occurred only in areas of soft plaque or superficial tissue disruption of calcified plaque. This study confirmed that there was no significant damage to the media and no dissections were caused by the procedure. A residual plaque load of 54% was reported indicating that athero-ablation using a burr strategy of 70–80% of the reference vessel lumen by angiography still resulted in a significant residual plaque even with adjunctive balloon dilatation in the majority of patients.[32]

A subsequent study of sequential ultrasound imaging before and after rotational atherectomy did confirm dissection planes in 26% of cases following rotablation increasing to 76% of cases after adjunct balloon dilatation with spread of the dissection plane to areas not only with the calcified plaque but also adjacent to the plaque, in part contributing to the expansion of the lumen area.[33] There was a reduction in plaque area from 15.7 ± 4.1 to 13.0 ± 4.7 mm^2 after initial rotablation, but still a residual percent cross-sectional narrowing of 74% indicating the need for adjunct balloon angioplasty to achieve an adequate final lumen area. In this study, the arc of calcium decreased significantly with full thickness calcium removal in some patients. Even without a measurable decrease in calcium arc, significant calcium ablation still occurred as evidenced by an increase in lumen area, uncovering of deeper calcium deposits, and the uncovering of deeper adventitial structures not seen pre-rotational atherectomy. In everyday practice, pre-interventional ultrasound scanning can direct athero-ablation appropriately. Superficial calcium not apparent by angiography is amenable to successful rotablation if the calcium arc is > 180 degrees and extends to more than half of the lesion length. This preliminary debulking may then be supplemented by balloon angioplasty or intra-coronary stenting.

One particular complementary role of IVUS and rotablation may be in the treatment of in-stent restenosis. Although several small studies exist, it is only within the last 2 years that a randomised controlled trial has been conceived – ARTIST (Angioplasty versus Rotablation for Treatment of Intra-STent Stenosis/Occlusion).[34] This is a multicentre trial randomising patients with intra-stent restenosis or occlusion to balloon angioplasty or rotablation in restenosed or occluded stents in native vessels. Important exclusion criteria are coil stents, stents deployed distal to or at bend points > 45 degrees, and stents not fully expanded by angiography or pre-procedure ultrasound. The primary endpoints of the study are acute success with quantitative angiographic assessment after the procedure (diameter stenosis < 30% visually without additional stenting is defined a procedural success) and at 6 months follow-up. Preliminary data has reported an angiographic restenosis rate of 42% with a clinical restenosis rate of 36%.[34] The acute and long-term outcome in 100 patients was recently reported and confirmed slow-flow in only 3% with only 2% sustaining an enzyme rise of > 3 × creatine-kinase.[35] With quantitative IVUS, 77% of acute gain occurred through rotablation and 23% through adjunctive balloon dilatation. At a mean of 13 months follow-up, repeat in-stent restenosis occurred in 28% with a target vessel revascularisation (TVR) of 26%.

SUMMARY

The use of intravascular ultrasound to answer questions not adequately addressed by angiography has established it as an important technology in the catheter laboratory, both in a diagnostic setting and as a support to intervention. The extent of IVUS use has been defined by existing studies with several clinical trials on the use of intravascular ultrasound in optimising both balloon angioplasty and intra-coronary stenting completed. The initial data from CLOUT confirms that the adjunctive use of IVUS improves the acute result of balloon angioplasty with no increase in major acute complications. The improvement in procedural success and reduction in early adverse events from SIPS suggests that IVUS is of value when used with balloon angioplasty alone. The MUSIC trial confirmed a reduction in stent restenosis rate using IVUS to direct high-pressure inflation, but with the objective comparison with angiography alone in OPTICUS, the expected improved clinical outcome did not materialise. Initial results from CRUISE confirm superior IVUS-guided stent expansion with a better clinical outcome compared to angiographic guidance. Based on the AVID trial, certain subgroups may be identified as having particular benefit – saphenous vein grafts, more severe stenoses (implying a greater plaque load) and smaller vessels. Although initial studies suggested a role for IVUS earlier in the decision-making process after balloon angioplasty, with the hope of an IVUS-defined 'stent-like' result from balloon dilatation leading to a policy of provisional stenting, the near universal use of stents in interventional practice has diminished this practice. IVUS will allow a superior deployment of a stent in many cases. In addition to its important role in clinical research, and its utility in defining unusual or ambiguous angiographic appearances, the evidence suggests that it is of additional benefit in improving the medium-term clinical outcome in selected patients at increased risk of restenosis.

REFERENCES

1. Yock PG, Fitzgerald PJ, Popp RL. Intravascular ultrasound. Sci Am 1995;2:68–77.

2. Waller BF. The eccentric coronary atherosclerotic plaque: morphologic observations and clinical relevance. Clin Cardiol 1989;12:14.

3. Picano E, Landini L, Lattanzi F et al. Time domain echo pattern evaluations from normal and atherosclerotic arterial walls: a study in vitro. Circulation 1988;3:654.

4. Fitzgerald PJ, St. Goar FG, Connolly RJ et al. Intravascular ultrasound imaging of coronary arteries. Is three layers the norm? Circulation 1992;86:154–8.

5. Maheswaran B, Leung CY, Gutfinger DE et al. Intravascular ultrasound appearance of normal and mildly diseased coronary arteries – correlation with histologic specimens. Am Heart J 1995;130:976–86.

6. Nishimura RA, Edwards WD, Warnes CA et al. Intravascular ultrasound imaging: in vitro validation and pathologic correlation. J Am Coll Cardiol 1990;16:145–54.

7. St. Goar FG, Pinto FJ, Alderman EL et al. Intra-coronary ultrasound in cardiac transplant recipients: *in vivo* evidence of 'angiographically silent' intimal thickening. Circulation 1992;85:979–87.

8. St. Goar FG, Pinto FJ, Alderman EL et al. Detection of coronary atherosclerosis in young adult hearts using intravascular ultrasound. Circulation 1992;86:756–63.

9. Tobis JM, Mallery J, Mahon D et al. Intravascular ultrasound imaging of human coronary arteries in vivo: analysis of tissue characterization with comparison to in vitro histological specimens. Circulation 1991;83:319–26.

10. GUIDE trial investigators. IVUS-determined predictors of restenosis in PTCA and DCA: final report from the GUIDE trial, Phase II. J Am Coll Cardiol 1996;27:156A (Abstract).

11. Farb A, Virmani R, Atkinson JB, Kolodgie FD. Plaque morphology and pathologic changes in arteries from patients dying after coronary balloon angioplasty. J Am Coll Cardiol 1990;16:1421–9.

12. Mintz GS, Douek P, Pichard A et al. Target lesion calcification in coronary artery disease: an intravascular ultrasound study. J Am Coll Cardiol 1992;20:1149–55.

13. Siegel RJ, Ariani M, Fishbein MC et al. Histopathologic validation of angioscopy and intravascular ultrasound. Circulation 1991;84:109–117.

14. Metz JA, Preuss P, Komiyama N et al. Discrimination of soft plaque and thrombus based on radiofrequency analysis of intravascular ultrasound. J Am Coll Cardiol 1996;27(Suppl. A);200A (Abstract).

15. Glagov S, Weisenberg E, Zarins CK, Stankunavicius R, Kolettis GJ. Compensatory enlargement of human atherosclerotic arteries. N Engl J Med 1987;316:1371–5.

16. Kakuta T, Currier JW, Haudenschild CC, Ryan TJ, Faxon DP. Differences in compensatory vessel enlargement, not intimal formation, account for restenosis after angioplasty in the hypercholesterolemic rabbit model. Circulation 1994;89:2809–15.

17. Post MJ, Borst C, Kuntz RE. The relative importance of arterial remodeling compared with intimal hyperplasia in lumen renarrowing after balloon angioplasty. Circulation 1994;89:2816–21.

18. Currier JW, Faxon DP. Restenosis after percutaneous transluminal coronary angioplasty: have we been aiming at the wrong target? J Am Coll Cardiol 1995;25:516–20.

19. Ellis SG, Popma JJ, Buchbinder M et al. relation of clinical presentation, stenosis morphology, and operator technique to the procedural results of rotational atherectomy-facilitated angioplasty. Circulation 1994;89:882–92.

20. Mintz GS, Pichard AD, Kovach JA et al. Impact of pre-intervention intravascular ultrasound imaging on transcatheter treatment strategies in coronary artery disease. Am J Cardiol 1994;73:423–30.

21. Stone GW, Linnemeier T, St. Goar FG, Mudra H, Sheehan H, Hodgson JMcB. Improved outcome of balloon angioplasty with intra-coronary ultrasound guidance – core lab angiographic and ultrasound results from the CLOUT study. J Am Coll Cardiol 1996;27(Suppl. A):155A (Abstract).

22. Frey AW, Dörfer K, Lange W, Hodgson JB. The impact of vessel size on long-term outcome after intra-coronary ultrasound guidance on provisional stenting. Circulation 1998;98(Suppl. I):1494 (Abstract).

23. Tobis JM, Mallery JA, Gessert J et al. Intravascular ultrasound cross-sectional arterial imaging before and after balloon angioplasty in vitro. Circulation 1989;80:873–82.

24. Fitzgerald PJ, Ports TA, Yock PG. Contribution of localized calcium deposits to dissection after angioplasty. an observational study using intravascular ultrasound. Circulation 1992;86:64–70.

25. Kuntz RE, Safian RD, Levine MJ, Reis GJ, Diver DJ, Baim DS. Novel approach to the analysis of restenosis after the use of three new coronary devices. J Am Coll Cardiol 1992;19:1493–9.

26. de Jaegere P, Mudra H, Figulla H et al. for the MUSIC Study Investigators. Intravascular ultrasound-guided optimized stent deployment. Immediate and 6 months clinical and angiographic results from the Multicenter Ultrasound Stenting in Coronaries Study (MUSIC study) Eur Heart J 1998;19:1214–23.

27. Mudra H, Macaya C, Zahn R et al. Interim analysis of the Optimization with ICUS to reduce stent restenosis. Circulation 1998:98(Suppl. I):1908 (Abstract).

28. Fitzgerald PJ, Oshima A, Hayase M et al. Final results of the Can Routine Ultrasound Influence Stent Expansion (CRUISE) study? Circulation 2000;102:523–30.

29. Russo RJ, Attubato MS, Davidson CJ, DeFranco AC, Fitzgerald PJ, Iaffaldano RA et al. Angiography versus intravascular ultrasound-directed stent placement: final results from AVID. Circulation 1999;100(Suppl. I);I–234(Abstract).

30. Stone GW, St. Goar F, Fitzgerald PJ et al. The optimal stent implantation trial – final core lab angiographic and ultrasound analysis. J Am Coll Cardiol 1997:29 (Suppl. A);369A (Abstract).

31. Stone GW, Bailey S, Roberts D *et al.* Long-term results following maximal stenting using ultrasound guided focal balloon stent overexpansion – the second Optimal Stent Implantation study. Circulation 1998;98(Suppl. I):826 (Abstract).

32. Mintz GS, Potkin BN, Keren G *et al.* Intravascular ultrasound evaluation of the effect of rotational atherectomy in obstructive atherosclerotic coronary artery disease. Circulation 1992;86:1383–93.

33. Kovach JA, Mintz GS, Pichard AD *et al.* Sequential intravascular ultrasound characterization of the mechanisms of rotational atherectomy and adjunct balloon angioplasty. J Am Coll Cardiol 1993;22:1024–32.

34. Radke PW, Hoffmann R, Haager PK, Janssens U, vom Dahl J, Klues HG. Predictors of recurrent restenosis after rotational atherectomy of diffuse in-stent retenosis at 6 month angiographic follow-up: a serial intravascular ultrasound study. Circulation 1998;98(Suppl. I):3772 (Abstract).

35. Sharma SK, Duvvuri S, Dangas G *et al.* Rotational atherectomy for in-stent restenosis: acute and long-term results of the first 100 cases. J Am Coll Cardiol 1998;32:1358–65.

Section Four

Acute MI
and Shock

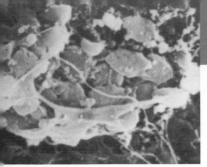

24

Angioplasty for acute myocardial infarction

KEITH D. DAWKINS

KEY POINTS

▪ Intravenous thrombolytic therapy is widely used as primary treatment in acute myocardial infarction.

▪ There are a number of contraindications to thrombolytic therapy.

▪ Acute angiography and primary PTCA has a number of advantages over 'blind' thrombolysis.

▪ Trials of primary angioplasty/stenting are reported.

▪ Routine use of stents (rather than simple balloon angioplasty) should be the norm for myocardial infarction except for exceptional circumstances.

EPIDEMIOLOGY OF MYOCARDIAL INFARCTION

The Health Survey for England suggests that 0.5% of adults have had a myocardial infarct within the last 12 months, which equates to 246 000 people. Deaths from coronary heart disease, the majority of which result from acute myocardial infarction accounted for 150 000 cases in the UK in 1995. The incidence and mortality of acute myocardial infarction is improving with time as a result of efforts targeted at primary prevention and risk factor reduction, patient awareness, paramedic ambulance personnel, coronary care units, drug therapy (e.g. aspirin, β-blockade, angiotensin converting enzyme [ACE] inhibitors), thrombolysis, rehabilitation, post infarct risk stratification and revascularisation (percutaneous transluminal coronary angioplasty [PTCA], coronary artery bypass grafting [CABG]).

This chapter will focus on the restoration of blood flow in an occluded coronary artery, in particular, comparing mechanical (PTCA/stenting) with pharmacological (thrombolytic) strategies.

PATHOGENESIS OF ACUTE MYOCARDIAL INFARCTION

Acute myocardial infarction usually results from thrombotic occlusion of a coronary artery. Angiographic and post-mortem studies of patients very early after the onset of symptoms demonstrate a high (> 85%) incidence of occlusive thrombus in the culprit artery. Other rare causes of coronary occlusion include spasm, spontaneous dissection or flap occlusion (e.g. in aortic dissection). Thrombus may either deposit on a pre-existing atheromatous flow-limiting stenosis, or suddenly de novo on a minor plaque that has ruptured (plaque-fissure). Rapid restoration of blood flow in the culprit artery by whatever means improves left ventricular function

303

and ultimately reduces mortality. Maximum benefit is achieved in the first hour after the occlusion; with later treatment the mortality benefit is attenuated. In the early hours after occlusion, there is a 1% reduction in mortality for each hour saved. Early mortality and long-term outcome following acute myocardial infarction relate to early and complete reperfusion as judged by *normal* (TIMI-3) flow in the target coronary artery (Fig. 24.1).

THROMBOLYSIS

Coronary thrombus is a mixture of white (platelet rich) and red (fibrin/erythrocyte rich) clot. Even without treatment, the incidence of thrombosis falls to 65% by 24 hours indicating that spontaneous thrombolysis occurs in some, if the patient survives the acute event. Intravenous thrombolytic therapy is widely used as primary treatment in the patient suffering an acute myocardial infarct. Despite the development of newer more specific agents (e.g. tissue plasminogen activator [t-PA]), there is little evidence that there has been a significant improvement in efficacy, despite an increase in expense, when compared with the earlier drugs (e.g. streptokinase) (Fig. 24.2). Clinical trials in more than 100 000 patients have shown that intravenous thrombolytics improve prognosis in Q-wave myocardial infarction by limiting infarct size, improving ventricular function and reducing mortality. The best reported patency rates are in the region of 80%, with TIMI-3 (normal) flow observed in only 50–60% of patients; early re-occlusion occurs in 10% of patients. Thrombolytic agents do not appear to improve prognosis in acute myocardial infarction complicated by cardiogenic shock or intractable

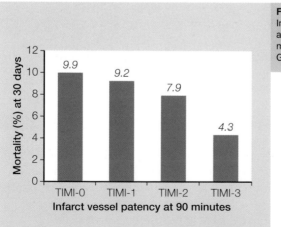

Figure 24.1:
Infarct vessel patency status at 90 minutes related to mortality at 30 days in the GUSTO-I angiographic trial.

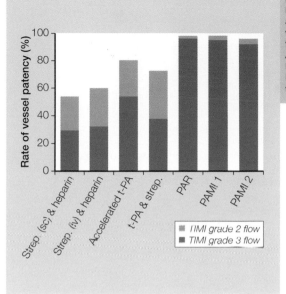

Figure 24.2:
Patency of infarct-related arteries in patients treated with primary angioplasty or thrombolysis. (PAR: Primary Angioplasty Registry. PAMI: Primary Angioplasty in Myocardial Infarction. t-PA: tissue plasminogen activator).

arrhythmias. Furthermore, many patients with non Q-wave myocardial infarct and other acute ischaemic syndromes do not benefit from thrombolytics. Haemorrhagic stroke can be anticipated in 1% of patients, and other major bleeding complications in 8%; the elderly appear to be particularly prone to haemorrhage. There are a number of contraindications to thrombolytic therapy (Table 24.1), such that 30% of patients may be ineligible for thrombolytics, either due to a contraindication, late presentation or non-diagnostic electrocardiogram [ECG] changes (Table 24.2). In many series, thrombolytic agents have only been prescribed in < 50% of eligible patients. The administration of thrombolytic agents does not require a catheterisation laboratory or specialist personnel, but can be administered by a nurse, paramedic, junior doctor, physician or cardiologist, either in hospital, in the ambulance or at the patient's home.

PRIMARY ANGIOPLASTY

The strategy of acute angiography and primary PTCA has a number of advantages over 'blind' thrombolysis. It is important to realise that the clinical (bedside) assessment of reperfusion following thrombolysis is unreliable. Normalisation of the ST segment is a poor surrogate for arterial patency, although this combined with the resolution of chest pain and a 'reperfusion' arrhythmia (e.g. accelerated idioventricular rhythm)

TABLE 24.1 – CONTRAINDICATIONS TO THROMBOLYSIS

ABSOLUTE

- Previous haemorrhagic stroke (at any time)
- Other strokes or cerebrovascular events (within 1 year)
- Intra-cranial neoplasm
- Active internal bleeding
- Suspected aortic dissection

RELATIVE

- Severe or uncontrolled systemic hypertension (BP > 180/110)
- History of previous cerebrovascular event
- Current use of anticoagulants
- Known bleeding diathesis
- Recent major trauma, including head injury (within 4 weeks)
- Recent major surgery (within 4 weeks)
- Prolonged cardiopulmonary resuscitation
- Non-compressible vascular punctures (especially arterial)
- Recent internal bleeding (within 4 weeks)
- Prior administration (within 2 years) or allergic reaction to streptokinase or anistreplase
- Active peptic ulceration
- Pregnancy

TABLE 24.2 – ECG CRITERIA FOR THROMBOLYSIS

- Sinus tachycardia segment elevation (> 0.1 mV in at least two contiguous leads)
- New bundle branch block (LBBB, RBBB)
- Time from symptom onset < 12 hours (> 12 hours in selected patients, but diminishing benefit)

may be highly suggestive of a restoration of arterial patency. Coronary angiography allows an accurate determination of arterial anatomy and left ventricular function, and patients may be risk stratified to allow early hospital discharge (Fig. 24.3). Early observational studies of primary PTCA in acute myocardial infarction indicated high recanalisation rates (> 90%), in association with a low in-hospital mortality (~ 8%) (Fig. 24.4), and a satisfactory late (1 year) survival of > 90%. Predictors associated with a favourable outcome included early reperfusion (within 2 hours of the onset of chest pain), a patent culprit artery at hospital discharge, well-preserved ventricular function, and single vessel coronary disease. Nevertheless, simple PTCA was associated with recurrent ischaemia prior to hospital discharge in 10–15% of patients, sufficient to result in reinfarction in 3–5% of patients. The predictable limitations of simple balloon angioplasty were all seen in the setting of acute myocardial infarction, including platelet activation as a consequence of intimal disruption, vessel recoil, intimal hyperplasia and late remodelling. Platelet activation resulting in a large thrombus burden proved to be a particular problem before the advent of the newer antiplatelet regimens (see below). Overall, angiographic restenosis (≥ 50% diameter) was demonstrated in

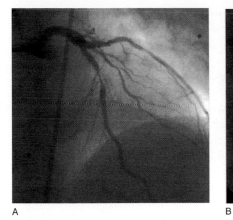 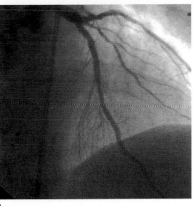

A   B

Figure 24.3:
Angiogram before (a) and after (b) angioplasty in a patient with acute lateral MI secondary to sub-acute circumflex occlusion.

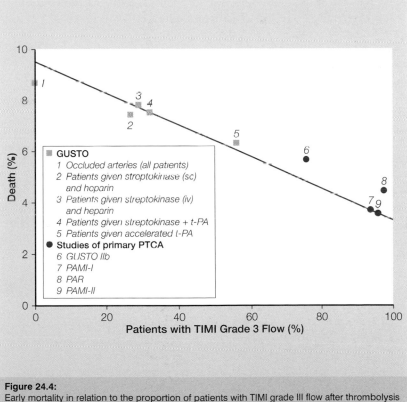

Figure 24.4:
Early mortality in relation to the proportion of patients with TIMI grade III flow after thrombolysis or primary PTCA.

30–50% of patients at 6-month follow-up, as a result of which ~ 20% of patients required target vessel revascularisation by redo PTCA or conventional CABG.

PRIMARY ANGIOPLASTY VS THROMBOLYSIS (TRIALS)

Ten trials have been published comparing simple balloon angioplasty (PTCA) with intravenous thrombolysis. Some are small (< 50 patients in each arm), inclusion criteria vary, and a variety of thrombolytic agents have been used including streptokinase (4), t-PA (3) and accelerated t-PA (3). A total of 1290 patients treated with PTCA were compared with 1316 patients in the thrombolytic group. Outcome measures included total mortality, non-fatal myocardial infarction, the composite endpoint of death and non-fatal infarction, total stroke, haemorrhagic stroke, and major bleeding (requiring blood transfusion).

Overall mortality in the PTCA group was 4.4% and 6.5% in the thrombolytic group; the reduction in mortality in the PTCA group was significant (odds ratio 0.66, 95% confidence limits 0.46–0.94, $p = 0.02$). The absolute risk reduction was 2.1% (95% CI 0.4–3.4%). In other words, 47 patients needed to be treated to save one life. Combining all trials and comparing the composite end point of death and reinfarction also favoured the PTCA arm. Death and reinfarction occurred in 7.2% of the PTCA group and 11.9% of the lytic group (odds ratio 0.58, 95% CI 0.44–0.76, $p < 0.001$). Deaths from both fatal and non-fatal reinfarction were significantly reduced in the PTCA group. Total stroke rate was significantly lower in the PTCA group (2.0% vs 0.7%, odds ratio 0.35, 95% CI 0.14–0.77, $p = 0.07$), with a ten-fold reduction in haemorrhagic stroke (1.1% vs 0.1%, odds ratio 0.07, 95% CI 0.0–0.43, $p < 0.001$). Of all the thrombolytic agents used, accelerated t-PA had a significantly worse haemorrhagic stroke rate compared with the other agents. Bleeding rates were similar for the PTCA and thrombolytic groups at 8.3% and 8.4% respectively (odds ratio 1.06, 95% CI 0.79–1.41, $p = 0.75$), and did not differ significantly between the lytic agents. It is likely that the contemporary bleeding rates for patients undergoing percutaneous intervention would be reduced by superior management of the femoral access site (including closure devices, etc). Two-year follow-up of the PAMI-I trial indicates less recurrent ischaemia in the PTCA group compared with the patients receiving t-PA (36.4% vs 48% respectively, $p = 0.026$), lower reintervention rates (27.2% vs 46.5% respectively, $p < 0.0001$), and a reduced hospital admission rate (58.5% vs 69% respectively, $p = 0.035$). The composite end point of death and reinfarction was 14.9% in the PTCA group and 23% in the lytic patients ($p = 0.034$). Multivariate logistic regression analysis found PTCA to be an independently predictive of a reduction in death, reinfarction and target vessel revascularisation ($p = 0.0001$) (Fig. 24.5).

Caution should be used when assessing the results of these trials. Most of the studies were small, patient selection was high, and many of the

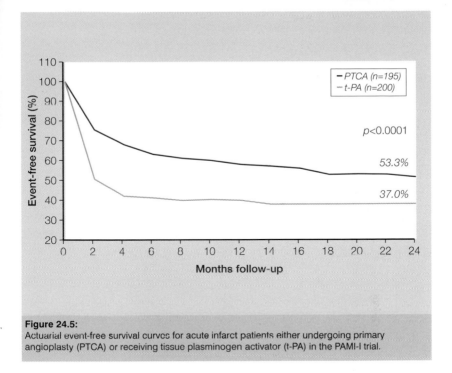

Figure 24.5:
Actuarial event-free survival curves for acute infarct patients either undergoing primary angioplasty (PTCA) or receiving tissue plasminogen activator (t-PA) in the PAMI-I trial.

reports came from high-volume operators working in single centres. The effects of delay in treatment in the PTCA arm needs further investigation. It appears that the benefit of thrombolysis is strongly dependent on time delay from the onset of symptoms, whereas this factor seems to be less critical in patients undergoing percutaneous intervention (Fig. 24.6). Furthermore, up to one-third of the mortality difference between the PTCA and lytic groups could be accounted for from death due to haemorrhagic stroke.

Changes in practice including the widespread use of intra-coronary stents and newer antiplatelet agents render the results from the simple PTCA trials largely of historical interest.

PRIMARY ANGIOPLASTY PLUS STENTING

Despite the enthusiasm for primary coronary angioplasty in selected centres and the favourable in-hospital results in the published trials, recurrent myocardial ischaemia requiring reintervention occurs in 10–15% of patients, with a reinfarction rate of 3–5%. These predictable complications occur when plain balloon angioplasty is used in a milieu of intense platelet activation resulting from both balloon induced barotrauma and the myocardial infarct per se. Furthermore unopposed vessel recoil and late remodelling results in an angiographic restenosis rate of 30–50% **309**

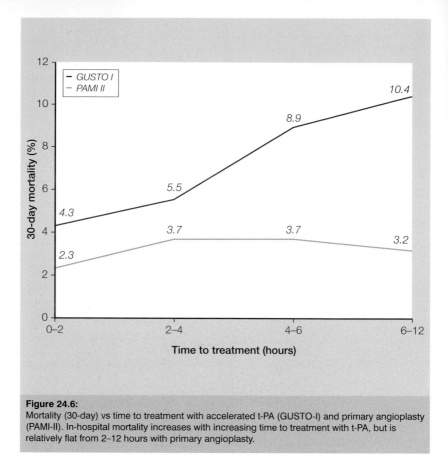

Figure 24.6:
Mortality (30-day) vs time to treatment with accelerated t-PA (GUSTO-I) and primary angioplasty (PAMI-II). In-hospital mortality increases with increasing time to treatment with t-PA, but is relatively flat from 2–12 hours with primary angioplasty.

at 6 months leading to a ~ 20% TVR (target vessel revascularisation) rate using either redo PTCA or CABG. Thus, the results of primary balloon angioplasty in the setting of acute myocardial infarction are rather less satisfactory than when balloon angioplasty is undertaken in the elective patient with stable angina.

In the major stent trials (e.g. BENESTENT and STRESS) comparing plain balloon angioplasty and elective intra-coronary stenting, patients with evolving myocardial infarction and the more severe forms of unstable angina (Braunwald IIIb) were excluded because of concerns over implanting a potentially thrombogenic stainless steel prosthesis into a thrombotic environment. Early reports using anticoagulant protocols based on warfarin showed an unacceptable early thrombosis rate (~ 5%) when stents were used in this subgroup of patients. An increase in operator experience leading to optimal stent sizing and deployment coupled with newer aggressive drug regimens based on antiplatelet rather than anticoagulant therapy has resulted in superior in-hospital results. In particular the more recent aspirin/ticlopidine or aspirin/clopidogrel

combinations are associated with an early subacute stent thrombosis rate of approximately 0.5%.

PRIMARY ANGIOPLASTY/STENTING (TRIALS)

The PAMI stent pilot trial studied 236 highly selected patients presenting with an acute myocardial infarct, who were treated with a mean of 1.4 ± 0.7 mainly Palmaz–Schatz stents (97%). During the follow-up period (7.4 ± 2.6 months), death occurred in only four patients (1.7%), reinfarction in five (2.1%) and target vessel revascularisation [TVR] in 26 (11.1%); angiographic restenosis occurred in 27.5% of patients. These favourable results were also reflected in three smaller studies.

PRIMARY ANGIOPLASTY VS STENTING (TRIALS)

In a small randomised study Suryapranata and colleagues compared the outcome of patients undergoing intra-coronary stenting (n = 112) with plain balloon angioplasty (n = 115) in a setting of acute myocardial infarction. Overall 6-month mortality for the study was a remarkably low 2%. Reinfarction was reduced in the stent group compared with the patients treated with PTCA alone at 1% and 7% respectively (p = 0.036) and target vessel revascularisation at 6 months was required in 4% of the stent group compared with 17% of the PTCA group (p = 0.0016) (Fig. 24.7). With a cardiac event-free survival rate of 95% in the stented patients compared with 80% in the PTCA group (p = 0.012), the authors concluded that primary stenting could be applied safely to selected patients following acute myocardial infarction.

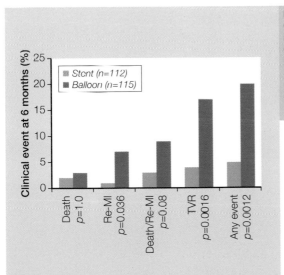

Figure 24.7:
Clinical outcome at 6 months in patients treated with intra-coronary stenting (Stent) and simple balloon angioplasty (Balloon). (Re-MI indicates recurrent myocardial infarction, TVR, target-vessel revascularisation).

PRIMARY PTCA/STENTING IN DISTRICT (COMMUNITY) HOSPITALS

In the UK and elsewhere, the majority of hospitals do not have the facilities for cardiac catheterisation. Where a cardiac catheter laboratory is available, personnel may not be experienced in interventional techniques, an out of hours service may not be available, and on-site surgery may not be provided. The resources necessary for treating large numbers of patients experiencing an acute myocardial infarct with thrombolytic drugs is minimal compared with the provision of a primary intervention service. In assessing the applicability and efficacy of offering primary intervention in a District (Community) hospital setting, it is important to be sure that the published results from large tertiary centres with experienced operators can be translated to patients presenting to local hospitals. If patients are to be treated in the District hospital, should these be highly selected (e.g. those ineligible for thrombolysis, or with extensive infarction, or cardiogenic shock)? Is it more appropriate to transfer patients to the local tertiary centre? Is surgical standby an issue in primary intervention? (Tables 24.3 & 24.4) A number of trials have addressed some of these issues.

In an observational study from the MITI investigators, early and late results were compared in a group of patients undergoing primary PTCA ($n = 1050$) and those treated with conventional balloon angioplasty ($n = 2095$) in a group of Seattle community hospitals. Primary angioplasty success rates appeared to be lower in a community setting (89%) compared with that achieved in a tertiary centre (e.g. 98% for PAMI). In-hospital mortality was similar in the primary angioplasty and thrombolytic groups at 5.5% and 5.6% respectively ($p = 0.90$); even in 'high-risk' patients

TABLE 24.3 – PATIENTS WHO SHOULD BE CONSIDERED FOR PRIMARY PTCA/STENTING

- Contraindication to thrombolysis
- Elderly
- Anterior myocardial infarction (MI)
- Tachycardia (large MI)
- Cardiogenic shock
- Intractable ventricular arrhythmias
- When experienced intervention team/catheter laboratory available

TABLE 24.4 – PATIENTS WHO SHOULD BE CONSIDERED FOR THROMBOLYSIS

- Patients in whom PTCA is of questionable benefit:
  - Young MI
  - Non-anterior MI
  - 'Small' MI
- Patients with contraindications to PTCA:
  - Severe peripheral vascular disease
  - Renal insufficiency
  - Contrast allergy
- Experienced intervention team/catheter laboratory not available

the results were similar for patients treated with PTCA (8.7%) and thrombolysis (8.1%) ($p = 0.70$). Interestingly, the results from patients treated at 'high-volume' centres were not significantly better. Mean in-hospital costs and costs at 3-year follow-up were higher in the patients treated with percutanous intervention, and patients treated with thrombolysis underwent 30% fewer angiograms and 15% fewer angioplasty procedures. Cumulative survival after 4 years follow-up was similar in the two groups (Fig. 24.8). They concluded that primary angioplasty cost more and offered no mortality advantage when compared with thrombolysis used for the treatment of acute myocardial infarction in a community setting. These disappointing results may be due to the fact that this study compared two groups of low-risk patients, who would be predicted to have a low mortality whatever the treatment strategy adopted.

In a retrospective report from The Netherlands, it was concluded that it was safe to transport patients for primary angioplasty to the local tertiary centre. Total ischaemic time (symptom onset to first balloon inflation) was similar for 'in-house' patients and those transferred from the community hospital, and late clinical outcome at 6 months (death, reinfarction, re-PTCA and CABG) was not significantly different.

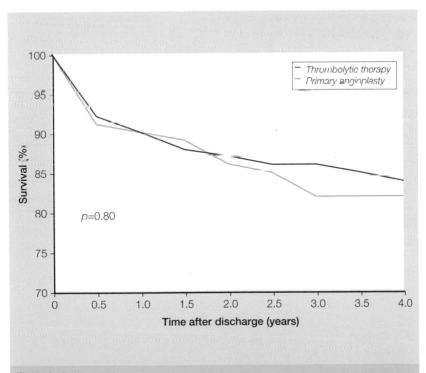

Figure 24.8:
Cumulative survival among 1050 patients treated by primary PTCA and 2095 patients treated with thrombolysis. There was no significant difference in unadjusted long-term survival between cohorts.

In that the majority of patients with myocardial infarction present to community hospitals, an alternative strategy would be for experienced interventional cardiologists based at the tertiary centre, to undertake primary PTCA in the community hospital – move the cardiologist rather than the patient. Wharton and colleagues reported on a series of 506 consecutive patients treated by experienced operators in two community hospitals without on-site surgery. Patients were unselected, 13.4% were in Killip Class III, and 11.3% in cardiogenic shock. Primary PTCA success (TIMI grade III flow and 50% residual stenosis) was achieved in 94.3% of patients, with an overall in-hospital mortality of 6.6% (cardiogenic shock 25%, no shock 3.8%). Reinfarction occurred in 2.5% of patients, and stroke or TIA in 0.4% (none of which were haemorrhagic). A total of 27 patients (5.3%) required CABG within 12 hours of presentation because of cardiogenic shock (eight patients) or critical multivessel disease (19 patients). No patient required CABG because of a procedural complication related to primary PTCA. No complication occurred during inter-hospital transfer, and 25/27 (93%) survived. With regard to surgical standby, an accompanying editorial concluded, '. . . interventional cardiologists have gained a consistent, dependable proficiency that should enable them to declare their independence from surgery'. The results from this trial are particularly impressive because they predate the stent era (only 17 stents were deployed), and only 12 patients received abciximab. Overall, stents or abciximab were only used in 4.2% of procedures.

ADJUVANT THERAPY

If primary angioplasty/stenting in acute myocardial infarction is regarded as a relatively high-risk coronary intervention, then the routine use of abciximab (ReoPro) may be beneficial. In the EPISTENT trial, comparing patients with stent plus placebo, stent plus abciximab and balloon plus abciximab, abciximab was clearly beneficial in terms of a reduction in the primary endpoint (a combination of death, myocardial infarction, or the need for revascularisation within 30 days) for patients receiving a stent. The primary end point occurred in 10.8% of the patients in the stent plus placebo group and 5.3% of the stent plus abciximab group (hazard ratio 0.48, 95% CI 0.33–0.88, $p < 0.001$). Death and myocardial infarction occurred in 7.8% of the stent placebo group and only 3.0% in the stent abciximab group ($p < 0.001$) (Fig. 24.9). At 6 months, there was a persisting relative risk reduction for death or myocardial infarction of 50% (placebo group 11.4%, abciximab group 5.6%, $p < 0.001$). Recently, the 12-month data presented in abstract form indicate a 57% relative reduction in death with abciximab.

The effect of abciximab on primary PTCA has been reported in the RAPPORT trial of 483 patients randomised within 12 hours of an acute myocardial infarct into treatment with primary PTCA and abciximab or placebo. Abciximab significantly reduced the incidence of death,

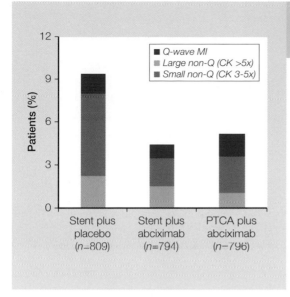

Figure 24.9:
EPISTENT trial: incidence and type of myocardial infarction for each treatment group.

reinfarction, or urgent TVR at 7 days (9.9% vs 3.3%, p = 0.003), 30 days (11.2% vs 5.8%, p = 0.03), and at 6 months (17.8% vs 11.6%, p = 0.05), when compared with placebo. The incidence of bail-out stenting was reduced by 42% (20.4% vs 11.9%, p = 0.008). However, major bleeding occurred significantly more frequently in the group treated with abciximab (16.6% vs 9.5%, p = 0.02), usually at the femoral access site.

The results of the CADILLAC trial are awaited in which 2000 patients with acute myocardial infarction are being randomised in a 2×2 factorial design to primary PTCA alone, primary PTCA plus abciximab, primary stenting alone and primary stenting plus abciximab. The ACS Multilink stent will be used in vessels as small as 2.5 mm diameter. Other features of the trial will be early (48-hour) discharge from hospital and an intravascular ultrasound [IVUS] sub-study. It should therefore be possible to separate the relative benefits and contribution of stents and abciximab in this trial.

RESCUE PTCA/STENTING

The strategy of rescue PTCA/stenting is used to refer to the use of percutaneous intervention in the patient who has failed to reperfuse using conventional thrombolytic therapy. In this setting, the early trial data favour mechanical opening of the infarct vessel rather than further thrombolysis. Early published series were small and pre-dated the routine use of stents and IIb/IIIa inhibitors, which is likely to favour the mechanical approach. The timing of angiography is important, as it is clear that early intervention improves late myocardial salvage.

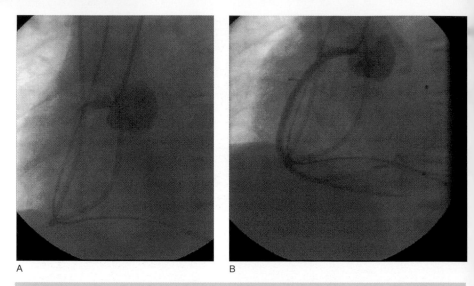

A   B

Figure 24.10:
A 56-year-old man. Acute inferior Q wave infarct complicated by cardiogenic shock and complete AV block. Intra-aortic balloon pump, temporary pacing wire. RCA reconstructed with 5 intra-coronary stents. Procedure covered with abciximab.

PTCA/STENTING FOR CARDIOGENIC SHOCK

More than 20 small published, non-randomised often retrospective series have reported on the use of PTCA in the setting of cardiogenic shock. Although most of the studies used PTCA alone without stenting, it seems that mortality can be reduced from > 80% in historical controls to ~45% in patients undergoing intervention (Fig. 24.10). This impressive figure is likely to improve still further using contemporary techniques. Reopening an infarct related vessel has also abolished intractable ventricular arrhythmias.

PRIMARY ANGIOPLASTY/STENTING – CATHETER LABORATORY SET-UP

The catheter laboratory team (cardiologist, scrub nurse/runner, radiography, technician) should be used to working together, and have wide experience in diagnostic catheterisation, elective coronary intervention, and be proficient at resuscitating a patient requiring haemodynamic or respiratory support. It is helpful (but not always possible) to have a second physician in attendance to assist in resuscitating the patient if necessary. The catheterisation laboratory should be equipped with a high quality digital imaging chain with data storage preferably on CD-ROM. Availability of an anaesthetic machine, defibrillator, and intra-aortic balloon counter pulsation are mandatory.

Diagnostic arteriography is undertaken via a standard femoral approach using 6 F–8 F catheters depending on physician preference. Many operators do not undertake routine ventriculography. Having

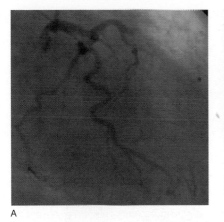
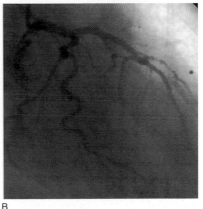

A   B

Figure 24.11:
A 60-year-old man. Six-hour history of chest pain. Acute anteroseptal infarct (peak CK 3170 iu/l). Treated with intravenous streptokinase. Pain continued and no resolution of ECG changes. Cardiac catheterisation demonstrated proximal occlusion LAD, occluded RCA, severe stenosis main circumflex. LAD reopened and stented (7 F FL4 guide, 0.014 inch Balance wire, 2.0 × 20 mm Ranger balloon, 3.0 × 23 mm NIR stent). Discharged home the following day with a view to elective CABG.

obtained the diagnostic images, the usual strategy is to reopen the infarct related vessel, leaving any distant disease for percutaneous or surgical revascularisation at a later date (Fig. 24.11). A standard technique is used for reopening the occluded vessel, with coated wires supported by a balloon if necessary. Occlusions are usually soft and thrombus containing, and therefore easy to open. Reperfusion arrhythmias should be anticipated and treated appropriately. Despite the enthusiasm for direct stenting, predilatation allows better visualisation of the distal vessel, and hence better sizing of the stent. Routine use of stents (rather than simple balloon angioplasty) should be the norm in the setting of myocardial infarction except in exceptional circumstances (diffuse disease, small caliber, poor runoff, etc.) (see Chapter 4). If thrombus and/or coronary dissection is extensive, abciximab should be administered in the usual manner (see Chapter 5 for details of antiplatelet therapy). Arterial closure devices (e.g. Angioseal™, Vasoseal™) are useful in these patients. Post-procedure monitoring is ideally undertaken in a high-care environment with early hospital discharge (48–72 hours) possible in the majority of patients.

FURTHER READING

Angelini P. Guidelines for surgical standby for coronary angioplasty: should they be changed? J Am Coll Cardiol 1999;33:1266–8.

Brener SJ, Barr LA, Burchenal JEB *et al*. On behalf of the ReoPro and Primary PTCA Organization and Randomized Trial (RAPPORT) Investigators. Circulation 1998;734–41.

Brodie BR. When should patients with acute myocardial infarction be transferred for primary angioplasty? Heart 1997;78:327–8.

Every NR, Parson LS, Hlatky M, Martin JS, Weaver WD. For the Myocardial Infarction Triage and Intervention Investigators. N Engl J Med 1996;335:1253–60.

Grines CL. Primary angioplasty – the strategy of choice. N Engl J Med 1996;1313–17.

Lange RA, Hillis LD. Should thrombolysis or primary angioplasty be the treatment of choice for acute myocardial infarction? N Engl J Med 1996;335:1311–12.

Lim R, Walters MI, Norell MS. Transferring patients for primary infarct angioplasty. Heart 1997;78:325–26.

Nunn CM, O'Neill WW, Rothbaum D et al. For the Primary Angioplasty in Myocardial Infarction I Study Group. Long-term outcome after primary angioplasty: report from the primary angioplasty in myocardial infarction (PAMI-I) trial. J Am Coll Cardiol 1999;33:640–46.

The EPISTENT Investigators. Randomised placebo-controlled and balloon-angioplasty-controlled trial to assess safety of coronary stenting with use of platelet glyocoprotein-IIb/IIIa blockade. Evaluation of Platelet IIb/IIIa Inhibitor for Stenting. Lancet 1998;352:81–2.

Smith D, Dean J. Transferring patients for primary angioplasty. Heart 1997;78:323–4.

Stone GW. Primary stenting in acute myocardial infarction: the promise and the proof. Circulation 1998;97:2482–5.

Stone GW, Brodie BR, Griffin JJ et al. For the PAMI Stent Pilot Trial Investigators. Clinical and angiographic follow-up after primary stenting in acute myocardial infarction: the primary angioplasty in myocardial infarction (PAMI) stent pilot trial. Circulation 1999;99:1548–54.

Suryapranata H, van't Hoff AWJ, Hoorntje JCA, de Boer M-J, Zijlstra F. Randomized comparison of coronary stenting with balloon angioplasty in selected patients with acute myocardial infarction. Circulation 1998;97:2502–2505.

The GUSTO angiographic investigators. The effects of tissue plasminogen activator, streptokinase, or both on coronary-artery patency, ventricular function and survival after acute myocardial infarction. N Engl J Med 1993;329:1233–8.

Weaver WD, Simes J, Betriu A et al. Comparison of primary coronary angioplasty and intravenous thrombolytic therapy for acute myocardial infarction. JAMA 1997;278:2093–8.

Wharton TP, McNamara NS, Fedele FA, Jacobs MI, Gladstone AR, Funk EJ. Primary angioplasty for the treatment of acute myocardial infarction: experience at two community hospitals without cardiac surgery. J Am Coll Cardiol 1999;33:1257–65.

Zijlstra F, van't Hoff AWJ, Liem AL, Hoorntje JCA, Suryapranata H, de Boer M-J. Transferring patients for primary angioplasty: a retrospective analysis of 104 selected high risk patients with acute myocardial infarction. Heart 1997;333–6.

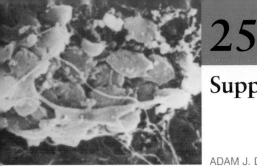

25

Supported angioplasty

ADAM J. DE BELDER

KEY POINTS

- Intra-aortic balloon pumping may be a useful adjunct to angioplasty for:
  - patients with poor LV function;
  - 'failed' thrombolysis;
  - cardiogenic shock;
  - ischaemic arrhythmias.

- Meticulous technique for insertion and removal with adequate nursing and technical support is essential to minimise complications associated with use of a balloon pump.

- IABP is best used prophylactically in 'high-risk' patients rather than waiting for problems to arise.

INTRODUCTION

Coronary angioplasty can be risky for the patient and the operator. Certain groups of patients can be considered to be at prohibitively high risk for coronary angioplasty. Typically, these patients have markedly impaired left ventricular function, a single target vessel supplying a large area of viable myocardium, or both, and the cardiac surgeons are not interested. While angioplasty is generally well tolerated in the low-risk setting, transient coronary occlusion induced by balloon inflations in these high-risk patients, may impose an intolerable ischaemic burden on marginally compensated myocardium and lead to haemodynamic collapse.

It is logical to propose that any reduction in risk that can be achieved in high-risk patients is worth the effort.

It is sometimes difficult to predict which patients will run into trouble in the catheter laboratory, but the following conditions should make one consider carefully before putting the gloves on:

- Cardiogenic shock
- Poor left ventricle (LV) function
- Ischaemic arrhythmias
- Unstable refractory angina.

There are a number of techniques available to support the myocardium under these circumstances.[1] Most of them are confined to the dustbin of history, but are worthy of a mention.

Anterograde coronary perfusion

There are a number of catheters designed to maintain anterograde coronary perfusion driven by central aortic pressure, in the presence of transient coronary occlusion. They are of limited benefit, particularly when there is systemic hypotension. Coronary stenting has also revolutionised the management of occlusive dissections.

Coronary haemoperfusion

Various techniques are described to provide haemoperfusion during coronary artery occlusion. After withdrawal of the sidearm of an oversized arterial sheath, blood is heparinised and reinfused using either hand injection, roller pump or power injector to provide adequate flow rates. The main limitation to this technique is that blood cannot be perfused to side branches that are occluded by the angioplasty balloon.

Perfluorocarbon coronary perfusion

Fluosol is a biologically inert perfluorocarbon emulsion with a high oxygen carrying capacity and a low viscosity, and has been used as a distal coronary perfusate during coronary angioplasty. There is little convincing evidence that it has any clinical benefit, which, in addition to the preparation time and cost, has limited the use of fluosol in this setting.

Coronary sinus retroperfusion

Oxygenated blood is delivered via the coronary sinus to the great cardiac vein during ventricular diastole; a 10 mm balloon 1 cm from the coronary sinus distal tip inflates and deflates with each cardiac cycle, preventing escape of retroperfused blood into the right atrium.

There are disadvantages to this technique:

- It is only really feasible for left anterior descending (LAD) angioplasty, as the right coronary and circumflex vessels usually drain into the right atrium, ventricle or a portion of the coronary sinus.
- Coronary sinus cannulation is not easy, and setting up retroperfusion can take time.
- There are little data about the degree of myocardial protection offered during high-risk angioplasty.

Cardiopulmonary support

Total circulatory support with cardiopulmonary bypass can now be performed percutaneously. This does require the use of large stiff cannulae (18–20 F) inserted into the femoral vein and artery. This has limited its use due to a very high femoral access site complication rate.

INTRA-AORTIC BALLOON PUMP

The one device that has survived and is in regular use is the intra-aortic balloon pump (IABP).

History

A failing heart poses a therapeutic dilemma – the increased aortic pressure required for adequate myocardial perfusion produces an unfavourable increase in afterload on the failing left ventricle. Ross[2] pointed out that peripheral vasoconstrictors often made the failing heart worse and proposed that mechanical assistance to the circulation would help. Since then a number of means to temporarily support the circulation have been devised, all with the same purpose to provide diastolic augmentation with increased coronary perfusion and to decrease left ventricular work.

In 1961, Clauss et al. reported the use of a 'proportioning pump' placed on the arterial side of the circulation.[3] The original paper highlighted the potential benefits and many of the problems associated with the use of such a device. In dog experiments, they elegantly demonstrated that the greatest and most consistent relief of heart work, with the highest diastolic perfusion were achieved by very accurate timing of counterpulsation in co-ordination with direct arterial pressure measurement, or even triggered to the electrical output from the ECG machine. They showed the inefficiency of the pump with improper synchronisation with the cardiac cycle.

The first paper to report the use of balloon inflation (using CO_2) as a means of providing aortic counterpulsation came from Moulopoulos et al.[4]. Using a human cadaver, the balloon catheter was inserted into the ascending aorta of a patient half an hour after death, and radio-opaque dye injected which showed movement of dye toward the coronary tree, augmented by the balloon.

In 1967, Nachlas and Siedband reported that intra-aortic counterpulsation in a dog model diminished the size of experimentally-induced myocardial infarction.[5] Kantrowitz and colleagues[6] described the use of a helium-filled balloon placed within the aorta to support the failing heart in a number of patients. One of these patients died, but not before substantial physiological data had been obtained to support its use.

Since then, improvements have made the ABP a standard piece of equipment for most catheterisation laboratories. The following section describes how to use the device safely, and then the relevant literature is reviewed in order to summarise those situations in which the IABP might be helpful.

Insertion technique for placing the IABP

It is important to establish that the patient has good peripheral circulation mainly to determine if limb ischaemia develops.

Ideally, an IABP should be inserted in the appropriate surroundings with easy access to imaging and where strict sepsis can be maintained. It is possible to insert balloon pumps at the bedside, but it is not ideal.

Choosing the size of balloon is important. Generally, balloon capacity varies between 34 and 40 cc helium, and are now available in as small as 8 F. The principle is to use bigger balloon capacity on taller patients (>5′ 6″). If possible, I insert the IABP without a sheath, as this reduces the risk of limb ischaemia.

The femoral artery is approached using the Seldinger technique.

The femoral artery is dilated over a J tipped guidewire. If the procedure is performed without a sheath, the IABP is inserted directly over the wire. The slender polyurethane balloon is very low profile and has a blunt end. Passage of the IABP into the femoral artery is best done with gentle manual rotation as the balloon enters the femoral artery. The tip of the balloon is radio-opaque – this helps position it within the descending aorta, with the distal tip placed just below the origin of the left subclavian artery.

The IABP has only two connections. The first is for the measurement of arterial pressure, and the other is to attach to a console that shuttles helium in and out of the balloon for rapid inflation and deflation.

Augmentation is best achieved with timing of the inflation/deflation to the arterial waveform, but timing can also accurately be co-ordinated with the ECG waveform.

Thrombosis is a potential problem with a large artificial structure within the aorta, and I like to anticoagulate my patients with heparin to keep an ACT of approximately 200 seconds.

It is always sensible to monitor patients using staff accustomed to looking after sick cardiac patients. In addition, technical support from perfusionists or similar staff helps prevent complications and optimises the effectiveness of the device.

Removal of the IABP

Once the decision to withdraw the IABP is made, the rate of augmentation is gradually decreased. Once augmentation is decreased to 1 in 4 or 1 in 8, the device can be removed. The heparin is tailed off such that when the activated clotting time (ACT) is < 150 seconds, the balloon can be taken out. It is important to aspirate the balloon before removal. Manual pressure is then applied to the groin, until haemostasis is achieved.

Complications

Patients requiring an IABP tend to have a higher incidence of concomitant disease, and it is not uncommon for problems to arise with peripheral ischaemia. It is therefore very important to assess limb vessel patency before placement and have regular checks during placement.

Other complications have been reported, such as aortic dissection and traumatic injury to the femoral artery, but these are fortunately rare.

PATIENTS WHO WOULD BENEFIT FROM IABP TO COVER ANGIOPLASTY PROCEDURE

Patients with acute myocardial infarction (AMI)

Brodie *et al.*[7] reported their experience with the IABP in the management of 1490 patients undergoing primary angioplasty for AMI from 1984–1997. Catheter laboratory events occurred in 88 (5.9%) patients (ventricular failure, cardiopulmonary arrest, prolonged hypotension). Retrospective analysis of this group compared the incidence of these

events with or without an IABP. There were fewer adverse events in the
IABP group compared with no IABP:

■ Cardiogenic shock (14.5% vs 35.1%, $n = 119$).

■ Congestive heart failure or low ejection fraction (0% vs 14.6%, $n = 119$).

■ In all high-risk patients combined (11.5% vs 21.9%, $n = 238$).

There are obvious limitations to this study with selection bias, but it
suggests that patients who have low blood pressure (BP) or malignant
arrhythmias during an acute MI should be considered for prophylactic use
of an IABP.

IABP as adjunctive therapy to rescue angioplasty after failed thrombolysis for anterior AMI

This was a non-randomised study[8] of 60 patients who had successful
reperfusion performed to a blocked LAD after unsuccessful thrombolysis.
The results are presented as before ($n = 20$ group A) and after ($n = 40$
group B) the decision to prophylactically insert an IABP. Before discharge
all patients had a repeat angiogram.

	GROUP A	GROUP B	
Reinfarction	3	1	
Reocclusion	2	0	
In-hospital mortality	20%	5%	
LVEF	No difference	44.3 ± 8.2% to 51.0 ± 14.21%	**p** < 0.01

LVEF: left ventricle ejection fraction.

This is a small non-randomised study, but supports the possibility that
IABP as adjunctive therapy to percutaneous transluminal coronary
angioplasty (PTCA) for rescue angioplasty reduces reocclusion and
improves left ventricular function.

Use of IABP in 'high-risk' patients with AMI

Within the PAMI-II trial was a subgroup randomisation concerning the
use of IABP in 'high-risk' patients.[9] These were defined as patients who:

■ Were aged > 70 years.

■ Had three vessel disease.

■ LVEF < 45%.

■ Vein graft occlusion.

■ Malignant arrhythmia.

■ Suboptimal PTCA result.

This group were randomised to receive 36–48 hours of IABP ($n = 211$) or
traditional care ($n = 226$).

There was no significant difference in death, reinfarction, infarct-related artery reocclusion, stroke or new-onset heart failure or sustained hypotension seen between the two groups.

It might be argued that any beneficial effects of IABP were not seen because of the soft inclusion criteria for 'high-risk' patients. Whatever, this chapter would not support the blanket use of IABP for so-called 'high-risk' patients with AMI.

AMI – cardiogenic shock treated with thrombolysis and IABP insertion

This was a retrospective analysis of 335 patients with cardiogenic shock over a 10-year period from two community hospitals in the USA.[10] Forty-six patients underwent thrombolysis within 12 hours of acute infarction with established cardiogenic shock (27 underwent IABP, 19 did not). There was a remarkable community hospital survival rate in the IABP group (93% vs 37%) with a significant improvement in overall hospital and 1-year survival rate (67% vs 32%).

This study also emphasised the benefit of using the IABP when transferring high-risk patients for revascularisation.

It has been difficult to enrol patients with cardiogenic shock into prospective randomised studies, and there is no definitive study to direct practice. However, I feel there is sufficient evidence to warrant a strategy of IABP support and revascularisation by PTCA in these patients who otherwise have a very grim outlook.

Patients with poor left ventricular function undergoing PTCA

This is a group who, I believe, benefit most from the use of prophylactic balloon pumping, yet there are no randomised studies examining this issue. A retrospective analysis of 28 patients undergoing 'high-risk' angioplasty with IABP support with a mean LV ejection fraction of 24%, showed that despite systolic BP falling to < 70 mmHg in 39% cases, the augmented diastolic pressure was > 90 mmHg at all times. There were no deaths or myocardial infarctions complicating these procedures, but three patients required surgical repair of the femoral artery.[11]

There seems little doubt that in patients undergoing angioplasty to the last remaining conduit, which perhaps supply collaterals to other areas of a heart, which is already significantly impaired, the use of an IABP is sensible.

There are a number of interventional cardiologists who have never used an IABP on the grounds that it is:

■ cumbersome;

■ a potential threat to the peripheral circulation;

■ of little clinical value;

■ inconvenient ('by the time the balloon pump is in, I could have done the angioplasty').

More fool them. I have heard a number of stories where the cardiologist has mourned the fact that an IABP was not inserted before a case. Occasionally, its insertion can help a dire situation, but its presence when trouble starts is gratefully received.

CASE REPORT 1

A 53-year-old man presented with chest pain at rest. He reported a myocardial infarction 15 years ago since when he had been free of symptoms. On admission he was hypotensive and tachycardic. His resting ECG showed left bundle branch block.

He underwent urgent angiography. This revealed poor left ventricular function (EF: 20%). The LAD was chronically occluded. The circumflex was free of significant disease, and the right coronary artery revealed a critical lesion at the ostium and in the proximal segment (see Fig. 25.1A).

He developed ventricular tachycardia with loss of output requiring multiple DC shocks. After restoration of sinus rhythm, a 40 cc 8 F IABP was placed via the left femoral artery, which settled the ST segment shift and ventricular ectopy. Angioplasty with stenting was performed to restore blood flow to the right coronary artery (see Fig. 25.1B) after which there were no further complications.

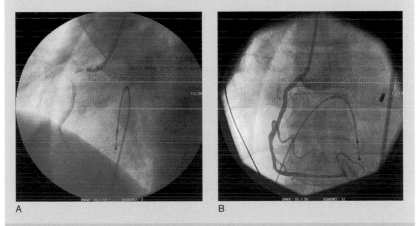

A   B

Figure 25.1:
Case Report 1. (a) Angiogram revealing critical lesion at the ostium of the right coronary artery and in the proximal segment. (b) After IABP, angioplasty and stenting.

CASE REPORT 2

A 68-year-old man presented with severe chest pain and was in cardiogenic shock. Seventeen years previously he had four vein coronary artery vein grafts applied. Over the last 3 years, he had developed mild angina which had responded to medical therapy.

A coronary angiogram revealed poor LV function (EF: 15–20%). All his native vessels were occluded (see Fig. 25.2A). Three of the vein grafts were occluded. A vein graft supplied the LAD, which back-filled the distal right coronary artery.

A 40 cc 8 F IABP was placed via the left femoral artery and the balloon augmentation set to 1:1. The native circumflex artery was reopened and a stent inserted at the site of occlusion (see Fig. 25.2B). He made a good recovery with resolution of his shock and complete alleviation of his angina. He remains well.

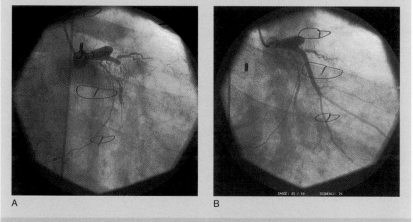

A   B

Figure 25.2:
Case Report 2. (a) Coronary angiogram revealing poor LV function. (b) After IABP, angioplasty and stenting.

REFERENCES

1. Lincoff AM, Popma JJ, Ellis SG, Vogel RA, Topol EJ. Percutaneous support devices for high risk or complicated coronary angioplasty. J Am Coll Cardiol 1991;17:770–80.

2. Ross J Jr. Left ventricular contraction and the therapy of cardiogenic shock. Circulation 1967;35:611–13.

3. Clauss RH, Birtwell WC, Albertal G et al. Assisted circulation. I. The arterial counterpulsator. J Thoracic Cardiovasc Surg 1961;41:447–58.

4. Moulopoulos SD, Topaz S, Kolff WJ. Diastolic balloon pumping (with carbon dioxide) in the aorta – a mechanical assistance to the failing circulation. Am Heart J 1962;63:669–75.

5. Nachlas MM, Siedband MP. The influence of diastolic augmentation on infarct size following coronary artery ligation. J Thoracic Cardiovasc Surg 1967;53:698–706.

6. Kantrowitz A, Tjønneland S, Freed PS et al. Initial clinical experience with intra-aortic balloon pumping in cardiogenic shock. JAMA 1968;203:113–17.

7. Brodie BR, Stuckey TD, Hansen C, Muncy D. Intra-aortic balloon counterpulsation before primary percutaneous transluminal coronary angioplasty reduces catheterization laboratory events in high-risk patients with acute myocardial infarction. Am J Cardiol 1999;84:18–23.

8. Ishihara M, Sato H, Tateisha H *et al*. Intra-aortic balloon pumping as adjunctive therapy to rescue coronary angioplasty after failed thrombolysis in anterior wall acute myocardial infarction. Am J Cardiol 1995;76:73–5.

9. Stone GW, Marsalese D, Brodie BR *et al*. A prospective, randomized evaluation of prophylactic intra-aortic balloon counterpulsation in high risk patients with acute myocardial infarction treated with primary angioplasty. J Am Coll Cardiol 1997;29:1459–67.

10. Kovack PJ, Rasak MA, Bates ER, Ohman EM, Stomel RJ. Thrombolysis plus aortic counterpulsation: improved survival in patients who present to community hospitals with cardiogenic shock. J Am Coll Cardiol 1997;29:1454–8.

11. Kahn JK, Rutherford BD, McConahay DR *et al*. Supported 'high risk' coronary angioplasty using intra-aortic balloon pump counterpulsation. J Am Coll Cardiol 1990;15:770–80.

Section Five

New Techniques in
Vascular Access

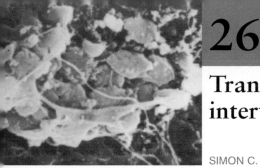

26

Transradial coronary intervention

SIMON C. ECCLESHALL AND JAMES NOLAN

KEY POINTS

- The percutaneous transradial approach is currently the safest route available for coronary interventional procedures.

- Cost benefit, improved short-term quality of life and patient preference all favour the radial approach.

- A learning curve exists for the technique but the long-term gain outweighs this short term disadvantage.

- Careful attention to specific technical factors are required to successfully perform interventional procedures via the transradial approach.

- For experienced transradial operators, radiation exposure, total procedure times and PTCA success rates are comparable to those obtained with other access sites.

INTRODUCTION

Coronary intervention requires access to the aorta and coronary ostia, obtained by retrograde cannulation of a peripheral artery. The arterial access site chosen for an interventional coronary procedure significantly influences procedural costs, quality of life and the morbidity and mortality rates associated with vascular access site complications.[1] Until recently, the most commonly used access sites have been the femoral and brachial arteries. The femoral artery has been the preferred route of access ever since the percutaneous Seldinger technique superseded the more technically challenging brachial cut-down approach. The exponential rise in stent implantation rates combined with the use of more aggressive antithrombotic therapy in some patients has, however, resulted in an important increase in femoral artery vascular complications. Although the antiplatelet regimes currently employed after routine stent implantation have improved the situation, major bleeding complications following percutaneous transluminal coronary angioplasty (PTCA) with concurrent use of glycoprotein IIb/IIIa inhibitors can occur in up to 23% of patients.[2] It has therefore become increasingly apparent that a safer route of arterial access would be highly desirable.[1]

The radial artery has been widely used for many years for haemodynamic monitoring with a low risk of significant neurovascular complications.[3] Two important anatomical features contribute to reducing the risk profile of this access site. First, the vessel is superficial and, in the majority of patients, is not an end artery. Radial artery occlusion does not therefore result in major ischaemic complications. Haemostasis is easily achieved by pressure over the point of arterial puncture, while any bleeding is easily recognised allowing prompt action. Second, no major veins or nerves lie close to the radial artery, limiting the risk of neurological damage or arterio-venous fistula formation. The development of small calibre diagnostic catheters facilitated the use of the radial artery for coronary angiography, first described by Campeau in 1989.[3] The success of these diagnostic cardiac procedures has led other cardiologists to explore the use of the radial artery as an access site for PTCA.[4]

A COMPARISON OF ARTERIAL ACCESS SITES FOR CORONARY INTERVENTION

When a surgical cut down approach to the brachial artery is employed for cardiac procedures, major neurovascular complications (resulting in acute arm ischaemia or median nerve palsy) occur in around 5% of patients (Fig. 26.1). Operator skill and experience are important factors in limiting the rate of complications associated with this technically demanding approach, with reported major complication rates ranging from 1.4% to 20%.[1,5] An alternative method to access the brachial artery employs a percutaneous Seldinger technique to position a sheath in the brachial artery. This technique is technically much simpler than a surgical cut down, but is associated with a similar continuing risk of important neurovascular complications.[1] When the percutaneous femoral access site is employed, the rate of significant neurovascular complications ranges from 1% following a simple diagnostic procedure to 15% when large bore catheters are employed in association with anticoagulant therapy.[1] Femoral artery occlusion leading to major lower limb ischaemia will require urgent vascular surgical repair to avoid amputation. Concealed retroperitoneal bleeding is an ominous complication that has a reported mortality rate of 15%.[6] One-third of patients who sustain an iatrogenic femoral nerve

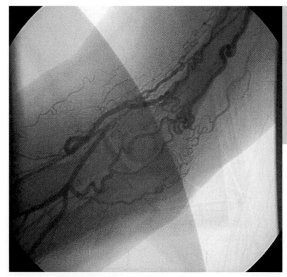

Figure 26.1:
Arteriogram in a patient with arm claudication following a PTCA performed via a surgical cut down approach to the brachial artery. There is total occlusion of the brachial artery at the level of the antecubital fossa with collateral formation limiting forearm ischaemia at rest.

injury related to a cardiac procedure have a permanent neurological
deficit.[7] Because of the favourable anatomical relations of the radial artery,
performing cardiac procedures via this access site can minimise the risk of
these major iatrogenic complications. In addition, in 5–10% of patients
requiring cardiac procedures, access via a brachial or femoral access site is
impossible due to anatomical variation, peripheral vascular disease or
obesity, and the radial access site may allow such patients to be
investigated and treated.[8]

A large prospective randomised study has examined the relative merits
of the percutaneous brachial, femoral and radial access sites in patients
undergoing elective PTCA. The Access Trial demonstrates that the radial
approach is the safest, with no significant vascular complications
occurring, compared to rates of 2% in the femoral group and 2.3% in the
brachial group.[9] Failure to gain vascular access occurred in 4.6% of the
radial group and 2.3% of the percutaneous brachial group. The rates of
successful coronary artery cannulation for the different access sites were
93% (radial), 95.7% (brachial) and 99.7% (femoral). The procedural
success rates of PTCA and stent deployment were comparable between the
access sites. More recent reports have demonstrated improved primary
success rates via the radial approach related to improvements in
equipment and technique, with important vascular access complications
occurring in only 0.06% of more than 5000 patients.[10] There is no
increase in total procedure duration or radiation exposure when
transradial procedures are compared with percutaneous femoral
procedures.[9] When compared with the radial access site, patients
undergoing diagnostic angiography via a surgical approach to the brachial
artery have an increase in procedure time and radiation exposure.[11]

Given the demonstrated reduction in the risk of vascular
complications, the radial artery is a particularly attractive option in the
setting of thrombolytic or aggressive antiplatelet therapy. In a recent
comparison of vascular access site complications in patients undergoing
PTCA with adjunctive intravenous IIb/IIIa receptor therapy, 7.4% of the
transfemoral patients had a major vascular access site complication
(despite the use of weight adjusted heparin, small calibre guiding catheters
and femoral artery closure devices in the majority of these patients),
compared to none of the similarly treated radial patients.[12]

Patient comfort and preference are important considerations in the
comparison of these access sites. Delayed mobilisation after transfemoral
procedures is common, due to inguinal pain, while bed rest itself has been
shown to have an adverse effect on outcome.[13,14] Patients undergoing
transradial PTCA can be mobilised immediately after the completion of
these procedures with no adverse effects or risks, which allows PTCA to
be performed on a day case basis.[15] Coronary angiography via the radial
artery as opposed to the femoral artery is associated with short-term
improvements in quality of life, whilst at the same time reducing hospital
costs by 10–15%.[1] The radial approach for intervention was preferred by

73% of patients in whom preceding diagnostic films were performed by the femoral route.[4] As a result of the shorter hospital stay and reduced complication rates associated with transradial procedures, hospital costs of coronary stent deployment can be reduced by 23% when compared with the femoral route.[4] The transradial technique therefore fulfils the requirements for a safer access site for interventional procedures with the added advantages of cost savings and improved quality of life.

CASE SELECTION

The radial artery is a superficial vessel palpable in the forearm proximal to the flexor retinaculum of the wrist. Any patient with good radial pulsation and a positive Allen test may be considered to be suitable for a transradial approach.[16] The Allen test is performed by completely occluding the radial and ulnar arterial supply to the hand using digital pressure. The patient is then asked to repeatedly flex and extend their fingers, producing a blanched palmar surface when the hand is opened. With the hand in the open position, the occlusive pressure applied to the ulnar artery is released. If palmar flushing appears within 10 seconds the Allen test is regarded as positive. A positive Allen test (present in over 90% of the population) confirms that an adequate collateral supply to the hand is present, and that occlusion of the vessel after cannulation will not result in major distal ischaemia. Asymptomatic occlusion of the radial artery has been reported to occur in 5% of patients following a coronary procedure, with spontaneous recanalisation in half of these cases.[17] Performing a transradial procedure does not preclude the use of the radial artery as a surgical conduit. If required, the contralateral artery can be utilised. Since procedure related occlusion is rare (and usually localised to a small distal segment of the artery) both arteries will be available in almost all patients if required.

RADIAL ARTERY CANNULATION

The patient's right arm is prepared by removing all hand and wrist jewellery before shaving and disinfecting the wrist. The design of most catheterisation laboratories and operator preference dictate the use of the right arm, but the left radial artery can be utilised if required or preferred. Any intravenous lines should be placed in the opposite arm. The right arm is supported on an arm board and a small volume of local anaesthetic (2 ml of 1–2% lignocaine) infiltrated over the radial artery proximal to the wrist skin creases and the styloid process. Care should be taken at this stage not to obliterate the pulse by injecting a large volume of anaesthetic, or to puncture the artery (which may induce spasm).

Radial artery puncture can be performed using either a dedicated transradial introducer system (ARROW International Inc., Reading, PA) or an open needle. The ARROW system consists of an outer plastic cannula mounted over a small calibre puncture needle. The puncture needle is co-axial with an integrated guidewire housed within a clear barrel. The system must be checked prior to arterial puncture to ensure that the guidewire is engaged within the needle hub and that it exits the needle smoothly. The guidewire should then be fully retracted using the actuating lever to ensure that the distal end of the puncture needle is not obstructed by partial engagement of the guidewire. The radial artery is then palpated using the left hand and the skin punctured directly under the left index finger at the point of maximal pulsation. The system is advanced at an angle of 45 degrees to the skin with a lateral to medial approach. The puncture site must be at least 1 cm proximal to the styloid process to ensure that the fibrous flexor retinaculum is avoided and to reduce the risk of entering small superficial branches of the distal radial artery. When the anterior wall of the radial artery is punctured, arterial blood flows back into the clear barrel, and the integrated guidewire can be easily advanced into the radial artery to achieve initial stabilisation of the access device. If resistance is felt at the point of guidewire entry into the vessel (as indicated by a marker on the barrel) then the wire should be fully withdrawn and the angle of entry into the vessel changed slightly before re-advancing the wire. After successful introduction of the wire into the artery, the integral soft plastic outer cannula is advanced over the wire and into the radial artery with gentle rotation. The needle, wire and delivery tube are then removed at which point successful cannulation is confirmed by free passage of arterial blood from the proximal end of the cannula. A 'cocktail' of anti-spasmolytic drugs such as verapamil and nitrates are then given through the cannula (after warning the patient to expect a short lived burning sensation in their forearm and hand), and a long guidewire advanced. An open needle technique can also be employed to cannulate the radial artery. A hollow bore needle is advanced through the skin until arterial blood flows freely from its proximal end, indicating successful puncture of the radial artery. A guidewire is then introduced directly into the radial artery through the needle. Although it is possible to achieve a high success rate with an open needle technique, it may be difficult to adequately stabilise the needle during guidewire introduction.

The choice of guidewire used to secure access to the radial artery is dictated by the technique used, with most open needles accommodating a 0.035 inch wire while the ARROW needle system will require use of a smaller 0.025 inch wire. A curved tip to the guidewire helps in the manipulation of the wire past side branches and through tortuous vessels, but if resistance is repeatedly encountered an injection of contrast may be helpful to visualise the anatomy. An exchange wire is useful, particularly during the learning process, to aid repeated negotiation of the peripheral vessels and to guarantee access to the aortic root. Entrance into the ascending aorta can be difficult and may be facilitated by asking the patient to take a deep breath, which straightens out the angle between the subclavian artery and the aorta. Once the guidewire has been advanced into the proximal vessels, a vascular access sheath can be positioned in the radial artery. The choice of sheath length is between short (50 mm), or long (230 mm). Many operators use long sheaths with the aim of reducing the occurrence of radial spasm due to catheter manipulation, but shorter sheaths may have the advantage of being easier to remove. A skin incision to facilitate insertion of the sheath reduces the chance of damage to the vessel wall or tip of the sheath.

GUIDING CATHETER SELECTION AND MANIPULATION

The majority of patients will have an adequate radial lumen to accommodate a 6 F sheath, which is currently compatible with kissing balloon techniques or the use of adjunctive devices such as intravascular ultrasound. The reduction in size of guide catheters from 8 to 6 F can cause problems with the recognised techniques of acquiring adequate guiding catheter back-up. The selection of an optimal catheter configuration is vitally important when using the transradial technique. The guiding catheter must provide support from the opposite aortic wall, whilst being co-axial with the coronary ostium. Deep intubation of the catheter may be necessary (Fig. 26.2), in which case the guide catheter must have a soft, atraumatic tip and be flexible enough to be inserted into the vessel. The use of coronary stents requires the guide catheter to have blunt, flexible curves to allow the passage of the stent system with a minimum of friction. The left internal mammary artery is easily engaged from the left radial artery and is the shortest route available, eliminating the problems encountered with accessibility of the grafted distal vasculature. The guide catheters available include those designed for the femoral approach and dedicated radial catheters.[17] The left coronary artery may be engaged with the left Judkins, Extra backup, left Amplatz and Multipurpose catheters, the Kimny Radial or MUTA radial left. The right

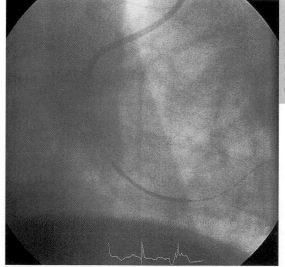

Figure 26.2:
Deep intubation of a 6 F guiding catheter in the right coronary artery, facilitating distal delivery of a stent despite tortuous proximal anatomy and a proximal stent.

coronary is similarly approached with the right Judkins, Multipurpose, right (or left) Amplatz, the Kimny Radial or MUTA radial right.

Some complex PTCA procedures require the use of large calibre devices or adjunctive supportive therapy such as balloon pumping and coronary pacing. Recent data suggests that many individuals have a radial artery capable of accommodating large calibre sheaths, and 7 F or 8 F sheaths can be used in many patients.[18] Where necessary, an arm vein can be percutaneously punctured to allow access to the right side of the heart for pacing or pressure measurement. Simultaneous positioning of a radial and femoral sheath will allow PTCA to be performed with balloon pump support, without the necessity for bilateral groin punctures.

THE LEARNING CURVE

Performing percutaneous transradial procedures provides new technical challenges. During the learning phase, the operator must reliably puncture the relatively small calibre radial artery, successfully manipulate catheters from a distal access site in the right arm, and perform interventions utilising a different range of guiding catheter configurations, calibres and operating techniques. Initial failure rates for radial artery cannulation of 3.8% improving to 1.2% have been reported during a 650 patient series.[19]

One common problem during the initial part of the learning curve is radial artery spasm (Fig. 26.3) which occurs in up to 10% of cases in an initial series making successful cannulation less likely and catheter manipulation more difficult, as well as causing pain during the procedure and making sheath removal extremely unpleasant.[20] The occurrence of spasm is probably related to operator experience and to the degree of patient anxiety, such that a successful, painless first pass will be least likely

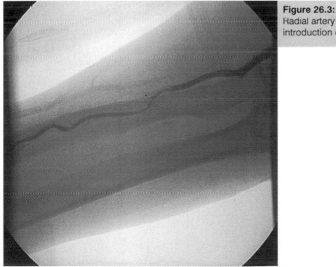

Figure 26.3:
Radial artery spasm prior to introduction of a guidewire.

to provoke spasm. The following points may help reduce the occurrence of spasm:

- Adequate patient sedation if necessary.
- Effective local anaesthetic.
- Successful first pass cannulation (avoiding haematoma formation and the initiation of spasm before cannulation).
- Use of an anti-spasmolytic, either via the cannula or after insertion of a short length of the sheath. Verapamil and nitrates are commonly used.
- Use of a long sheath to protect the vessel wall during catheter movement.
- Use of an exchange length guidewire to minimise vessel trauma.
- Operator experience is important (more frequent successful first punctures and shorter procedure times).

If spasm occurs, the patient should be warned that sheath removal would be painful. Extreme spasm (and pain) may make immediate withdrawal impossible, in which case patient sedation and analgesia is required, and sublingual nifedipine should be administered. Intra-arterial nitrates and verapamil can be re-administered, whilst warm compresses applied to the arm may reduce the spasm. If the problem persists, increased analgesia and an hour's wait may be sufficient, but if this is unsuccessful, an axillary block will rapidly remove radial spasm. Ongoing research to quantify radial artery spasm and allow comparisons of sheath length and coating and the use and composition of anti-spasmolytic cocktails are currently underway.

CONCLUSIONS

Coronary intervention performed via a brachial or femoral access site is associated with significant risk of important neurovascular complications. The use of aggressive antithrombotic regimes in association with PTCA procedures will increase this risk, which cannot be eliminated by the use of vascular access closure devices. Transradial PTCA almost eliminates the risk of arterial access site complications. In addition, patients prefer transradial procedures, and hospital costs can be significantly reduced compared with procedures performed via the femoral or brachial artery. The major limitation to widespread clinical use of this access site is the learning curve associated with reliably puncturing the radial artery, and performing PTCA from a distal upper limb access site. With improvements in technique and equipment the learning curve has been considerably shortened, and a committed interventionist should have no difficulty in developing a transradial service.

REFERENCES

1. Eccleshall S, Muthusamy T, Nolan J. The transradial access site for cardiac procedures: A clinical perspective. Stent 1999;2(3):74–9.

2. Sundlof D, Rerkpattanapitat P, Wongpraparut N *et al*. Incidence of bleeding complications associated with abciximab use in conjunction with thrombolytic therapy in patients requiring percutaneous transluminal angioplasty. Am J Cardiol 1999;83:1569–71.

3. Campeau L. Percutaneous radial artery approach for coronary angiography. Cathet Cardiovasc Diagn 1989;16(1):3–7.

4. Kiemeneij F. Transradial artery coronary angioplasty and stenting: History and single centre experience. J Invas Cardiol 1996;8 (Suppl. D):3D–8D.

5. Nolan J, Batin P, Welsh C *et al*. Feasibility and applicability of coronary stent implantation with the direct brachial approach: Results of a single-centre study. Am Heart J 1997;134(939–44).

6. Sreeram S, Lumsden AB, Miller JS, Salam AA, Dodson TF, Smith RB. Retroperitoneal hematoma following femoral arterial catheterization: a serious and often fatal complication. Am Surg 1993;59(2):94–8.

7. Kent KC, Moscucci M, Gallagher SG, DiMattia ST, Skillman JJ. Neuropathy after cardiac catheterization: incidence, clinical patterns, and long-term outcome. J Vasc Surg 1994;19(6):1008–13.

8. Al-Allaf K, Eccleshall S, Muthusamy T, Nolan J. Selection of arterial access sites for cardiac procedures. Br J Cardiol 2000;7:422–5.

9. Kiemeneij F, Laarman GJ, Odekerken D, Slagboom T, van der Wieken R. A randomized comparison of percutaneous transluminal coronary angioplasty by the radial, brachial and femoral approaches: the Access study. J Am Coll Cardiol 1997;29(6):1269–75.

10. Black A, Cortina R, Aoun A, Lucas G, Fajadet J, Marco J. Efficacy and safety of transradial coronary angioplasty. a report of 5354 consecutive cases. Eur Heart J 1999;20 (Abstract Suppl.):268.

11. Hildick-Smith D, Ludman P, Lowe M *et al*. Comparison of radial versus brachial approaches for diagnostic coronary angiography when the femoral approach is contraindicated. Am J Cardiol 1998;81:770–2.

12. Choussat R, Black A, Bossi I, Fajadet J, Marco J. Vascular complications and clinical outcome after coronary angioplasty with platelet IIb/IIIa receptor blockade. Eur Heart J 2000;21:662–7.

13. Allen C, Glasziou P, Del Mar C. Bed rest: a potentially harmful treatment needing more careful evaluation. Lancet 1999;354:1299–33.

14. Foulger V. Patients' views of day-case cardiac catheterisation. Prof Nurse 1997;12:478–80.

15. Laarman GJ, Kiemeneij F, van der Wieken LR, Tijssen JG, Suwarganda JS, Slagboom T. A pilot study of coronary angioplasty in outpatients. Br Heart J 1994;72(1):12–5.

16. AlAllaf K, Eccleshall S, Kaba R, Nolan J. Arterial access for cardiac procedures utilising the percutaneous transradial approach. Br J Cardiol 2000;7;548–52.

17. Kiemeneij F. Transradial approach for coronary angioplasty and stenting. Stent 1998;1:83–88.

18. Saito S, Ikei H, Hosokawa G, Tanaka S. Influence of the ratio between radial artery inner diameter and sheath outer diameter on radial artery flow after transradial coronary intervention. Cathet Cardiovasc Intervent 1999;46:173–8.

19. Louvard Y, Harvey R, Pezzano M, Bradai R, Benaim R, Morice M. Transradial complex coronary angioplasty: The influence of a single operator's experience. J Invas Cardiol 1997;9 (Suppl. C):647–9.

20. Barbeau G, Carrier G, Ferland S, Létourneau L, Gleeton O, Larivière M. Right transradial approach for coronary procedures: Preliminary results. J Invas Cardiol 1996;8 (Suppl. D):19D–21D.

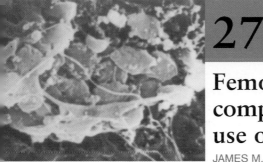

27

Femoral artery complications and the use of closure devices

JAMES M. McLENACHAN

KEY POINTS

■ The femoral artery is the preferred access site to the arterial system for most percutaneous coronary interventions.

■ Two major complications following sheath removal are haematoma and false aneurysm.

■ Closure of the femoral artery puncture site may be achieved by puncture site compression, sealing devices, or suturing devices.

■ Femoral artery closure devices are relatively new; it is inevitable that novel and improved devices will be developed.

INTRODUCTION

The femoral artery is the preferred access site to the arterial system for the vast majority of percutaneous coronary interventions. Other sites, such as the brachial artery or the radial artery, are used if the femoral artery is unavailable and may be the preferred access site for some interventionists. These arteries, however, are smaller than the femoral artery and their instrumentation carries a higher risk of dissection and occlusion. Percutaneous puncture of the brachial artery is more likely to require surgical repair than percutaneous femoral puncture while brachial arteriotomy under direct vision can be technically challenging for the inexperienced operator and is time-consuming. Percutaneous radial artery puncture appears to be safe but results in occlusion of around 5% of radial arteries; this may become an increasing cause for concern as the radial artery becomes established as a conduit for coronary artery bypass grafting. In contrast, percutaneous puncture of the femoral artery is relatively straight-forward and occlusion of this vessel is rare, even if inadvertently dissected by a coronary catheter. The challenge, therefore, is to remove the arterial sheath without complications.

COMPLICATIONS FOLLOWING SHEATH REMOVAL

The two major complications following removal of the arterial sheath are haematoma formation and false aneurysm. These are variants of the same process since both result from a failure to 'seal' the hole in the arterial wall resulting in the flow of blood from the artery into the surrounding tissues. A haematoma implies that the puncture site has eventually sealed, and does not usually require active intervention. The blood in the tissues around the artery will break down and resorb but the patient may have extensive bruising for weeks or even months. If the patient loses a lot of blood into the surrounding tissues, then transfusion may be required.

False aneurysm (or pseudo-aneurysm) implies that the puncture site is still allowing flow between the artery and the extra-arterial collection. False aneurysms are usually pulsatile and are generally more tender than haematomas. The diagnosis is made by ultrasound with colour flow doppler which demonstrates flow through the narrow neck of the false aneurysm. Fortunately, compression of the neck of the false aneurysm under ultrasound control is often successful in converting the false aneurysm into a haematoma and surgical repair is now rarely required.

THE NEED FOR PUNCTURE SITE DEVICES

Following diagnostic coronary angiography, manual compression of the femoral artery puncture site by a trained individual for around 5 to 10 minutes usually results in satisfactory haemostasis without complications. In interventional procedures, the arterial sheath may be larger and the patient is usually heparinised. Manual compression will eventually achieve haemostasis but this may take 20 to 30 minutes. As a result, sheath removal is often delayed for 2–3 hours to allow the effects of the heparin to wear off. In many cardiac units, however, there is considerable pressure on catheter laboratory time and on bed availability. Early sheath removal, early ambulation and early discharge (or transfer) have all become priorities and have been the driving force behind the development of femoral artery closure devices.

CLASSIFICATION OF DEVICES TO TREAT THE PUNCTURE SITE

The approaches to closure of the femoral artery puncture site can be divided as follows:

1. Puncture site compression
   – manual
   – mechanical
2. Sealing devices
3. Suturing devices

Puncture site compression

The traditional treatment of a femoral artery puncture site is to apply manual compression locally for a period of 10 to 20 minutes. Opinion varies as to how this is best achieved; some operators use a large number of swabs and apply pressure to a large area but most operators prefer one or two swabs (or none) with pressure applied locally over the arterial puncture site which is cranial to the skin puncture site. This way, the puncture area can be kept under review and significant external bleeding or haematoma formation can be detected early. The disadvantages of manual compression are that it is time-consuming and uncomfortable for the operator since a reasonable degree of force is required. As a result, a number of mechanical devices have been tried. These include sandbags, C-clamps, stasis buttons and pneumatic devices. Sandbags do not appear to reduce vascular complications and may even increase patient discomfort.[1] Mechanical clamps have been shown to be as effective as manual compression in terms of preventing complications although the compression time may be longer.[2] The Colapinto compression device[3] and the FemoStop pneumatic device[4] both involve wrapping a device tightly around the patient's upper thigh and lower torso and then directing the compressor force into the puncture site area using either a polystyrene button or a pneumatic chamber; the latter has the advantage that the pressure can be gradually reduced without removing the device. The pneumatic device (FemoStop) has been shown in a large study to be as effective as a clamp device.[4] These devices, however, are no more effective than manual compression, may be less safe, and, by their nature, cannot shorten the time to haemostasis.

Sealing devices

Most of the clinical experience in this area has been gained using two devices which employ bovine collagen to seal the arterial puncture; the prototype was the vascular haemostatic device (VHD or VasoSeal), which was followed by the haemostatic puncture closure device (HPCD or AngioSeal). Both have undergone considerable improvement since the original devices were developed. In addition, a third device (Duett) is now available in the UK.

Vascular haemostatic device (VasoSeal)

The VasoSeal acts by deploying a collagen plug on to the external arterial wall after dilatation of the skin puncture site and subcutaneous tissues. Early versions required multiple different devices to be kept in stock depending on the depth of the artery but the latest device (VasoSeal ES) is advertised as 'one size fits all'. With this version, the arterial sheath is first replaced by a 'locator' device. The locator is then advanced to deploy a 'J segment' in the artery. The locator is then pulled back until resistance is felt. This ensures that the J segment is pulled back against the arteriotomy. A dilator sheath is then advanced over the locator down to the arterial surface. The device is then withdrawn allowing the collagen cartridge to deploy.

  The VasoSeal device is easy to use and, when successfully deployed, allows early mobilisation of the patient. Several studies of this device have been reported.[5,6,7] In an early British study of 63 patients, the device was successfully deployed in 90% of patients[6] with a mean insertion time of less than 2 minutes. About 95% of those in whom the device was deployed were mobilised without complication within 2 hours. However, the device could not be deployed in six patients (9.5%), the most common reason for this being perforation of the femoral artery by the dilator ($n = 3$). Furthermore, three of the 57 who received the device could not be mobilised at two hours because of a sizeable haematoma. A larger multicentre study reported similar results with failure to deploy the collagen plug in around 13% of patients.[7] One prospective randomised study of 124 patients has compared immediate sheath removal and VasoSeal use with delayed sheath removal and mechanical compression.[5] The incidence of false aneurysm was the same in both groups (4%); however, there were two other complications in the 62 patients in the VasoSeal group (one arterial occlusion, one venous thrombosis). Although the numbers are small, these are worrying complications that are rarely seen in patients treated by manual compression. In a review, major complications from the VasoSeal range from 0% to 3.2%.[8]

Haemostatic puncture device (AngioSeal)

The AngioSeal, like the VasoSeal, uses bovine collagen to seal the arterial puncture site. However, the AngioSeal also deploys an anchor on the inside of the artery which provides a mechanical block and holds the collagen in the tract. Attached to the anchor is a suture which carries a small collagen sponge. The principle of the device is that the anchor and the collagen sponge, retained by the suture, form a mechanical sandwich around the arteriotomy. The anchor, the suture and the collagen sponge are all fully bio-resorbable. To deploy the device, a short guidewire is inserted through the existing arterial sheath which is then replaced by an 8 F (or 6 F) AngioSeal sheath containing a modified dilator. The dilator, in addition to the usual guidewire channel, has a 'locator' channel which starts just beyond the end of the arterial sheath and opens proximal to the proximal end of the sheath. By moving the sheath and dilator backwards and forwards, the operator can determine the position of the arteriotomy by the free flow of blood through the locator channel. Once the site of the arteriotomy has been determined, the sheath is advanced by approximately 1 cm to ensure that the distal end of the sheath is free in the lumen of the artery. The dilator and guidewire are then removed. The sheath is then held firmly and the carrier tube is pushed through the haemostatic valve and into the artery. Still fixing the sheath, the carrier is then pulled backwards until resistance is felt. This resistance is caused by the anchor being pulled against the arterial wall. Once the anchor has been deployed, the carrier tube and insertion sheath are held firmly and withdrawn together. As they are withdrawn, a 'tamper' tube appears. Still maintaining the tension on the suture, the tamper tube is used to 'tamp down' the collagen plug. A tension spring is then applied to the suture to maintain gentle pressure on the tamper tube for 20 to 30 minutes. At this point, the tension spring is removed and the suture is cut at skin level.

As with the VasoSeal, the AngioSeal is quick and easy to use[9,10,11] and allows for early mobilisation of the patient. One recent study reported successful deployment in 88% of patients although most studies have shown successful deployment in 90 to 100% of cases.[8] The risk of major complications has varied from 0% to 2.6% in different series, the range being similar to reported complications for the VasoSeal.

The Duett sealing device

Unlike the VasoSeal and Angioseal, the Duett is deployed through the existing introducer sheath; this eliminates the need to enlarge the tissue tract and arterial puncture prior to deployment. A catheter is inserted through the sheath and a small balloon inflated with saline. The sheath is then withdrawn until the balloon is pulled against the arterial wall. A procoagulant liquid (a mixture of collagen and fibrin) is then delivered via the side-arm of the sheath onto the adventitial surface of the artery. The balloon is then deflated and removed while moderate pressure is maintained on the access site for 2–5 minutes. The potential advantages of this device are that no foreign material is left inside the artery and that the artery can be repunctured immediately if this proves necessary. In the small series published to date, this appears to be an effective sealing device.[12]

Suturing devices

The 'Perclose' system is an ingenious device which allows 'surgical' closure of a femoral arteriotomy without direct vision of the artery. After pre-dilating the sub-cutaneous tissues, the suture-containing device is advanced into the artery; four needles (or two in the case of the smaller 6 F device) are then retracted back through the arterial wall and delivered to the surface; the needles are then removed, the knots are tied and these knots are then pushed against the arterial wall using a knot-pushing tool. Some studies have been encouraging[13] but the device requires more time and greater expertise than the sealing devices described above. Furthermore, the use of the device even in a centre with high volume experience still resulted in a need for vascular repair in over 2% of cases while another large series has reported a rate of failed deployment of over 10%. Problems are particularly likely to occur if there is steep angulation of the puncture tract.[14]

FUTURE DIRECTIONS

Femoral artery closure devices are relatively new: it is inevitable that there will be evolution of existing devices and the development of new devices. The ideal device should be quick and easy to use, should achieve haemostasis even in patients treated with anticoagulants and antiplatelet drugs, should have an extremely low incidence of major complications such as vessel occlusion, distal embolisation and late bleeding and should, if possible, allow early repuncture of the artery.

REFERENCES

1. Christensen B, Lacarella C, Manion R, Bruhn-Ding B, Meyer S, Wilson R. Sandbags do not prevent complications after catheterization. Circulation 1994;90:1–205.

2. Simon A, Bumgarner B, Clark K, Israel S. Manual versus mechanical compression for femoral artery haemostasis after cardiac catheterization. Am J Crit Care 1998;7:308–13.

3. Colapinto RF, Harty PW. Femoral artery compression device for outpatient angiography. Radiology 1988;166:890–1.

4. Janerot-Sjoberg B, Broquist M, Fransson SG. Femoral artery haemostasis with a pneumatic compression device versus a clamp after coronary angiography. Scand Cardiovasc J 1998;32:281–4.

5. Camenzind E, Grossholz M, Urban P, Dorsaz PA, Didier D, Meier B. Collagen application versus manual compression: a prospective randomized trial for arterial puncture site closure after coronary angioplasty. J Am Coll Cardiol 1994;24:655–62.

6. Foran JP, Patel D, Brookes J, Wainwright RJ. Early mobilisation after percutaneous cardiac catheterization using collagen plug (VasoSeal) haemostasis. Br Heart J 1993;69:424–9.

7. Ernst SM, Tjonjoegin RM, Schrader R et al. Immediate sealing of arterial puncture sites after cardiac catheterization and coronary angioplasty using a biodegradable collagen plug: results of an international registry. J Am Coll Cardiol 1993;21:851–5.

8. Sibler S. Rapid haemostasis of arterial puncture sites with collagen in patients undergoing diagnostic and interventional cardiac catheterisation. Clin Cardiol 1997;20:981–92.

9. O'Sullivan GJ, Buckenham TM, Belli AM. The use of the angio-seal haemostatic puncture closure device in high risk patients. Clin Radiol 1999;54:340–1.

10. Beyer-Enke SA, Soldner J, Zeitler E. Immediate sealing of arterial puncture site following femoropopliteal angioplasty: a prospective randomized trial. Cardiovasc Intervent Radiol 1996;19:406–10.

11. Henry M, Amor M, Allaoui M, Tricoche O. A new access site management tool: the Angio-Seal haemostatic puncture closure device. J Endovasc Surg 1995;2:289–96.

12. Silber S, Gershony G, Schon B et al. A novel vascular sealing device for closure of percutaneous arterial access sites. Am J Cardiol 1999;83:1248–52.

13. Gerckens U, Cattelaens N, Lampe EG, Grube E. Management of arterial puncture site after catheterization procedures: evaluating a suture-mediated closure device. Am J Cardiol 1999;83:1658–63.

14. Duda SH, Wiskirchen J, Erb M et al. Suture-mediated percutaneous closure of antegrade femoral arterial access sites in patients who have received full anticoagulation therapy. Radiology 1999;210:47–52.

Section Six

Current Practice and Future Perspectives

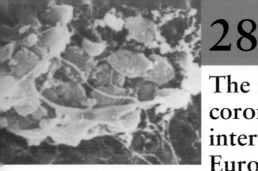

28

The future of coronary catheter intervention from a European perspective

BERNHARD MEIER

KEY POINTS

- PTCA is a derivative of peripheral catheter angioplasty, based on Grüntzig's form-constant polyvinyl chloride balloon.

- Grüntzig invented the method for early coronary disease, for which it is still mostly used.

- Europe lagged behind the USA for 15 years, but is now about to catch up, with Germany in the lead (in 1996 125 804 PTCAs were reported).

- The need for coronary revascularisation will continue to grow because of the general ageing of the population.

- Surgical and non-surgical methods are moving closer together, as are the cardiac specialists performing these procedures. However, PTCA is still less invasive.

PLACE IN MEDICAL HISTORY

Percutaneous transluminal coronary angioplasty (PTCA), also called percutaneous coronary intervention (PCI), is a derivative of peripheral catheter angioplasty, introduced by Dotter and Judkins in 1964[1]. It is based on the invention by Andreas Grüntzig of a form-constant polyvinyl chloride balloon[2].

Grüntzig was born on 25 June 1939 in Dresden at the beginning of the Second World War. His widowed mother raised two sons to become fine medical doctors. The socialist German regime had planned for Grüntzig to become a mason, but the mother intervened and emigrated to Heidelberg where Grüntzig studied medicine. In 1969 Grüntzig moved to Switzerland to take up a job at the University Hospital of Zurich in the recently founded Division of Angiology. The German Zeitler taught him Dotter's dilatation method of treating peripheral arteries. Grüntzig liked the idea of non-surgical treatment of arterial stenoses but not the technique. With the help of his wife, a befriended couple, and a plastic expert from the nearby Technical University of Zurich, Grüntzig developed a catheter with a cylindrical, form-constant balloon at the tip.

After encouraging results in several hundred peripheral arteries, Grüntzig moved to the cardiology section and so did his balloon. A small Swiss firm (Schneider Medintag) helped to miniaturise the balloon catheters to prepare them for use in coronary arteries. Everything was ready by early 1976, but a suitable case could not be found. Coronary angiography, being reserved for patients late in their course of coronary artery disease, generally revealed multivessel disease. Yet Grüntzig was

349

looking for an isolated stenosis. On 22 March 1976, a compassionate attempt to save a dying patient with end-stage coronary artery disease who had been turned down by cardiac surgery, failed due to technical problems before a balloon ever got close to the heart. Catherization had to be done from the arm, but the only guiding catheter available could not reach the left coronary ostium[3].

After a small series of successful intra-operative applications of his coronary balloon catheter in San Francisco, Grüntzig finally found the ideal patient for the world's first PTCA. It took place on 16 September 1977 in Zurich. The patient was 38 years old, as was Grüntzig. The successful dilatation of a proximal stenosis of the left anterior descending coronary artery freed the patient of a debilitating angina before an infarction could occur. The result has remained stable ever since. As Grüntzig's assistant I participated in this first intervention and I have kept contact with the patient who had a splendid subsequent course. I carried out the latest angiographic control in April 2000 (almost 23 years after the treatment). It showed a pristine long-term result of the dilated site and only minimal progression of atherosclerosis elsewhere.

In the late autumn of 1980, the centre of PTCA activity and interest shifted with Andreas Grüntzig from Europe to the United States, where the disease was more prevalent and disease awareness among the population and resources for diagnosis and treatment were further developed.

Grüntzig never expected the method to be universally successful and without complications. Nonetheless, he predicted a good potential for it. Little did he know how significant this potential was going to be. The true size of the importance of PTCA was not even apparent when Grüntzig died in a plane crash on 27 October 1985. The stent, for example, was only to be clinically introduced 5 months later (28 March 1986) by Jacques Puel in Toulouse.[4]

CURRENT STATUS OF PTCA

In contrast to the widespread opinion that indications for PTCA never ceased to expand, indications basically remained unchanged from the very beginning. Grüntzig invented the method for early coronary artery disease, ideally implying only one vessel. Up to the current day, this is where it is mostly used. Multivessel PTCA in a single session amounts to 15–20% in Europe and around 10% in the United States. The huge increase of absolute and population-adjusted numbers of PTCA procedures is explained by the earlier invasive assessment of the disease, thanks to the easier accessibility of cardiac catheterisation laboratories in industrialised countries.

Calculating an investment of roughly 6000 Euros per intervention and multiplying this with the estimated 1 million cases done worldwide to date per year, the enormous economic impact of PTCA can be grasped. Investments in publications, training, and associated professional and private tourism have to be added.

While Europe was lagging behind the USA for about 15 years, it is about to catch up, with Grüntzig's country of origin, Germany, in the lead. In 1996 a total of 125 804 PTCAs were reported from Germany, accounting for about 1600 per million inhabitants.[5] Estimated figures from the US for 1996 were 476 000 and 1800, respectively.

In countries without significant waiting lists for diagnostic coronary angiography, examination will yield no significant disease, single vessel disease, double vessel disease or triple vessel disease in equal quarters.[6] Two-thirds of these patients will have a PTCA, one-fifth a coronary bypass operation and only one-seventh medical therapy exclusively. Considering only single vessel disease, the percentage of PTCA is about 90%. Even in triple vessel disease PTCA will be used in 30%. The application of PTCA to true triple vessel disease where all three main arteries are significantly narrowed remains rare, however. Such patients fare better with coronary bypass surgery, particularly if they are diabetic.

ALTERNATIVES AND COMPLEMENTS TO BALLOON ANGIOPLASTY

In the 1980s, a strange phenomenon was observed. The restenosis rate hovered around 50% in American series but was only around 30% in European series. My interpretation is that in this era Americans dilated more lesions less and Europeans dilated fewer lesions more. The fee per service system in the United States invited Americans to dilate as many lesions in a patient that they could possibly find an indication for. The fear of liability claims forced them to keep the complications to a minimum. Underdilatation, avoiding dissections prone to acute occlusion, was the solution. This engendered the high restenosis rate. Europeans usually worked in a less profit-oriented system. They stuck to the truly significant lesions but tried to achieve a good result, trading a slightly elevated acute risk for a significantly lower restenosis rate.

The American background was ideal for new methods such as atherectomy and laser. These methods found fairly wide distribution in the United States where the competitive situation forced interventional cardiologists to apply them, not to fall behind their peers. European operators shunned them, recognising before long their lack of efficacy and their increased potential of complications.

The balloon-complementing stent differed from the other new devices from the beginning.[7] The results of stenting were first overshadowed by the fact that stents (in contrast to other new devices) were only used when a complication already had occurred (bail-out situation). Therefore, infarctions and mortality were high in stent cases. Nevertheless, the individual operator rapidly became aware of the salutary effect of stenting in the face of poor balloon, atherectomy, or laser results. An objective analysis of cases performed during live demonstration courses showed that the other new devices were initially used to show-off, but were quickly abandoned when things got tough, whereas the stent was introduced at that moment to save the day.[8]

In the meantime the Americans have also recognised the importance of stenting and have again taken the lead in the world. Elective stenting and even direct stenting have become the trend because evidence-based medicine proves a reduction of restenosis after stenting. The consequence is that acute and subacute vessel occlusions have increased to a level above that which was known before stenting was available. It is difficult to say what the ideal proportion of stenting would be, but it should be borne in mind that before stenting about 70% of lesions neither had an acute problem nor a restenosis. Consequently, stents can only be beneficial in the remaining 30%. These 30% should be concentrated on as far as possible. Stenting 100% of patients is not only dangerous, but also cost-inefficient.

During the past 10 years, the eternal question of whether a surgical back-up has to be organised and ready under the same roof for every PTCA case, has been settled for good. The stent has played an important role in this. Currently it is almost universally accepted that a PTCA done by an experienced team does not need an organised surgical back-up. This has also opened the door for an increased combination of diagnostic coronary angiography and PTCA in one session (ad hoc PTCA). This is a blessing for patients and catheterisation laboratories with limited resources in terms of time and money.

Currently, much focus is on other methods to reduce acute problems and in particular restenosis. Brachytherapy is the most sophisticated of them and also the most advanced in terms of available data. Its effect is undisputed if it is applied at adequate dose. The cloud of possible late effects looms over this method, as does the fact that in order to prevent one reintervention, about 10 patients have to be subjected to brachytherapy. This is not really a bargain in terms of time and money invested.

REMAINING LIMITATIONS

The accumulated risks, the patience of the usually awake patient, the amount of contrast medium, and to a lesser degree the aggregated radiation dose place a boundary on the possibilities of PTCA. The problem of restenosis is a further concern, which, however, is less on the mind of the operator than the other limitations. Restenosis is a nuisance but rarely dangerous. Restenotic lesions hardly have a potential for myocardial infarction as the initially rupture-prone plaque is sealed by a smooth neo-endothelium.[9]

Chronic total occlusions remain the major reason to opt for bypass surgery rather than for PTCA in patients with double or triple vessel disease.[10] Some progress has been made with special wires, but the technical failure rate for chronic occlusions stays at about 30% compared with <2% for stenoses.

CURRENT PREREQUISITES

A modern catheterisation laboratory with digital image treatment, backed up by a second fluoroscopy unit for the case of system failure, is the backbone of every PTCA service. It is complemented by a comprehensive stock of guiding catheters, guidewires, balloon catheters, and stents. A small but specialised pharmacy with drugs used for the cardiovascular system (anticoagulants, antiplatelet drugs, pain medications, tranquillisers, inotropic agents, antibiotics, etc.) is important.[11] The laboratory has to be equipped with mobile monitoring equipment. An intra-aortic balloon pump is recommended but not mandatory. Other PTCA devices such as atherectomy catheters, laser catheters, intra-coronary ultrasound equipment, flow or pressure measuring wires, clot lysers or catchers, local delivery catheters, or a percutaneous left ventricular assist device or cardiac-pulmonary bypass machine are not essential and can remain reserved for high volume centres.

The prime quality factor of a PTCA laboratory is the team. At least the principal operator must have had thorough training at a high volume institution including a fellowship dedicated to interventional cardiology of at least 1 year. A second fully trained cardiologist should be in the house. The auxiliary personnel must have profound knowledge of the procedure and all available material. Professional care for the patient has to start before the procedure and continue until hospital discharge. Dedicated cardiac services extending from the emergency department to the rehabilitation programme are the ideal setting.

Regular morbidity and mortality rounds and inter-operator statistics are important. So is a comprehensive data bank maintained by professionals who are not at the same time responsible for the patients. A structured training programme for doctors and medical personnel should be individually enhanced by regular study of the literature and participation in cardiology congresses and dedicated practical courses for PTCA.

PERSPECTIVES

The age-corrected prevalence of coronary heart disease is receding in industrialised countries thanks to preventive measures. Notwithstanding, the need for coronary revascularisation will continue to grow because of the general ageing of the population engendering more overall prevalence of coronary artery disease.[12]

Performing PTCA provides a professional challenge with a high overall satisfaction and prestige topped in many countries by a handsome remuneration. Catheterisation laboratories abound and are not fully exploited in many European countries, let alone the United States. The awareness among the population of the disease and the possibility to treat it effectively without surgery continues to increase in Europe also. This leads to high expectations of the population, readily met by an ever-growing number of trained interventional cardiologists eager to help (and to prosper).

This evolution will only be halted, if at all, by rationing in terms of budget restrictions or politically imposed indication limits (e.g. age barrier).

As politicians tend to think of the next election, it is unlikely that they will impose such drastic restrictions when there is a growing proportion of voters with coronary artery disease.

Cost can be contained without necessarily reducing the number of patients treated by curbing incentives to utilise fancy but unnecessary gadgets. The fee per case or even more the fee per patient (capitation) will prompt the physicians to stick to the essential. Atherectomy, laser treatment, brachytherapy, embolus protection, intra-coronary ultrasound, and even direct stenting will be out of the question. The patients will be grateful.

The remarkable progress of our fellow cardiac surgeons, awakened by our evolution from the scolded and misbehaving child to a partner casting an ever bigger shadow, may shift the indication line slightly back to the surgical side. Bypass surgery with all arterial grafts implanted without the use of the heart–lung machine comes close to PTCA. However, it only comes close and PTCA is still less invasive. A PTCA patient can leave the same day or at least the next morning after perhaps even having done a reassuring exercise test. Surgery will never match that. An off-pump arterial bypass operation is a formidable alternative for a cumbersome multi-lesion angioplasty often requiring several sessions. It remains to prove, however, that working on the beating heart can parallel the anastomotic results attained on the resting heart.

The fact is, that surgical and non-surgical methods are moving closer together and so are the protagonists performing these procedures. The overlap of indications has grown again. It prompts us to meet with our surgical colleagues more often, only to find out once more that we are stronger together as 1 + 1 may be greater than 2.

REFERENCES

1. Dotter CT, Judkins MP. Transluminal treatment of arteriosclerotic obstruction: description of a new technique and a preliminary report of its application. Circulation 1964;3:654–70.

2. Grüntzig A, Hopff H. Perkutane Rekanalisation chronischer arterieller Verschlüsse mit einem neuen Dilatationskatheter. Dtsch Med Wochenschr 1974;99:2502–5.

3. Meier B. Balloon angioplasty. In Topol EJ (ed) Textbook of cardiovascular medicine. Philadelphia: Lippincott-Raven, 1998, pp. 1977–2009.

4. Puel J, Joffre F, Rousseau H et al. Endo-prothèses coronariennes auto-expansives dans la prévention des resténoses après angioplastie transluminale. Arch Mal Coeur 1987;8:1311–12.

5. Maier W, Windecker S, Lablanche JM, Mühlberger V, Wijns W, Meier B. The European registry of cardiac catheter interventions 1996. For the Working Group Coronary Circulation of the European Society of Cardiology. Eur Heart J 2001 (in press).

6. Delacrétaz E, Meier B. Use of coronary angioplasty, bypass surgery, and conservative therapy for treatment of coronary artery disease over the past decade. Eur Heart J 1998;19:1042–6.

7. Meier B. New devices for coronary angioplasty: The Emperor's new clothes revisited. Am J Med 1995;98:429–31.

8. Chatelain P, Meier B, De la Serna F et al. Success with coronary angioplasty as seen at demonstrations of procedure. Lancet 1992;340:1202–5.

9. Meier B, Ramamurthy S. Plaque sealing by coronary angioplasty. Cathet Cardiovasc Diagn 1995;36:295–7.

10. Delacrétaz E, Meier B. Therapeutic strategy with total coronary artery occlusions. Am J Cardiol 1997;79:185–7.

11. Meier B, Bonzel T, Heyndrickx G et al. For the Study Group Clinical Issues, Working Group Coronary Circulation of the European Society of Cardiology. Recommendations for training and quality control in coronary angioplasty. Eur Heart J 1996;17:1477–81.

12. Levin PJ, Sassouni C. The potential world market for cardiovascular and medical devices. J Invas Cardiol 1997;9:138–43.

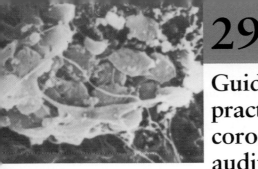

29

Guidelines for good practice and training in coronary angioplasty, audit and device regulation

MICHAEL S. NORELL

KEY POINTS

- Interventional centres should undertake a minimum of 200 cases per year and provide 24-hour catheter laboratory availability.

- Whether emergency surgical cover is provided on or off-site, the facility should exist to enable cardiopulmonary bypass to be established within 90 minutes of referral for urgent CABG.

- The primary operator is defined as an individual actively involved in a case and taking overall responsibility for its outcome.

- In order to maintain skills, operators should undertake a minimum of 75 cases annually.

- A PTCA trainer should have performed at least 500 cases as first operator and undertake 125 cases per year, 50 of these directly supervising the trainee.

- Trainees should assist in at least 25 interventional cases in their first 4 years as Specialist Registrar, and be involved in at least 200 cases in their last 2 years of subspecialty training, 125 of these as first operator.

- A minimum dataset for audit in cardiac intervention has been defined; operators and their institutions should be committed to data collection and reporting to a central registry (UKCCAD).

- The British Cardiac Society, in conjunction with the British Cardiovascular Intervention Society (BCIS), will set up a systematic peer review process involving a site visit to all interventional centres every 3 years.

- The Medical Devices Agency (MDA) exists to monitor and regulate the introduction and performance of all interventional technology; early reporting of adverse device-related events is encouraged.

- The recommended target for annual UK interventional activity is 500 cases per million to be achieved by the year 2002.

In 1996 a joint working group of the British Cardiac Society and the British Cardiovascular Intervention Society (BCIS) published guidelines which addressed good practice and training in coronary angioplasty.[1] These were based on a consensus of professional judgement, acknowledging similar publications from other countries,[2] and have now been updated. This chapter only summarises these guidelines; a complete description is to be found in the latest publication,[3] which also describes the means by which interventional activity may be properly audited. The process regulating the introduction of new devices, is also described here.

357

STANDARDS FOR CENTRES AND OPERATORS

In order to ensure the highest standards of practice, interventional centres and operators undertaking angioplasty must focus on safety and the best possible outcome for patients. The factors that directly influence this process are the facilities, staff and equipment in the interventional centre itself, the skill and experience of the operator, and the selection of cases thought suitable for percutaneous intervention.

Institutional standards

In addition to equipment found in facilities for diagnostic angiography, cardiac catheter laboratories undertaking intervention should also have the availability for oxygen saturation monitoring and intra-aortic balloon counterpulsation. The X-ray imaging may need to be superior to that used for diagnostic work and attention paid to guidelines covering radiation exposure to operators, staff and patients.

Acknowledging that complications during PTCA may be unpredictable, a comprehensive range of interventional equipment must be available. Allowing for the rapidly increasing knowledge in this field, this should include adjunctive pharmacology as well as hardware, and will need to be upgraded as interventional research advances. Centres undertaking PTCA for acute coronary syndromes should provide 24-hour catheter laboratory availability. Even in facilities doing only elective intervention, the laboratory should be available within 60 minutes of being notified, in order to treat patients who may require emergency repeat PTCA.

In order to ensure continuity in the provision of an interventional service, each centre should have at least three, and preferably five trained operators. When diagnostic angiography is undertaken at a site remote from the PTCA centre, there should be close liaison between that cardiologist and the centre to which the patient is referred for revascularisation. This will allow patients to benefit from the latest advances in percutaneous techniques. Regular meetings between the referring cardiologist, interventionist and cardiac surgeon are to be encouraged, and audited results of activity circulated.

Data have been reported suggesting that centres with high intervention volumes may have better results. Although not conclusive it is felt nevertheless that institutions should undertake a minimum number of cases annually in order to maintain the skills of all the staff involved with patients having PTCA (Figs 29.1 and 29.2). A minimum volume of 200 cases per year has been suggested but this is not to be rigidly applied; in 1996, five centres in the UK were doing less than this figure. It is felt that in these instances, accepting that peer review indicates good practice, then such centres should be supported and encouraged to increase their volume.

In the UK there has been a long running discussion as to the need to have standby surgery on-site, which has been regarded as the 'strongly

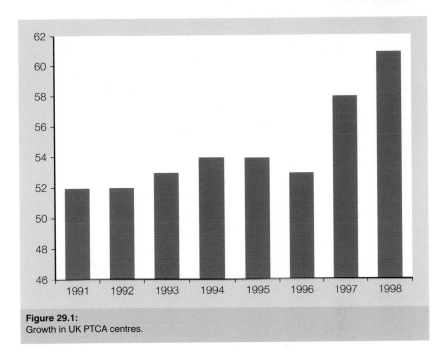

Figure 29.1:
Growth in UK PTCA centres.

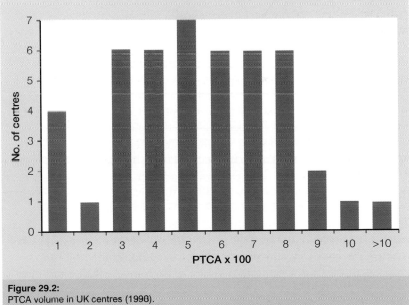

Figure 29.2:
PTCA volume in UK centres (1998).

preferred option'. The exponential growth in coronary stenting has not negated this requirement. In a small minority of patients, a pre-procedural decision may be made (after full discussion) that access to emergency CABG is not required. Otherwise, emergency CABG should be available (whether on or off-site) such that cardiopulmonary bypass can be established within 90 minutes of a referral for surgery being made. In centres with off-site surgical support, case selection may need to be modified. There will also need to be close liaison between the operator and the surgical centre providing cover, to ensure rapid transfer of patients when necessary.

Care after the interventional procedure can also directly influence patient outcome. The ward in which patients are observed after PTCA should be staffed by personnel experienced in the management of such patients and particularly familiar with the care of the femoral arterial puncture site so as to minimise complications related to bleeding or vasovagal reactions. There should also be ready access to pathology laboratory services (including blood transfusion) and to vascular surgical advice when necessary.

Operator standards

The results of interventional activity relate predominantly to the experience, skill and judgement of the operator. It would therefore be reasonable to conclude that such qualities can be maintained at a high standard only by practitioners undertaking a minimum number of cases annually. Setting such a figure has tended to produce intense debate. Low volume operators will demonstrate that their results are as good as those undertaking higher volumes. Indeed, they may even be superior if their case mix comprises fewer high-risk or complex cases. By attempting to increase their volume in order to comply with updated guidelines there is concern that more demanding cases are approached, the complexity of which may be beyond their expertise. Similarly, such interventionists may tend to refer more complex cases for surgery even though a percutaneous approach might still be feasible in the hands of a higher volume operator.

In 1996 the Working Group settled on a figure of 60 cases per year with the understanding that this was likely to increase. The latest guidelines are now in accord with those from the USA[2] and indicate a figure of 75 cases annually as a minimum undertaken by a primary operator. This individual is determined after the procedure and defines that person who is actively involved in, and assumes principal responsibility for, the outcome of the case. Operators should also be committed to continuing education and professional development in order to keep up with the rapidly changing technology and adjunctive pharmacology involved with percutaneous intervention. They should also be committed to a process of audit, on both a personal and departmental level, which should be presented locally and on a regular basis to other cardiologists, cardiac surgeons, nursing staff and interested non-medical disciplines.

TRAINING

Trainees

With the introduction of a formalised 6-year Specialist Registrar training programme in cardiology,[4] trainees should have been involved in at least 25 interventional cases during their first 4 years. Specific subspecialty training in PTCA begins formally in their final 2 years.

As with the volume of cases required to maintain expertise, defining a number at which an individual is deemed to be trained, is also a matter of debate. Previous recommendations restricted PTCA training only to the final year and advised involvement in at least 100 cases, of which the trainee was recorded as primary operator in 50. Allowing for interventional training over the 2 years, this level has been increased such that the trainee should assist in a minimum of 200 cases of which 125 should be as first operator.

Importantly, the trainee should not confine him or herself only to the execution of the case, but also be familiar with catheter laboratory and angioplasty equipment, and issues related to radiation protection. They should be involved with case selection, aftercare and follow-up of patients, and take an active part in departmental data collection and audit. A logbook of cases should be maintained and appropriate interventional meetings attended in order to ensure a comprehensive and up-to-date education.

Trainers

Operators who undertake the role of trainer should have performed at least 500 cases as first operator and themselves perform a minimum of 125 cases annually of which at least 50 should involve direct supervision of the trainee. The centre should be performing as wide a range of interventional cases as possible and should designate one individual who is primarily responsible for the organisation and appraisal of interventional trainees, as well as confirming their satisfactory completion of training.

Future demand for PTCA in the UK

The number of operators in training has to take account of the anticipated need for interventional services. The level of PTCA activity in the UK (437 cases per million in 1998) was considerably less than that in other European countries (Figs 29.3 and 29.4), and there is now a recommended target of 750 cases per million to be attained by the year 2002. Whether this target is achieved by expansion of existing PTCA centres or devolving activity to district general hospitals remains to be seen. The issue of surgical standby is likely to become less important than a unit's volume of activity and the experience of their interventional team.

It is clear however that the UK will need to modify its view of a PTCA service. In addition to recognising the need for more trainees, practitioners will need to focus more of their time on interventional practice (for which they have been specifically trained) and working in teams, and perhaps less on more general cardiological activities.

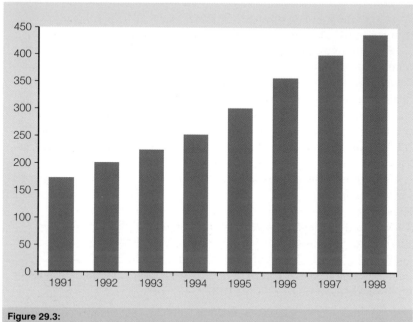

Figure 29.3:
PTCA activity in the UK. (Rates per million population.)

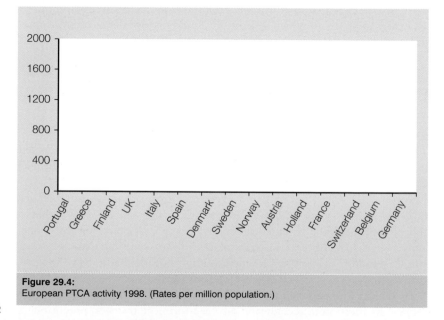

Figure 29.4:
European PTCA activity 1998. (Rates per million population.)

AUDIT

Data collection

Since BCIS grew from its predecessor, the British Angioplasty Group, it has striven to collect data related to numbers of procedures and outcomes, from all active interventional centres. These results were then published intermittently in the British Heart Journal. Because the process was voluntary, the information presented was incomplete, its validity and reliability being frequently open to question. Furthermore, because information systems in most centres were either basic or non-existent, there could be little if any attempt to relate outcome to pre-procedural risk. Nevertheless, the information did provide a valuable insight into interventional activity in the UK. The slow but steady growth of PTCA in this country could thus be monitored, and its risk and success rates assessed as we moved into the realms of unstable ischaemic syndromes, the introduction of new devices and increasingly complex coronary anatomy.

BCIS always anticipated that a formalised and reliable system would emerge, by which results are reported to a central site and thus enable a unit's practice to be compared anonymously with others. This development had to await the arrival of sufficiently sophisticated software, and agreement as to what information was essential, rather than desirable, to collect. Recent events surrounding cardiac surgical outcomes have brought these issues into sharp focus and now require progress to be made. Furthermore, a voluntary commitment to provide such information cannot be seen as sufficient.

Reviewing previous publications, it can be seen that along with slow but steady growth in interventional activity, the volume and variety of data collected has also increased.[5,6] The simple recording of the numbers of patients treated and crude outcome measures confined only to major complications (emergency CABG, myocardial infarction and death), is far from sufficient to describe the quality of care and thereby set national standards for PTCA. Data related to patient characteristics, clinical presentation, angiographic variables and the long-term results of intervention, are just as important as PTCA procedural information and immediate ('in-lab') outcomes.

For these reasons a dataset has been defined, which identifies the core information required from interventional centres in the UK. Individual operators or departments may wish to collect additional data, which may be locally relevant, but the fields defined by BCIS represent the minimum information to be collected. In order for centres to compare their performance to others and to agreed benchmarks, the information collected needs to be transferred to a central site for collation and analysis. It is anticipated that the UK Central Cardiac Audit Database (CCAD) will provide this service.[7] This project is designed to collect information on patients undergoing a variety of cardiological and cardiac surgical procedures, the data being transferred to a central server electronically using appropriate encryption to ensure confidentiality.

Peer review

In order to reinforce public and professional confidence, a formal system of peer review is to be set up by the British Cardiac Society to which BCIS, as a specialist group, is affiliated. The cornerstone of this process is the requirement for systematic collection and reporting of interventional data. It is envisaged that each interventional centre will receive a site visit and formal external review every 3 years. A report will be produced intended to support centres and help them plan or improve services in order to meet published guidelines and standards.[8]

REGULATION OF NEW DEVICES

As interventional knowledge has advanced, operators and the institutions in which they work are increasingly exposed by industry to an array of updated, modified or new devices. The large variety of available stents is an example of this scale and complexity. In order to keep up with these developments and to ensure that new technology is appropriately tested and standardised, the European Union has established the Medical Devices Agency (MDA) which is based in London.

This body is analogous to the Food and Drugs Administration in the USA, and serves a similar function for European countries. It examines the pre-marketing development and testing of materials and devices used in all branches of medicine, and thus the field of PTCA represents a significant focus for its activities. Importantly it also serves as a body to which suspected device malfunction can be reported and in this way acts in a similar role as the Committee on Safety of Medicines (CSM).

Unexpected or untoward events related to device use are not infrequent during percutaneous coronary intervention; dislodgement or misplacement of a manually crimped stent, represented a familiar example in the early experience of stenting before balloon mounted stents became commonplace. Similar circumstances continue to occur, albeit perhaps less frequently, and then cause operators to question whether events are related to a device fault or to the particular way in which they were using it. The common assumption of the latter possibility tends to result in under reporting of adverse events and thereby could delay the appropriate withdrawal of potentially dangerous technology.

For this reason the MDA encourages the reporting of all adverse events involving medical devices, whether or not thought to be operator related, using a system similar to that employed by the CSM for drug reactions. Only in this way can device use be properly monitored. Any design or manufacturing faults be recognised rapidly, and appropriate action taken in order to ensure patient safety.

A representative of the MDA sits on the Council of BCIS, whose members serve as its advisers when necessary. Contact details for the MDA are to be found in Appendix B.

REFERENCES

1. Parker DJ, Gray HH, Balcon R *et al*. Planning for coronary angioplasty: guidelines for training and continuing competence. Heart 1996;75:419–25.

2. Hirshfeld JW Jr, Ellis SG, Faxon DP. Recommendations for the assessment and maintenance of proficiency in coronary interventional procedures. Statement of the American College of Cardiology. J Am Coll Cardiol 1998;31(3):722–43.

3. Gray H *et al*. Coronary angioplasty: guidelines for good practice and training. Heart Suppl. 1999.

4. Guidelines for specialist training in cardiology. Report of the Specialist Advisory Committee in Cardiovascular Medicine of the Royal College of Physicians and Council of the British Cardiac Society. Br Heart J 1995;73 (Suppl. 1):1–24.

5. Gray H. Cardiac interventional procedures in the UK 1992–1996. Heart 1999;82 (Suppl. II):II10–II17.

6. de Belder M. Cardiac intervention procedures in the United Kingdom 1997: developments in data collection. Heart 1999;82(Suppl. II):II2–II9.

7. Rickards A, Cunningham D. From quantity to quality: the central cardiac audit database project. Heart 1999;82(Suppl. II)II18–II22.

8. Perrins J. Quality assurance in interventional cardiology. Heart 1999; 82(Suppl. II):II23–II26

Appendix A

Major trials in interventional cardiology

ANGELA HOYE AND MARK WALTERS

ABACUS: Adjunct Balloon Angioplasty Coronary Atherectomy Study

214 patients with a >74% coronary stenosis in a vessel >2.7 mm diameter suitable for IVUS-guided optimal atherectomy were randomised to undergo the procedure with or without additional balloon angioplasty. At 6 months further angiography with IVUS evaluated evidence of restenosis in 84 patients.

RESULTS:		DCA alone (n=43)	DCA+PTCA (n=41)	p value
Lumen cross sectional area (mm²)	Pre-	3.3 ± 2.7	3.5 ± 3.0	NS
	Post-	8.6 ± 6.4	10.1 ± 9.7	0.01
	6 months	6.1 ± 10.1	6.1 ± 10.8	NS
Angiographic restenosis at 6 months		16%	17%	NS

CONCLUSIONS: After aggressive IVUS-guided DCA additional balloon PTCA achieves a larger lumen. However there was no significant reduction in restenosis rates at 6 months.
JACC 1999 Oct; 34(4):1028–35.

ACME: Angioplasty Compared to MEdicine Study

212 patients with stable angina who had an abnormal exercise test or thallium scan, or a history of myocardial infarction within 3 months. All had single vessel coronary artery disease with a stenosis of >70%. They were randomised to medical therapy alone, or intervention with PTCA with a calcium channel blocker given for 1 month. All patients were on aspirin 325 mg/day. Follow-up at 6 months reassessed exercise time and use of sublingual nitroglycerin.

RESULTS:		Medical therapy (n=107)	PTCA (n=105)	p value
Exercise test criteria	Change in exercise time (min)	+0.5 ± 2.2	+2.1 ± 3.1	< 0.0001
	Maximal HR-BP (×10 − 3)	−2.8 ± 5.8	+1.8 ± 6.0	< 0.0001
	Change in time to onset of angina (min)	+0.8 ± 3.8	+2.6 ± 4.1	< 0.01
Clinical criteria	Mean change episodes angina/month	−7 ± 22	−15 ± 39	0.06
	Percent angina-free at 6 months	46%	64%	< 0.01
	Mean change in use NTG tablets/month	−5 ± 25	−9 ± 30	0.25

Two patients in the PTCA group needed emergency CABG, a total of seven patients (7%) in the group had CABG within 6 months compared to none of the medically treated group (p < 0.01). 16 PTCA patients (16%) had repeat

Appendix A

PTCA procedure, 11 medically treated patients (10%) crossed over to PTCA in the first 6 months.

CONCLUSIONS: Intervention with PTCA improved symptoms and exercise time compared with medical therapy. However it initially costs more and is associated with a higher frequency of complications.

NEJM 1992;326:10–16.

ADMIRAL

300 pateints with acute myocardial infarction undergoing primary PTCA and stenting were randomised to abciximab 0.25 mg/kg bolus +0.125 µg/kg/min infusion, or placebo prior to intervention. All received aspirin, heparin and ticlopidine.

RESULTS:	Abciximab (n = 150)	Placebo (n = 150)
TIMI 3 flow pre-intervention (%)	21.0	10.3*
TIMI 3 flow at 24 hours (%)	92.0	82.5*
30-day death, MI, urgent target vessel revascularisation (%)	7.3	14.7*
Major bleeding (%)	4.0	2.6 ($p = 0.50$)
Minor bleeding (%)	6.7	1.3 ($p = 0.02$)

*Significant difference

CONCLUSIONS: Abciximab administered prior to intervention in primary stenting for acute myocardial infarction significantly improved early angiographic and 30-day clinical outcomes.

Results presented at AHA meeting Atlanta 1999.

ALKK: Arbeitsgemeinschaft Leitender Kardiologischer Krankenhausarzte

300 patients who were stable following a myocardial infarction were randomised to medical therapy versus percutaneous intervention of the infarct vessel. Patients had to have little or no angina and single vessel disease. The mean stenosis in both groups was about 88%, with total occlusion in 30%. PTCA was successful in 85% with a relatively low use of stents in just 20%.

RESULTS:		PTCA (n = 149)	Medical therapy (n = 151)	p value
1 year	Event-free survival	90%	82%	NS
	Death	1	4	NS
	Reinfarction	4	6	NS
	Reintervention	8	20	0.01
Mean	Event-free survival	67%	76%	0.1
follow-up of	Death	8 (5.3%)	16 (10.7%)	NS
53 months	Nitrate use	38%	67%	0.001

Appendix A

CONCLUSIONS: Routine PTCA in stable postinfarction patients showed only a non-significant trend towards reducing mortality although there was significantly less nitrate use at follow-up.
Results presented at ACC meeting Anaheim 2000.

ARTS: Artery Revascularisation Therapy Study

1205 patients with multivessel coronary artery disease were randomised to receive revascularisation with either CABG or percutaneous angioplasty. Patients were excluded if there was evidence of overt heart failure, ejection fraction < 30%, or history of vascular accident. Rates of major adverse cardiac events to be reviewed at 1 and 5 years.
RESULTS: at 1 year there was no significant overall difference in major cardiac event rates. However, the PTCA group required significantly more repeat revascularisation procedures than the surgical group (26.3% vs 12.2%). Analysis of the 1 year DIABETIC subgroup (n = 208) is below:

RESULTS:	PTCA	CABG
Mortality (%)	6.3	3.1
Mortality from stroke (%)	1.8	6.3
Freedom from death, stroke, MI, repeat revascularisation (%)	60.7	82.3

CONCLUSIONS: Patients in the PTCA group were more likely to undergo a further revascularisation procedure. Diabetic patients overall did worse and fared significantly better with bypass surgery than PTCA.
Data presented in AHA meeting Atlanta 1999.

AVID: Angiography versus Intravascular Ultrasound Directed Coronary Stent Placement

800 patients undergoing stent implantation were randomised to angiography alone or in conjunction with IVUS. All received aspirin and ticlopidine.

RESULTS: overall target lesion revascularisation rate (TLR) at 1 year was 32% lower in the IVUS group. Below are the TLR rates for different subgroups:

	IVUS and angio	Angiography alone	p value
Full cohort	8.4	12.4	0.08
SVG patients	5.4	21.0	0.03
Those with >70% stenosis	3.4	14.4	0.003
Small vessels	2.8	4.9	

CONCLUSIONS: IVUS-guided PTCA results in significantly less repeat target lesion revascularisation procedures particularly in patients with severe stenosis and saphenous graft lesions.
Results presented at Transcatheter Cardiovascular Therapeutics symposium (TCT) 1999.

Appendix A

BARI: Bypass Angioplasty Revascularisation Investigation

1796 patients took part and were randomised to either balloon PTCA or CABG in severe angina due to multivessel coronary disease. Follow-up of primary endpoints of mortality and event-free survival.

RESULTS:		CABG (n = 892)	PTCA (n = 904)	p value
All patients	In-hospital mortality (%)	1.3	1.1	
	In-hospital Q wave MI (%)	4.6	2.1	< 0.01
	In-hospital stroke (%)	0.8	0.2	
	5-year survival (%)	89.3	86.3	0.19
	5-year free of Q wave MI (%)	80.4	78.7	
	5-year repeat PTCA (%)	7.0	34	
	revascularisation CABG (%)	1.0	31	
	7-year survival (%)	84.4	80.9	0.043
Diabetic subgroup	5-year survival (%)	80.6	65.5	0.003
	7-year survival (%)	76.4	55.7	0.0011

CONCLUSIONS: In multivessel disease, an initial treatment of PTCA as compared to CABG does not influence overall survival except in the diabetic population who fared significantly better with CABG. Over follow-up, there was an increased need for a further revascularisation procedure in the PTCA group (54.5% vs 8.0%). Most repeat PTCA procedures were carried out during the first year, 11% patients had both a repeat PTCA and bypass surgery.
NEJM 1996; 335: 217–225.
Circulation 1997;96:2162–70.
JACC 35(5) April 2000.

BENESTENT I: Belgium–Netherland STENT Investigators

516 patients with stable angina due to single vessel coronary disease were randomised to receive balloon PTCA with or without a stent. The lesion had to be suitable for PTCA, <15 mm in length and the vessel size > 3 mm diameter. Patients were excluded if the lesion was ostial, or at a bifurcation. All patients were followed up over 7 months and then had repeat angiography to reassess luminal diameter.

RESULTS:		Angioplasty (n = 257)	Stent (n = 259)	p value
Bleeding + vascular complications		3.1%	13.5%	< 0.001
Mean hospital stay (days)		3.1	8.5	< 0.001
Minimal luminal	Pre	1.08 ± 0.31	1.07 ± 0.33	NS
diameter (mm)	Post	2.05 ± 0.33	2.48 ± 0.39	< 0.001
	At 7 months	1.73 ± 0.55	1.82 ± 0.64	0.09[†]
50% restenosis rate		32%	22%	0.02
Clinical outcomes	Any event*	76 (29.6%)	52 (20.1%)	0.02
at 7 months	Repeat PTCA	60 (23.3%)	35 (13.5%)	0.005

*death, CVA, Q-wave MI, non-Q wave MI, CABG, repeat PTCA
[†]p = 0.08 and p = 0.03 when pre-intervention lumen and vessel size respectively were used as covariates

Appendix A

CONCLUSIONS: Stenting during angioplasty increases the risk of vascular problems at the access site and requires a longer hospital stay, however there is improvement in clinical and angiographic results at 7 months.
NEJM 1994: 331:489.

BENESTENT II: Heparin coated Palmaz–Schatz stents in human coronary arteries II

823 patients with stable angina due to single vessel coronary disease were randomised to receive balloon PTCA with or without a heparin coated Palmaz–Schatz stent. The lesion had to be suitable for PTCA, < 18 mm in length and the vessel size > 3 mm diameter. Patients were excluded if the lesion was ostial, at a bifurcation, or if there was impaired left ventricular function (EF < 30%). All patients were followed up over 12 months with 50% patients in each group having repeat angiography at 6 months to reassess luminal diameter.

RESULTS:		PTCA (*n* = 410)		Stent (*n* = 413)	
		6 months	12 months	6 months	12 months
Death		0.5%	1.0%	0.2%	1.0%
CABG		1.5%	1.5%	1.5%	1.9%
Repeat PTCA		13.7%	15.6%	8.0%*	9.4%*
Major adverse cardiac event		19.3%	22.4%	12.8%*	15.7%*
Minimal luminal	Pre	1.08 ± 0.31		1.08 ± 0.28	
diameter (mm)	Post	2.13 + 0.39		2.69 ± 0.37*	
50% restenosis		31.0%		16.0%*	

*Significant difference with stent versus PTCA

CONCLUSIONS: 55 patients (13.4%) in the PTCA group required 'bailout' stenting. Over 12 months follow-up, stenting was superior to balloon angioplasty alone.
Lancet 1998;352:673–81.

BERT-1: Beta Energy Restenosis Trial-1

64 consecutive patients undergoing balloon angioplasty were also treated with beta radiation (strontium[90]) using the Novoste delivery system. All patients had lesions < 15 mm in length, in a vessel 2.5–3.5 mm diameter and evidence of ischaemia. They were excluded if ejection fraction < 40%, visible thrombus was seen, creatinine > 2, or if vessel angle > 45% at lesion. Repeat angiography was carried out at 6 months.
RESULTS and CONCLUSIONS: Beta-radiation after angioplasty was safe and reduced treatment time and operator exposure compared with a gamma emitter. Its use resulted in low rate of clinical events and restenosis at 6 months (15%).
Circulation 1998;97:2025–30.

Appendix A

BESMART

381 patients undergoing PTCA to vessel < 3 mm diameter (mean 2.2 mm) were randomised as to whether they routinely had stenting. Those with ostial or bifurcation lesions, and impaired left ventricular function were excluded (EF < 30%). All had heparin 80 units/kg, aspirin, and a 1 month course of ticlopidine. Primary endpoint was restenosis rates at 6 months.

> **RESULTS: Initial success rates in both groups > 98% with a 24% crossover rate from balloon alone to stenting, and 3% crossover from stent to balloon. There was no difference in in-hospital major adverse event rates or rate of MI or death at 6 months.**

	With stent	Without a stent	p value
> 50% restenosis	22.7%	48.5%	< 0.0001 (RR 0.48)
Target lesion revascularisation	13%	25%	0.016

CONCLUSIONS: Stenting in these small vessels is feasible and safe. Risk of restenosis in small vessel angioplasty procedures is reduced by using a stent. Results presented at ACC meeting 2000.

BOAT: Balloon versus Optimal Atherectomy Trial

989 patients who had a history of stable or unstable angina, or who were at least 5 days post-acute myocardial infarction were enrolled. All had a focal de novo non-calcified coronary lesion in an artery at least 3.0 mm in diameter. They were randomised to either balloon angioplasty alone or optimal atherectomy and aggressive PTCA. Angiography was repeated at 6 months to reassess luminal diameter.

RESULTS	DCA (n = 497)	PTCA (n = 492)	p value
MLD post (mm)	2.82 ± 0.45	2.33 ± 0.49	< 0.0001
MLD 6 months (mm)	1.86 ± 0.71	1.68 ± 0.68	0.002
Restenosis 6 months (%)	40.1 ± 20.8	45.6 ± 20	0.002
Death 1 year (%)	31.4	39.8	0.016
Target vessel revascularisation (TVR) at 1 year (%)	0.6	1.6	0.14
Death, Q wave MI, or TVR 1 year	21.1	24.8	0.17

CONCLUSIONS: Optimal atherectomy and PTCA resulted in a significantly increased luminal diameter and reduced rate of restenosis at 6 months compared with balloon angioplasty alone. However there was no significant difference in event rates at 1 year.
Circulation: 1998;97:322–31.

CABRI: Coronary Angioplasty vs Bypass Revascularisation Investigation

1054 patients with one or more coronary artery lesions were randomised to either PTCA or CABG as first line intervention. The vessel size had to be

Appendix A

> 2.0 mm distal to the lesion and left ventricular EF >35%. Patients were followed up for 1 year with primary endpoints of mortality and symptoms of angina.

RESULTS:	PTCA (*n* = 541)	CABG (*n* = 513)	*p* value
Death	21 (3.9%)	14 (2.7%)	NS
Repeat revascularisation	33.6%	6.5%	< 0.001
Angina > CCS class 1	75 (13.9%)	52 (10.1%)	0.012

CONCLUSIONS: There was no significant difference in mortality however, at 1 year, those who underwent PTCA were more likely to require repeat intervention, were more symptomatic of angina, and required more anti-anginal medication ($p < 0.001$). The results were more significant in females. Lancet 1995;346:1179–84.

CADILLAC: Controlled Abciximab and Device Investigation to Lower Late Angioplasty Complications

2081 patients within 12 hours of acute myocardial infarction were randomised to one of four strategies (a) primary PTCA; (b) primary PTCA + abciximab; (c) primary stenting; (d) primary stenting + abciximab. Patients were mean age 60 years though many were elderly including > 90 years old. Patients were excluded if they were in cardiogenic shock or if the vessel had had previous stenting.
RESULTS: There were no significant differences in in-hospital mortality (1.4%), disabling stroke (0.4%), reinfarction (0.4%), or need for blood transfusion (5%) between the four groups.

	PTCA (*n* = 517)	PTCA + abciximab (*n* = 528)	Stenting (*n* = 511)	Stenting + abciximab (*n* = 525)
TIMI-3 flow (%)	94	92	92	96.7
Recurrent ischaemia (%)	4.5	1.45	3.9	1.2
Need for ischaemic target vessel revascularisation (%)	2.3	0.2	Not specified	Reduced from stenting

CONCLUSIONS: The overall rate of adverse events was low. Stenting was associated with a lower rate of TIMI-3 flow but this did not affect mortality. Use of abciximab in addition to stenting improved TIMI-3 flow
Presented at 72nd AHA meeting 1999.

CAPTURE: Chimeric c7E3 AntiPlatelet Therapy in Unstable REfractory Angina

1265 patients with unstable angina refractory to standard medical therapy underwent PTCA and were randomised to receive either Abciximab bolus (0.25 mg/kg) + infusion (0.1 mg/kg/min) 12–24 hours before PTCA until

1 hour after PTCA, or placebo. They were followed up over 30 days with primary endpoints of death, MI, or urgent reintervention.

RESULTS	Placebo (n = 635)	Abciximab (n = 630)	p value
Death, infarction, or urgent intervention	101 (15.9%)	71 (11.3%)	0.012
Death	8 (1.3%)	6 (1.0%)	>0.1
MI before PTCA	13 (2.1%)	4 (0.6%)	0.029
MI during PTCA (< 24 hours)	34 (5.5%)	16 (2.6%)	0.009
After PTCA (2–30 days)	5 (0.9%)	6 (1.0%)	>0.1
All myocardial infarction	52 (8.2%)	26 (4.1%)	0.002
Urgent intervention	69 (10.9%)	49 (7.8%)	0.054
All major bleeding	12 (1.9%)	24 (3.8%)	0.043

CONCLUSIONS: In unstable angina, patients who undergo PTCA have a significant reduction in early (30-day) complications especially risk of MI if treated with abciximab.
Lancet 1997;349:1429–35.

CAVEAT I: A comparison of directional atherectomy VErsus Coronary Angioplasty Trial

1012 patients with de novo coronary lesions of < 12 mm in length were randomised to receive either PTCA or directional atherectomy. They were followed up over 6 months and then had repeat angiography. Primary endpoints were of early complications related to the initial procedure, death, MI, CABG and restenosis.

RESULTS:		DCA (n = 512)	PTCA (n = 500)	p value
In-hospital complication (%)		11	5	<0.001
At 6 months	Death (%)	1.6	0.6	0.22
	MI (%)	7.6	4.4	0.04
	CABG (%)	8.2	6.8	0.39
	Restenosis (%)	50	57	0.06
	Freedom from adverse events (%)	60	63	0.49

CONCLUSIONS: directional atherectomy resulted in a higher early complication rate and was more expensive. At 6 months there was no significant difference between the two groups.
NEJM 1993;329:221.

CAVEAT II: Coronary Angioplasty Vs Excisional Atherectomy Trial for patients with saphenous vein graft lesions

305 patients with SVG lesions of < 12 mm in length in a vein > 3.0 mm diameter were randomised to either balloon PTCA or directional atherectomy. Angiography was repeated at 6 months to assess evidence of restenosis.

RESULTS:		DCA (n = 149)	PTCA (n = 156)	p value
In-hospital	Procedural success (%)	89	79	0.019
	Acute adverse event (death, MI, CABG, or acute closure) (%)	20	12	0.059
6 months	Angiographic restenosis (%)	46	51	NS
	Adverse event, i.e. death, MI, CABG, repeat PTCA (%)	40	44	0.199

CONCLUSIONS: Compared with angioplasty, DCA achieved a higher procedural success rate but with an increased risk of early complications. At 6 months there was no significant difference between the two groups. Circulation 1995;91:1966–74.

CLASSICS: CLopidogrel ASpirin Stent International Cooperative Study

1005 patients undergoing PTCA with stenting were randomised to one of three treatment options. All received 325 mg aspirin od and in addition had either ticlopidine 250 mg bd for 28 days, clopidogrel 75 mg od for 28 days, or clopidogrel 300 mg on day one then clopidogrel 75 mg for 27 days.

RESULTS:	300 mg clopidogrel then 75 mg/day (n = 335)	75 mg clopidogrel daily (n = 335)	Ticlopidine 250 mg/day (n = 335)
Major side effects (%)	2.9	6.3	9.1*
MI, sudden cardiac death, or subacute thrombosis (%)	1.2	1.5	0.0[†]

* Ticlopidine significantly less well tolerated compared to combined clopidogrel data p = 0.005
[†] No significant difference p > 0.05

CONCLUSIONS: Clopidogrel was better tolerated than ticlopidine with no increase in bleeding complications when given the loading dose. Adverse cardiac event rates were comparable between the three groups.
Not yet published, results presented at ACC meeting 1999.

CLOUT: Clinical Outcomes with Ultrasound Trial

102 patients had PTCA then IVUS was used to assess results and some patients had a further balloon angioplasty using balloons sized to average of lumen and vessel diameter.

RESULTS:	Standard PTCA (n = 27)	IVUS-guided PTCA (n = 75)	p value
QCA reference segment diameter (mm)	2.72 + 0.47	2.71 ± 0.48	0.80
QCA lesion MLD (mm)	1.95 ± 0.49	2.21 ± 0.47	< 0.0001
QCA lesion % DS ???	28.3 ± 14.9	18.1 ± 14.4	< 0.0001
IVUS lesion MLD (mm)	1.75 ± 0.30	2.10 ± 0.32	< 0.0001
IVUS lesion lumen area (mm^2)	3.16 ± 1.04	4.56 ± 1.14	< 0.0001
Angiographic dissection	37	40	0.67
Major in-hospital complication/death	0/0	2/0	NS

CONCLUSIONS: IVUS-guided PTCA balloon upsizing allowed a greater initial luminal diameter without increasing angiographic or in-hospital complications. Circulation 1997;95:2044–52.

CRUISE: Can Routine Ultrasound Influence Stent Expansion

499 patients undergoing PTCA and stenting were randomised as to whether they received guidance with IVUS (patients were a subgroup of those in STARS trial). Vessel size was 3.0–5.0 mm with either a single or two lesions per patient and the lesion had to require < 3 stents. All had IVUS luminal diameters measured blinded immediately post-procedure. Follow up was over 9 months with a primary endpoint of need for target vessel revascularisation.

RESULTS	IVUS guidance (n = 270)	Angiographic guidance (n = 229)	p value
IVUS reference luminal area (mm²)	9.92 ± 2.94	9.62 ± 3.12	NS
IVUS minimal stent diameter (mm)	2.82 ± 0.55	2.59 ± 0.43	0.038
IVUS minimal stent area (mm²)	7.76 ± 1.72	7.11 ± 2.13	0.001
Target vessel revascularisation	8.9%	14.8%	0.04

CONCLUSIONS: The use of IVUS resulted in a larger minimal stent diameter compared to angiographic guidance alone and at 9 months there was a significantly lower rate of revascularisation procedures.
JACC 1998;31(2):396A.

CUBA: Cutting Balloon vs Conventional Balloon Angioplasty

306 patients with single vessel coronary stenosis were randomised to either conventional balloon angioplasty or use of a cutting balloon. 96% had repeat angiography at 6 months to look for evidence of restenosis.

RESULTS:	Cutting balloon (n = 153)	Balloon PTCA (n = 153)	p value
Reference diameter (mm)	3.00 ± 0.4 mm	2.95 ± 0.4 mm	NS
Minimal luminal diameter gain	1.45 ± 0.5 mm	1.50 ± 0.4 mm	NS
Angiographic success without	89%	91%	NS
stent requirement or cross-over	(18 needed stents)	(12 needed stents)	
Major complication	2%	3%	NS
Restenosis at 6 months	30%	42%	0.047
6 month late loss (mm)	0.37 ± 0.8	0.52 ± 0.7	0.09

CONCLUSIONS: Compared with standard balloon angioplasty the cutting balloon results in similar initial angiographic results and in-hospital clinical outcome with no deaths. There was a slight reduction in restenosis at 6 months due to less late loss.

JACC 1998;31(2):223A.

Appendix A

DANAMI: DANish Trial in Acute Myocardial Infarction

1008 patients aged < 69 years were admitted with their first acute myocardial infarction and received thrombolysis. Prior to discharge they had evidence of recurrent or inducible ischaemia on exercise and were randomised to receive either conservative medical therapy or early coronary angiography within 2 weeks. Primary endpoints were the incidence of death, reinfarction or admission with unstable angina at follow up (median 2.4 years).

RESULTS:	Conservative (n = 505)	Invasive (n = 503)	p value
Revascularisation procedure in first 2 months	1.6%	53% had PTCA 29% had CABG	
Mortality	22 (4.4%)	18 (3.6%)	0.45
Reinfarction	53 (10.5%)	28 (5.6%)	0.0038
Unstable angina	149 (29.5%)	90 (17.9%)	< 0.00001
Combined endpoints	204 (40.4%)	135 (26.9%)	< 0.00001

CONCLUSIONS: Patients with evidence of spontaneous or inducible ischaemia following an AMI who undergo angiography with revascularisation when appropriate, have a significantly lower incidence of recurrent MI and unstable angina.
Circulation 1997;96(3):748–55.

DART: Dilation vs Ablation Revascularisation Trial

Patients with coronary disease were randomised to either standard balloon angioplasty or rotational atherectomy. Lesions were < 20 mm length in a vessel < 3.0 mm diameter. Angiography was repeated at 9 months to assess restenosis.

RESULTS:	Rotational (n = 222)	PTCA (n = 220)	p value
Death, Q-wave MI, or urgent CABG	1.3	0	NS
CKMB 1–3 × NML (%)	11.0	6.0	< 0.07
CKMB 3–8 × NML (%)	2.0	4.0	< 0.21
CKMB > 8 × NML (%)	3.0	1.0	< 0.12
Slow flow/no reflow (%)	8.0	0.5	< 0.01
Major dissection (%)	8.0	16.0	< 0.05
Bailout stenting (%)	6.0	14.0	< 0.01
Bleeding requiring transfusion (%)	4.0	0.5	< 0.04

CONCLUSIONS: Compared with standard balloon PTCA, rotational atherectomy was associated with significantly higher rates of slow flow/no reflow but no significant increase in CKMB or major cardiac complication. There were lower rates of major dissection and fewer bailout stents were required.
Circulation 1997;96(Suppl. A):I–467.

Appendix A

DEBATE I: Doppler Endpoints Balloon Angioplasty Trial Europe

225 patients with single vessel coronary disease and no previous history of MI had successful balloon angioplasty. Doppler flow velocity was measured to see whether they could predict early or late clinical outcomes. Repeat angiography at 6 months determined rate of restenosis.

RESULTS:	CFR > 2.5+ DS < 35%	CFR </= 2.5 Or DS > 35%	p value
Angina at 1 month (%)	10	19	0.149
Angina at 6 months (%)	23	47	0.005
Target vessel revascularisation	16	34	0.024
Angiographic restenosis	16	41	0.002

CONCLUSIONS: Coronary flow reserve (CFR) combined with % diameter stenosis (DS) after PTCA is predictive of angina, target vessel revascularisation and angiographic restenosis at 6 months. This may therefore help identify patients who would benefit from elective stenting.
Circulation 1997;96(10):3369–77.

DEBATE II: Doppler Endpoints Balloon Angioplasty Trial Europe II

410 patients having single vessel angioplasty to either a circumflex or left anterior descending artery stenosis were randomised to either primary stenting or doppler guided balloon angioplasty. These angioplasty patients were then randomised as to whether or not they received a stent.

RESULTS at 1 month:	Stent	PTCA only
DS </ = 35% and CFR > 2.5	0	0
DS > 35% or CFR </ = 2.5	10%	4%

CONCLUSIONS: Doppler can be used to identify patients in whom clinical outcome at 1 month is similar between stented and PTCA only patients.
Circulation 1998;98:Abstract 2622.

EAST: Emory Angioplasty vs Surgery Trial

392 patients with 2–3 vessel coronary disease suitable for either CABG or percutaneous revascularisation with stable or unstable angina were randomised to either intervention. They were followed up looking at rates of death, MI, and thallium scanning assessed residual ischaemia.

RESULTS:	CABG (n = 194)	PTCA (n = 198)	p value
3-year mortality	12 (6.2%)	14 (7.1%)	0.72
3-year Q wave MI	38 (19.6%)	29 (14.6%)	0.21
Large ischaemic defect on thallium	11 (5.7%)	19 (9.6%)	0.17
3-year composite primary endpoint	53 (27.3%)	57 (28.8%)	0.81

RESULTS:		CABG (n = 194)	PTCA (n = 198)	p value
3-year repeat revascularisation procedure	CABG	18%	13%	< 0.001
	PTCA	22%	41%	< 0.001
8-year mortality	All patients	17.3%	20.7%	0.40
	Diabetics	24.5%	39.9%	0.0011

CONCLUSIONS: At follow-up there was no overall significant difference in mortality, MI or incidence of large residual ischaemia on thallium scanning. Those who had PTCA were more likely to have needed a repeat revascularisation procedure. Those patients with diabetes fared significantly better with bypass surgery.
NEJM 1994;331:1044–50.
JACC 35(5) April 2000.

EPIC: Evaluation of c7E3 for the Prevention of Ischaemic Complications

2099 patients undergoing high risk coronary angioplasty or atherectomy were randomised to either bolus of abciximab (0.25 mg/kg) followed by infusion at 10 μg/min, or the bolus of abciximab followed by placebo, or placebo. All patients received aspirin and nonadjusted heparin. Patients were deemed to be high risk as they were within 12 hours onset of pain of acute MI, were early post-MI or unstable angina, and had high risk lesion morphology (AHA/ACC class B2 or C). Primary endpoints were of early (30-day) complications of death, MI, CABG or PTCA for acute ischaemia, stenting for procedural failure, IABP for refractory ischaemia.

RESULTS AT 30 DAYS	Placebo (n = 708)	c7E3 bolus (n = 695)	c7E3 bolus + infusion (n = 696)	p value
Composite (primary endpoint)	89 (12.8%)	79 (11.4%)	60 (0.3%)	0.009
Death	12 (1.7%)	9 (1.3%)	12 (1.7%)	0.96
Non-fatal MI	60 (8.6%)	43 (6.2%)	37 (5.2%)	0.013
Emergency CABG	25 (3.6%)	16 (2.3%)	17 (2.4%)	0.177
Emergency PTCA	31 (4.5%)	25 (3.6%)	6 (0.8%)	< 0.001
Major bleeding	46 (7.0%)	76 (11.0%)	99 (14.0%)	> 0.001

CONCLUSIONS: Abciximab increases the risk of bleeding complications but when given as a bolus and infusion significantly reduces the incidence of ischaemic events at 30 days.
NEJM 1994;330:956.
Am J Cardiol 1995;75:559–62.

EPILOGUE: Evaluation in PTCA to Improve Long Term Outcome with Abciximab GPIIb/IIIa Blockade Study Group

2792 patients undergoing elective or emergency PTCA for coronary stenosis of > 60% diameter were randomised to receive either weight-adjusted heparin

Appendix A

alone (100 units/kg) (goal ACT > 300), abciximab and standard-dose weight-adjusted heparin (100 units/kg) (goal ACT > 300), or abciximab and low-dose weight-adjusted heparin (70 units/kg) (goal ACT > 200). Abciximab was administered as a bolus of 0.25 mg/kg prior to PTCA procedure, followed by an infusion of 0.125 mcg/kg/hr (max 10 µg/hr) for 12 hours. Follow-up was for 30 days looking at incidence of death, MI, or urgent revascularisation.

RESULTS		Placebo + standard dose heparin (n = 939)	Abciximab + standard dose heparin (n = 918)	Abciximab + low dose heparin (n = 935)
30-day	Composite endpoint	11.7%	5.4%*	5.2%*
	Death	0.8%	0.4%	0.3%
	MI	8.7%	3.8%*	3.7%*
	Urgent revascularisation	5.2%	2.3%*	1.6%*
	Major bleeding	3.1%	3.5%	2.0%
	Minor bleeding	3.7%	7.4%*	4.0%
1 year composite endpoint		16.1%	9.5%	9.6%

*$p < 0.001$

CONCLUSIONS: The use of abciximab significantly reduces the risk of MI, and urgent revascularisation at 30 days. There was no evidence of an increase in major bleeding and when used in conjunction with low-dose weight adjusted heparin there was no difference in minor bleeding complications. NEJM 1997;336:1689–96.

EPISTENT: Evaluation in PTCA to Improve Long-Term Outcome with Abciximab GPIIb/IIIa Blockade Study Group – Stent

2399 patients undergoing elective or emergency PTCA for coronary stenosis of > 60% diameter were randomised to either stenting + abciximab, balloon angioplasty + abciximab, or stenting + placebo. Follow-up looked at incidence of death, MI, or urgent revascularisation.

RESULTS AT 30 DAYS:	Stent + placebo (n = 809)	PTCA + abciximab (n = 796)	Stent + abciximab (n = 794)
Composite (primary endpoint)	10.8%	6.9% ($p < 0.01$)	5.3% ($p < 0.001$)
Death or MI	7.8%	4.7% ($p < 0.01$)	3.0% ($p < 0.001$)
Major bleeding	2.2%	1.4%	1.5%

RESULTS AT 1 YEAR:	Stent + placebo	Stent + abciximab	p value
Death (%)	2.4	1.0	0.037
Death or MI (%)	11.0	5.3	< 0.001

Appendix A

CONCLUSIONS: The use of abciximab significantly reduced the composite endpoint of death, MI, or urgent revascularisation at 30 days, without adversely effecting the risk of bleeding. The use of a stent in addition to balloon angioplasty improved the results further.
Lancet 1998;352:87–92.
Lancet 1999;354:2019–24.

ERACI: ArgentinE Randomised Trial Coronary Angioplasty vs Bypass Surgery In Multivessel Disease

127 patients with multivessel coronary disease (> 70% stenosis in at least two epicardial arteries) and severe angina despite medical therapy were randomised to either PTCA or CABG. 3-year cardiac event rates were assessed as primary endpoints.

RESULTS:		PTCA (n = 63)	CABG (n = 64)	p value
In-hospital	Death (%)	1.5	4.6	NS
	Acute MI (%)	6.3	6.2	NS
	Stroke (%)	1.5	3.1	NS
1 year	Death (%)	3.2	0	NS
	Acute MI (%)	3.2	1.8	NS
	Repeat revascularisation (%)	32.0	3.2	< 0.001
3 years	Death (%)	1.5	4.6	NS
	Acute MI (%)	6.0	6.0	NS
	Repeat revascularisation (%)	1.5	1.5	NS
Event-free survival (%)		63.7	83.5	< 0.005

CONCLUSIONS: Incidence of death or acute MI were not significantly different in the two groups. However patients who initially had PTCA were much more likely to require a repeat revascularisation procedure within the first year, no difference at 3 years.
JACC 1996;27:1178–84.

ERACI-II: ArgentinE Randomised Trial Coronary Angioplasty vs Bypass Surgery In Multivessel Disease – II

450 patients with multivessel coronary disease suitable for either intervention were randomised to either angioplasty with stenting or CABG. 28% those in the PTCA group received abciximab. Follow-up was over 19.5 ± 6.4 months.

RESULTS:	PTCA + stent (n = 225)	CABG (n = 225)	p value
Death (%)	3.1	7.5	< 0.017
Myocardial infarction (%)	2.3	6.6	< 0.017
Repeat revascularisation procedure (%)	18.6	5.3	< 0.002

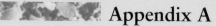

Appendix A

CONCLUSIONS: There was a significant difference in survival rates evident at 30 days but continued over follow-up in favour of the PTCA + stent group. However, this group needed more repeat revascularisation procedures. Only 6.2% PTCA group crossed over to the CABG group.
Results presented at ACC meeting 2000.

ERASER: Evaluation of Reopro And Stenting to Eliminate Restenosis

225 patients with coronary stenosis in an artery >/= 2.75 mm diameter underwent primary stenting. They were randomised to abciximab to be given as a bolus followed by infusion for either 12 or 24 hours, or placebo before coronary intervention. At 6 months they were reassessed for restenosis on quantitative angiography and using IVUS to look at in-stent intimal hyperplasia.

RESULTS			Abciximab bolus + infusion	
		Placebo (n = 75)	12 hours (n = 75)	24 hours (n = 75)
IVUS	In-stent tissue volume (%)	25 ± 15	27 ± 1	29 ± 14
	Minimal CSA (mm²)	4.82 ± 2.06	4.96 ± 2.40	4.64 ± 2.06
QCA	MLD (mm)	2.09 ± 0.64	1.96 ± 0.91	2.03 ± 0.68
	Diameter stenosis (%)	30 ± 19	34 ± 27	34 ± 20
	Binary restenosis (%)	11.6	18.9	19.4
Major	Death (%)	2.8	0	0
cardiac events	MI (%)	12.7	7.6	9.3
Target lesion revascularisation (%)		15.5	13.9	13.3

CONCLUSIONS: All results were not statistically significant suggesting Abciximab does not reduce incidence of in-stent restenosis.
Circulation 1997;96(Suppl. I):I–87.
Circulation 1999 Aug 24;100(8):799–806.

ERBAC: Excimer Laser, Rotational Atherectomy, and Balloon Angioplasty Comparison Study

685 patients with coronary lesions suitable for all three intervention arms were randomised to either conventional balloon angioplasty alone, laser angioplasty, or rotational atherectomy. Patients were excluded if there was angulation > 60%, or extreme tortuosity, thrombus, bifurcation lesion or total occlusion.

RESULTS	Balloon PTCA (n = 222)	Excimer laser atherectomy (n = 232)	Rotational atherectomy (n = 231)	p value
Post procedure DS (%)	35 ± 16	33 ± 15	33 ± 15	0.24
Procedural success (%)	79.7	77.2	89.2	0.002
In hospital event i.e. death, Q-wave MI, or CABG	3.1	4.3	3.2	0.71
Event within 1 year i.e. death, MI, CABG, re-PTCA, or TLR	36.6	47.9	45.9	ELCA vs PTCA 0.015 RA vs PTCA 0.057

Appendix A

CONCLUSIONS: Procedural success was significantly higher in those who had rotational atherectomy with adjunctive PTCA compared with laser atherectomy which was itself superior to balloon PTCA alone. However, at 1 year there was a higher adverse event rate in the patients who had undergone rotational or excimer laser atherectomy.
Circulation 1997;96:91–8.

ESPRIT: Enhanced Suppression of the Platelet Receptor glycoprotein IIb/IIIa using Integrilin Therapy

2064 patients undergoing elective stenting were randomised to integrilin 180 µg/kg bolus repeated after 10 minutes, then 2.0 µg/kg/min infusion for 18–24 hours or placebo.

RESULTS AT 48 HOURS:	Eptifibatide (n = 1040)	Placebo (n = 1024)	Relative risk reduction
Death and MI (%)	5.5	9.2	40%
Urgent revascularisation (%)	0.6	1.0	40%
Combined endpoint of death, MI, revascularisation or need for 'bailout' IIb/IIIa inhibitor (%)	6.6	10.5	37% (p = 0.0015)
Need for blood transfusion (%)	1.4	1.0	

CONCLUSIONS: The use of eptifibatide during stenting significantly reduces adverse cardiac events without significantly increasing the risk of severe bleeding (though there was more minor bleeding mainly at the femoral access site). Results presented at ACC Anaheim 2000.

FANTASTIC: The Full Anticoagulation Versus Aspirin and Ticlopidine study

485 patients undergoing PTCA who required stenting with a Wiktor stent were randomised to receive either heparin then oral full anticoagulation (INR 2.5–3.0) or aggressive antiplatelet therapy: 100–325 mg od aspirin longterm + 250 mg bd ticlopidine for 6 weeks.

RESULTS	Antiplatelet therapy (n = 249)	Anticoagulation (n = 236)	p value
Bleeding complications	33 (13.5%)	48 (21%)	0.03
Death	2 (0.8%)	5 (2.2%)	0.21
Acute MI	13 (5.4%)	16 (7.1)	0.44
CABG	3 (1.2%)	3 (1.3%)	0.93
Repeat PTCA	13 (5.4%)	11 (4.9%)	0.80

CONCLUSIONS: antiplatelet strategy reduces bleeding and rate of subacute stent occlusion.
Circulation 1998;98:1597–1603.

Appendix A

FLARE: Fluvastatin Angioplasty Restenosis

1054 patients underwent successful PTCA to a single coronary lesion. All had LDL levels of < 6 mmol/l and were randomised to receive either 40 mg twice daily of fluvastatin or placebo. They were followed up over 6 months and then underwent repeat angiography to assess evidence of restenosis. Primary endpoints were death, MI, CABG, or re-intervention at 40 weeks.

RESULTS:	Placebo (n = 528)	Fluvastatin (n = 526)	p value
Restenosis rate	31%	28%	0.42
Death/MI	4.0%	1.4%	0.025

CONCLUSIONS: 80 mg fluvastatin daily did not affect restenosis, however there was a significant reduction in mortality and rate of myocardial infarction at 40 weeks in the active treatment group.
Europ Heart J 1999;20(1):58–69.

FRISC II: Fragmin and Fast Revascularisation during InStability in Coronary artery disease Investigators

2457 patients with unstable coronary disease were randomised to early invasive or non-invasive strategy. All had 5 days of dalteparin and were then randomised to placebo or a further 3 months of subcutaneous injections of dalteparin.

RESULTS:	Dalteparin	Placebo	p value
30-day death or myocardial infarction (%)	3.1	5.9	0.002
3-month death or myocardial infarction (%)	6.7	8.0	0.17

RESULTS:	Invasive group	Non-invasive	p value
Death or myocardial infarction at 6 months (%)	9.4	12.1	0.031
Myocardial infarction (%)	7.8	10.1	0.045

Symptoms of angina and readmission rates were significantly reduced in the invasive group. All results were independent of the randomised dalteparin treatment. The greatest benefits were seen in the highest risk patients.
CONCLUSIONS: 3 months of dalteparin offered short-term protection with a reduction in 30-day events, however this was not sustained at 3 months. An early invasive strategy should be used in these patients with unstable angina who have ECG changes or raised biochemical markers of myocardial damage.
Lancet 28 August 1999;354(9180):701–715.

GABI: German Angioplasty Bypass Surgery Investigation

359 patients aged < 75 years with symptomatic (> = CCS class II) multivessel coronary artery disease were randomised to CABG or PTCA. At 1 year they were reassessed for symptoms of angina.

RESULTS	CABG (n = 177)	PTCA (n = 182)	p value
Reintervention (CABG or PTCA)	6%	44%	N/A
Freedom from angina	74%	71%	N/S
Needing no antianginal drugs	22%	12%	0.04

CONCLUSIONS: There was no significant difference in anginal symptoms at 1 year however, those who had PTCA were more likely to need more anti-anginal drugs or repeat revascularisation procedures. Those who had CABG were more likely to suffer AMI during the initial procedure.
NEJM 1994;331:1037–44.

GUSTO IIb Primary Angioplasty Substudy: Global Use of Strategies To Open Occluded Coronary Arteries in Acute Coronary Syndromes

1138 patients within 12 hours of onset of symptoms of acute MI associated with ECG changes were randomised to receive thrombolysis with accelerated t-PA or primary PTCA. Primary endpoints were early (30-day) mortality, reinfarction and stroke.

RESULTS	Accelerated t-PA (n = 573)	Primary PTCA (n = 565)	p value
Death	40 (7.0%)	32 (5.7%)	0.37
Reinfarction	37 (6.5%)	25 (4.4%)	0.13
Disabling stroke	5 (0.9%)	1 (0.2%)	0.11
Any of the above	78 (13.6%)	54 (9.6%)	0.033

CONCLUSIONS: Primary PTCA is safe and effective and provides moderate advantage over t-PA with respect to clinical outcome at 30 days.
NEJM 1997;336:1621–8.

GUSTO III (SUBSTUDY): Global Use of Strategies To Open Occluded Coronary Arteries in Acute Coronary Syndromes III

387 patients who presented within 6 hours of onset of acute MI had failed thrombolysis and underwent rescue PTCA within 24 hours. They were randomised to receive or not receive abciximab. Primary endpoint was 30-day mortality.

RESULTS:	Abciximab (n = 81)	No abciximab (n = 306)	p value
Intracranial bleed	0	2 (0.7%)	
Moderate bleed	13 (16.0%)	45 (15.0%)	
Severe bleeding	3 (3.7%)	3 (1.0%)	0.08
30-day mortality	3 (3.7%)	30 (9.8%)	0.04

Appendix A

CONCLUSIONS: Use of abciximab in rescue PTCA after failed thrombolysis is associated with a modest increase in the risk of bleeding. However, the 30-day mortality is significantly reduced.
JACC 1998;31:191A.

HELVETICA: Hirudin in a European Trial Versus Heparin In The Prevention of Restenosis after PTCA Trial

1141 patients with unstable angina underwent single or multivessel angioplasty and were randomised to one of three treatment groups. The first received 10 000 units heparin + 24 hour infusion of heparin + placebo SQ for 3 days, the second had hirudin 40 mg + hirudin infusion for 24 hours + placebo SQ for 3 days, and the third had hirudin 40 mg + hirudin infusion for 24 hours + hirudin SQ for 3 days. Patients were followed for 7 months and had repeat angiography at 6 months to compare mean luminal diameter.

RESULTS:	Heparin alone	Hirudin alone	Heparin + hirudin	p value
7-month event-free survival (%)	67.3	63.5	68.0	0.61
Early cardiac events (%)	11.0	7.9	5.6	0.023
Mean minimal luminal diameter at 6 months (mm)	1.54	1.47	1.56	0.08

CONCLUSIONS: Although hirudin reduced early cardiac event rates there was no apparent benefit clinically or angiographically at 6 months.
NEJM 1995;333:757–63.

IMPACT II: Integrilin to Minimize Platelet Aggregation and Prevent Coronary Thrombosis

Following a small preliminary trial (IMPACT I) 4010 patients with a history of stable or unstable angina underwent elective or emergency PTCA. All received aspirin and heparin and were then randomised to integrilin 135 µg/kg bolus + 0.5 µg/kg/min infusion for 20–24 hours, integrilin 135 µg/kg bolus + 0.75 µg/kg/min infusion for 20–24 hours, or placebo. Primary endpoints were events at 30 days – death, myocardial infarction, repeat revascularisation. Angiography was repeated at 6 months.

RESULTS:	Placebo	135/0.5 eptifibatide	135/0.75 eptifibatide
30-day composite endpoint (%)	11.4	9.2 $p = 0.063$	9.9 $p = 0.22$
Major bleeding (%)	4.8	5.1	5.2

CONCLUSIONS: Use of low dose integrilin (eptifibatide) during PTCA reduces risk of early abrupt closure and 30-day ischaemic events. This was not evident for the higher dose regime. There was no difference in the rates of bleeding.

Lancet 1997;349:1422–8.

Appendix A

ISAR: Intracoronary Stenting and Antithrombotic Regimen Trial

517 patients with successful PTCA and stenting (residual stenosis < 30%) were randomised to either aspirin and ticlopidine or aspirin, IV heparin, + phenprocoumon. Angiography was repeated to look for restenosis at 6 months.

RESULTS:		Antiplatelet (n = 257)	Anticoagulation (n = 260)	p value
In the high risk group at 30 days	Major adverse cardiac event	2.0%	12.6%	0.007
	Stent vessel occlusion	0%	11.5%	< 0.001
At 6 months	Mean luminal diameter (mm)	1.95 ± 0.86	1.90 ± 0.87	0.55
	Late lumen loss	1.10 ± 0.81	1.15 ± 0.75	0.54
	Restenosis rate (%)	26.8	28.9	0.70

CONCLUSIONS: Patients deemed to be high risk derived the most benefit from antiplatelet therapy. There was a significant reduction in rate of early thrombotic vessel occlusions although no significant difference in restenosis at 6 months or need for repeat revascularisation compared to standard anticoagulation therapy.
Circulation 1997;95:2015–21.
Circulation 1997;96:462–7.

ISAR-SMART

404 patients undergoing angioplasty to vessel 2–2.8 mm diameter (mean 2.5 mm) were randomised as to whether or not they had stenting. All received abciximab and ticlopidine for 2 weeks in the angioplasty group, and 4 weeks in the stent group. At 6 months the primary endpoint of restenosis was assessed on angiography.

RESULTS:	With stent	Without stent
>50% restenosis (%)	35.0	37.0
>70% restenosis (%)	22.2	18.8
Target vessel revascularisation (TVR) (%)	20.1	16.5

CONCLUSIONS: There was no significant difference between the groups, therefore there was no evidence that routine stenting reduces restenosis or need for TVR.
Results presented at ACC meeting 2000.

LONG WRIST: The Washington Radiation for In-Stent Restenosis Trial for Long Lesions

120 patients with in-stent restenosis of a long lesion (36–80 mm long, mean 31 mm) in a vessel 3–5 mm diameter, undergoing intervention (with use of directional atherectomy or laser ablation, etc. as needed) were randomised to Iridium[192] or placebo. All received either ticlopidine or clopidogrel.

Appendix A

RESULTS:		Ir^{192} (n = 60)	Placebo (n = 60)	p value
Minimal luminal	Pre-	0.78	0.68	
diameter (mm)	Post-	2.09	2.01	
	6 months	1.4	1.01	0.008
Late loss index		0.46	0.93	0.014
Major adverse cardiac event (%)		38.3	61.7	0.01
Death (%)		4.6	6.1	
Q-wave MI (%)		8.3	0	0.06
TLR (%)		30.0	60.0	0.001

CONCLUSIONS: Intra-coronary gamma radiation for the treatment of in-stent restenosis in long lesions is feasible and safe and reduces angiographic and overall adverse clinical events at 6 months with the exception of Q-wave MI. Results presented at ACC meeting 2000.

MUSIC: Multicentre Ultrasound Stenting in Coronaries Study

125 patients with a history of stable angina had coronary angioplasty and stenting with a single Palmaz–Schatz stent. IVUS was used to ensure full deployment of the stent with a mean luminal diameter > = 90% average proximal and distal reference cross sectional diameter or, a minimum stent cross sectional area >/= 9.0 mm^2. All patients were treated with aspirin and were followed-up with repeat angiography at 6 months to look at rates of restenosis (observational study).

RESULTS		
Procedural success		97.5%
At 1 month	Death	0%
	Q-wave MI	0%
	Non-Q-wave MI	3.2%
	CABG	0.6%
	Re-PTCA	1.3%
	Subacute thrombosis	1.3%
6-month restenosis		9.7%

CONCLUSIONS: IVUS-guided optimally deployed stents may be safely managed with aspirin alone.
Europ Heart J 1998;19:1214–23.

NIRVANA: NIR Vascular Advanced North American Trial

849 native vessel coronary artery lesions which were < 25 mm in length and in a vessel 3.0–4.0 mm diameter were included and randomised to stenting with either an NIR stent or Palmaz–Schatz. Repeat angiography at 6 months assessed in-stent restenosis. Primary endpoint of the study was clinical evidence of target vessel failure at 9 months.

Appendix A

RESULTS at 6 MONTHS:	NIR (n = 420)	Palmaz-Schatz (n = 429)	p value
Target vessel failure (%)	13.2	14.4	NS
Target lesion revascularisation (%)	7.4	9.0	NS
Angiographic restenosis (%)	20.0	21.7	NS

CONCLUSIONS: No statistically significant difference at 6 months between the two stents.
Circulation 1998;98:Abstract 3476.
JACC 1998;98:Abstract 80A.

OARS: Optimal Atherectomy Restenosis Study

199 consecutive patients with coronary disease underwent IVUS-guided directional atherectomy and were followed up over 1 year to assess clinical outcomes, with angiographic success reviewed at 6 months. All had at least 60% stenosis in a vessel > 2.8 mm, lesion length < 12 mm. Pre-procedure mean luminal diameter was 1.19 mm.

RESULTS	In-hospital (n = 199)	Angiographic follow-up at 6 months and clinical follow-up at 1 year (n = 176)
Post-MLD (mm)	3.16	2.01
Restenosis		28.9%
Death	0%	1.0%
Q-wave MI	1.5%	1.5%
Major complications	2.5%	
Target lesion revascularisation (TLR)		17.8%
Composite endpoint, i.e. death, Q-wave MI, or TLR		23.6%

CONCLUSIONS: IVUS-guided optimal direct coronary atherectomy resulted in high procedural success rates and a low rate of restenosis or complications.
Circulation 1998;97:332–9.

PAMI: Primary Angioplasty in Myocardial Infarction

395 patients within 12 hours of onset of symptoms of chest pain, with ECG confirming acute myocardial infarction were randomised to either t-PA or PTCA.

RESULTS	PTCA (n = 170)*	t-PA (n = 200)	p value
Stroke	0	7 (3.5%)	< 0.05
Reinfarction	5 (3%)	13 (6.5%)	0.06
Death in hospital	5 (3%)	13 (6.5%)	0.06
Death in 6 months	6 (4%)	16 (8%)	0.08

RESULTS	PTCA (n = 170)*	t-PA (n = 200)	p value
Unscheduled PTCA	12 (7%)	72 (36%)	0.001
CABG	16 (9%)	24 (12%)	0.21
LVEF at 6 weeks	53%	53%	NS
Non-fatal reinfarction or death	10 (6%)	24 (12%)	0.02
2-year freedom from death/MI/repeat PTCA/CABG	53.3%	37%	< 0.0001

*Of 195 patients randomised, 175 (90%) were candidates for PTCA, which was successful in 97%

CONCLUSIONS: PTCA in acute MI is associated with a lower risk of stroke and combined endpoint of in-hospital death and re-infarction compared with t-PA.
NEJM 1993;328:673–9.

PAMI II: Second Primary Angioplasty in Myocardial Infarction

908 patients within 12 hours of onset of acute MI with chest pain and ECG changes underwent PTCA. 437 patients were felt 'high-risk' because of one or more of the following: age >70 years, 3 vessel CAD, LVEF < 45%, or SVG occlusion and were randomised as to whether or not they received an intra-aortic balloon pump. The remaining 471 'low-risk' patients were randomised to either an early post-PTCA discharge or a longer traditional post-MI stay in hospital.

RESULTS of 'HIGH-RISK' GROUP:	IABP (n = 211)	No-IABP (n = 226)	p value
Recurrent ischaemia (%)	13.5	19.6	0.08
Congestive heart failure (%)	17.5	19.5	0.60
Haemorrhagic stroke (%)	1	0	0.23
Any haemorrhage – mostly at access site (%)	36	27.4	0.05
CABG (%)	11.9	10.7	0.70
Ejection fraction at 6 weeks (%)	47.6	46.0	0.60

RESULTS of 'LOW-RISK' GROUP:	Early discharge (n = 237)	Usual discharge (n = 234)	p value
In-hospital stay (days)	4.2 ± 2.3	7.1 ± 4.7	0.0001
Combined mortality, reinfarction, unstable angina, CHL (%)	15.2	17.5	0.49

CONCLUSIONS: In 'high-risk' patients, prophylactic use of an intra-aortic balloon pump does not significantly reduce adverse clinical events. In 'low-risk' patients an early discharge with shorter stay in hospital was safe.
JACC 1997;29:1459–67.
JACC 1998;31:967–72.

Appendix A

PAMI STENT PILOT: Primary Stenting in Acute Myocardial Infarction

312 patients within 12 hours onset of chest pains, with ECG criteria for acute myocardial infarction underwent immediate coronary angiography. Patients were included if vessel size > 2.75 mm and had primary PTCA with Palmaz–Schatz stent placement unless there was small vessel size, reduced flow, or diffuse distal disease.

RESULTS:	Stent (n = 231)	PTCA (n = 69)	p value
Pre-MLD (mm)	0.28 ± 0.46	0.38 ± 0.62	
Post-MLD (mm)	2.77 ± 0.59	1.86 ± 0.61	
In-hospital death	2 (0.8%)	0	0.99
In-hospital reinfarction	4 (1.7%)	0	0.58
In-hospital CABG	7 (2.9%)	9 (12.5%)	0.001
Target lesion revascularisation at 30 days	1 (0.4%)	5 (6.9%)	0.0004

CONCLUSIONS: Stenting compared to PTCA alone reduced the need for in-hospital CABG, and reduced target lesion revascularisation at 30 days. JACC 1998(31);1:23–30.

PAMI STENT: Primary Stenting in Acute Myocardial Infarction

900 patients with acute myocardial infarction and disease suitable for percutaneous intervention were randomised to angioplasty alone or with a Palmaz–Schatz stent. At 6 months they were assessed for recurrent angina and major adverse cardiac events.

RESULTS:	Stent (n = 452)	Angioplasty (n = 448)	p value
Angina (%)	11.3	16.9	0.02
Target vessel revascularisation (%)	7.7	17.0	< 0.001
Reinfarction (%)	2.4	2.9	1.0
Disabling stroke (%)	0.2	0.2	1.0
Death (%)	4.2	2.7	0.27

CONCLUSIONS: The use of a stent significantly reduced the need for a further revascularisation procedure and was associated with less angina. No significant impact on mortality (indeed a trend to worse mortality figures). NEJM 1999;341:1949–56.

PRISM: Platelet Receptor Inhibition in Ischaemic Syndrome Management

3232 patients with unstable angina, already receiving aspirin, were randomised to receive tirofiban or standard treatment with heparin. Primary endpoint was death, myocardial infarction, or refractory ischaemia at 48 hours.

Appendix A

RESULTS:	Tirofiban	Heparin	p value
Composite endpoint (%)	3.8	5.6	0.01
30-day composite endpoint (%)	15.9	17.1	0.34
30-day death (%)	2.3	3.6	0.02
Reversible thrombocytopenia (%)	1.1	0.4	0.04

There was no significant difference in rates of major bleeding.
CONCLUSIONS: tirofiban is well tolerated and reduces ischaemic episodes during the 48-hour infusion. There was a significant reduction in 30-day mortality.
NEJM 1998 May 21;338(21):1498–505.

PRISM-PLUS: Platelet Receptor Inhibition in Ischaemic Syndrome Management in Patients Limited by Unstable Signs and Symptoms

1915 patients with unstable angina or non-Q-wave infarction were randomised to tirofiban, heparin, or a combination of the two infused for 48 hours. After 48 hours, angiography and angioplasty was performed as indicated. Primary endpoint was death, myocardial infarction, or refractory ischaemia at 7 days.

RESULTS:	Tirofiban + heparin	Heparin alone	p value
7-day composite endpoint (%)	12.9	17.9	0.004
30-day composite endpoint (%)	18.5	22.3	0.03
6-month composite endpoint (%)	27.7	32.1	0.02
Major bleeding (%)	4	3	0.34

*The tirofiban alone arm was stopped prematurely because of excess deaths (4.6% vs 1.1% those treated with heparin alone

CONCLUSIONS: Tirofiban when given in addition to heparin and aspirin in this setting, significantly reduces adverse cardiac events without increasing the risk of bleeding. This effect was still significant at 6 months, and was seen in both the medically treated and angioplasty treated groups.
NEJM 1998 May 21;338(21):1488–97.

REDUCE: Low Molecular Weight Heparin, Reviparin, in the Prevention of Restenosis after PTCA

612 patients with single vessel coronary disease underwent PTCA and were randomised as to whether to receive reviparin 7000 units bolus and 24-hour infusion of 10 500 units + 28 days 3500 units bd SQ, or, unfractionated heparin 10 000 units bolus then 24-hour infusion of 24 000 units + 28 days placebo SQ. Primary endpoint was rate of adverse cardiac event, i.e. death, myocardial infarction, repeat revascularisation procedure. Follow-up was for 30 weeks.

RESULTS:	Control (n = 306)	Reviparin (n = 306)	p value
Acute events in 24 hours (%)	8.2	3.9	0.027
Primary endpoint (%)	32	33.3	0.7

There was no significant difference between the groups of rates of haemorrhage, or of late loss minimal lumen diameter.
CONCLUSIONS: Use of the low-molecular weight heparin reviparin reduced acute event rates compared with unfractionated heparin but there was no significant difference in 6 month rates of adverse cardiac events or of angiographically evident restenosis.
JACC 1996 Nov 15;28(6):1437–43.

RESIST: REStenosis after Ivus guided STenting

155 patients with symptomatic ischaemic heart disease were randomised to angioplasty and stenting with or without IVUS-guidance. After stenting, patients either had no further procedure or had additional balloon dilatation until achieving IVUS criteria for stent expansion. At 6 months angiography was repeated to look for restenosis.

RESULTS:	Stent alone	Stent + IVUS	p value
Initial cross sectional area (mm²)	7.16 ± 2.48	7.95 ± 2.21	0.04
Restenosis at 6 months (%)	28.8	22.5	0.25
6-month cross sectional area (mm²)	4.47 ± 2.59	5.36 ± 2.81	0.03

CONCLUSIONS: No significant difference was detected in restenosis rates but the number of patients having follow-up angiography was small and the study underpowered. IVUS did increase initial and 6-month cross sectional area.
JACC 32(2):320–8, 1998 Aug.

RESTORE: Randomised Efficacy Study of Tirofiban for Outcomes and Restenosis

2139 high risk patients undergoing PTCA who were at risk of abrupt vessel closure with unstable angina or recent MI. All received aspirin and heparin, and were then randomised to tirofiban 10 μg/kg bolus + 0.15 μg/kg/min infusion for 36 hours, or placebo. Primary endpoint was incidence of death, MI, or revascularisation procedure at 30 days. They had repeat angiography at 6 months to assess evidence of restenosis.

RESULTS:	Placebo (n = 205)	Tirofiban (n = 212)	p value
2-day composite endpoint (%)	8.7	5.4	0.005
7-day composite endpoint (%)	10.4	7.3	0.02
30-day composite endpoint (%)	12.2	10.3	0.16
6-month composite endpoint (%)	27.1	24.1	0.11
6-month >/= 50% diameter restenosis (%)	57.0	51.0	NS

Appendix A

CONCLUSIONS: Although tirofiban significantly reduced events over the first 7 days following PTCA when compared to standard therapy with heparin, the beneficial effects were not sustained at 6 months. Tirofiban therapy did not influence rate of angiographic evidence of restenosis.
NEJM 1997; 96:1445–53.

RITA: Randomised Intervention Treatment of Angina Trial

1011 patients with stable or unstable angina found to have suitable single or multivessel coronary artery disease with stenosis of greater than 50% on angiography were randomised to PTCA or CABG and followed up over 5 years.

RESULTS AT 2.5 YEARS		CABG (n = 501)		PTCA (n = 510)		p value
Death		18 (3.6%)		16 (3.1%)		NS
Non-fatal MI		26		34		NS
Reintervention	CABG	4		96		
	PTCA	16	11%	93	38%	0.001
	Coronary angiography	39		159		

CONCLUSIONS: Those in the PTCA group were significantly more likely to undergo revascularisation over the 5-year period compared to those who had CABG. However there was no significant difference in overall rates of death or MI.
Lancet 1993;341:573–80.

RITA-2: The Second Randomised Intervention Treatment of Angina

1018 patients with single or multivessel coronary artery disease with stenosis of at least 70% on angiography were randomised to medical therapy or balloon angioplasty. They were followed-up over 5 years to assess risk or death or MI.

RESULTS AT 2 YEARS	PTCA (n = 504)	Medical therapy (n = 514)	p value
Death or MI	6.3	3.3	0.02
Revascularisation (%)	19	23	NS
There was 16.6% excess, etc			

CONCLUSIONS: The group who had angioplasty had a higher risk of death or MI within 5 years, however there was a significant improvement in symptoms in this group.
Lancet 1997;350:461–8.

ROSTER: ROtablater vs Balloon for STEnt Restenosis

52 patients who had stent implantation > 6 weeks previously and then developed in-stent restenosis of >/= 50% diameter were randomised to high-

pressure balloon PTCA alone, or low-pressure PTCA and rotational atherectomy. Primary endpoint was the need for further target lesion revascularisation at 6 months.

RESULTS:	Rotational atherectomy (n = 26)	PTCA alone (n = 26)	p value
MLD pre (mm)	0.9 ± 0.4	0.9 ± 0.4	NS
MLD post (mm)	2.8 ± 0.4	2.5 ± 0.4	0.04
Dissection/stent use (%)	2 (8%)	13 (50%)	< 0.01
Clinical restenosis	1 (4%)	7 (27%)	0.03

CONCLUSIONS: Rotational atherectomy in addition to balloon angioplasty in the setting of in-stent restenosis resulted in improved luminal gain, lower stent use, lower dissection rate, and lower clinical restenosis compared to balloon angioplasty alone.
JACC 1998;40:142A.

SAVED: Saphenous Vein De Novo Trial

220 patients with objective evidence of ischaemia due to a stenosis in a vein graft > 3.0 mm and < 5.0 mm diameter were randomised to either PTCA alone or use of a Palmaz–Schatz stent. All had a left ventricular ejection fraction >25%. Repeat angiography at 6 months assessed restenosis. Follow-up over 8 months determined the clinical primary endpoint of major adverse cardiac event, i.e. death, MI, CABG, or repeat PTCA.

RESULTS:	PTCA (n = 107)	Stent (n = 108)	p value
Procedural success (%)	69	92	< 0.001
Restenosis (%)	46	37	0.24
Adverse cardiac event (%)	39	26	0.04

CONCLUSIONS: In SVG lesions, stenting significantly improved event-free survival despite similar rates of angiographic evidence of restenosis.
NEJM 1997;337:740–47.

SCRIPPS: Scripps Coronary Radiation to Inhibit Proliferation Post Stenting

55 patients with evidence of restenosis in either a native coronary or saphenous vein graft were randomised to stenting with or without catheter-based intracoronary gamma radiation (iridium[192]). All lesions were < 30 mm in length and were in a vessel 3.0–5.0 mm diameter. Follow-up at 6 months and then 3 years assessed adverse clinical event rates (death, MI, stent thrombosis, or target lesion revascularisation) and angiographic evidence of restenosis.

Appendix A

RESULTS:			Ir[192] (n = 26)	Placebo (n = 29)	p value
MLD (mm)	Pre-		1.10 ± 0.46	1.03 ± 0.46	0.60
	Post-		2.82 ± 0.60	2.88 ± 0.83	0.78
	6 months		2.43 ± 0.78	1.85 ± 0.89	0.02
Target lesion revascularisation		6 months	3/26	13/29	0.01
(TLR) (%)		3 years	15.4%	48.3%	< 0.01
Death, MI, or TLR (%)		6 months	4/26	14/29	0.01
		3 years	23.1%	55.2%	0.01
>50% restenosis (%)		6 months	8	36	0.02
		3 years*	33.3%	63.6%	< 0.05

*Angiography carried out in 43/55 patients

CONCLUSIONS: Catheter-based intracoronary radiotherapy overall, significantly reduced angiographic and IVUS evidence of restenosis, and adverse clinical events compared to placebo and this was sustained at 3 years. However, in those who did not undergo a TLR procedure, the radiation group showed a trend to greater late-lumen loss over time than the placebo group.

NEJM 1997;336:1697–703.

3-year results presented at ACC meeting 2000.

SHOCK: Should We Emergently Revascularize Occluded Coronaries for Cardiogenic Shock

302 patients with cardiogenic shock complicating recent (within 36 hours) acute myocardial infarction were randomised to medical stabilisation or emergency revascularisation with CABG or PTCA. 86% patients in both groups also had intra-aortic balloon counterpulsation. Primary endpoint was mortality at 30 days with a secondary endpoints of mortality at 6 months and 1 year.

RESULTS	Early revascularisation (n = 152)	Medical stabilisation (n = 150)	p value
Mortality at 30 days (%)	47	56	0.109
Mortality at 6 months (%)	50	63	0.027
Mortality at 1 year (%)	55	70	0.009

CONCLUSIONS: Although no significant difference in mortality was evident at 30 days, there was a significant improvement in mortality at 6 months and at 1 year for those who had early intervention. Results were significantly better for those aged < 75 years.

AHJ 1999;137:313–21.

1-year results presented at AHA meeting 1999.

Appendix A

269 consecutive patients undergoing angioplasty with elective stenting were randomised as to whether they had angiographic guidance, or used IVUS to achieve a lesion minimal lumen cross sectional area > 65% of the reference segment. Primary endpoint was adverse cardiac event rate or target lesion revascularisation, and angiographic evidence of restenosis at 6 months.

RESULTS:	IVUS-guided (n = 93)	Angiographic (n = 105)	p value
MLD follow-up (mm)	1.79 ± 0.84	1:52 ± 0.87	< 0.05
Restenosis (%)	21	41	< 0.001
Death	1	0	NS
MI	3 (2%)	5 (3%)	NS
PTCA	30 (18%)	52 (24%)	< 0.05
CABG	5 (3%)	4 (2%)	NS
Adverse cardiac event	38 (24%)	61 (33%)	0.096

CONCLUSIONS: IVUS-guided stent deployment reduces restenosis at 6 months and there was a trend towards fewer adverse cardiac events
Circulation 1997;96:1–222.

SMART: Study of AVE-Microstent Ability to Limit Restenosis Trial

662 patients undergoing PTCA and stent implantation for a single coronary stenosis requiring less than two stents and in a vessel 3.0–4.0 mm diameter, were randomised to either a Palmaz–Schatz stent or an AVE-Microstent II. Follow-up at 6 months looked at adverse clinical cardiac events including target lesion revascularisation, and angiography was repeated at 6 months to assess restenosis.

RESULTS:	AVE (n = 337)	Palmaz-Schatz (n = 325)	p value
MLD post (mm)	2.85 ± 0.44	2.77 ± 0.46	< 0.05
MLD at 6 months (mm)	1.86 ± 0.66	2.00 + 0.68	NS
DS at 6 months (%)	37 + 19	34 + 20	NS
Restenosis at 6 months (%)	24.8	22.9	NS
Adverse cardiac event at 6 months (%)	16.1	14.8	NS

CONCLUSIONS: Acute angiographic results were superior with the AVE stent with no significant difference in clinical events or rates of restenosis at 6 months.
JACC 1998;31:65A,80A.

SMASH: The Swiss EMergency Revascularisation for Acute Myocardial Infarction with SHock

55 patients within 48 hours of an acute myocardial infarction complicated by cardiogenic shock (high pulmonary capillary wedge pressure and hypotension)

Appendix A

were randomised to standard medical therapy or emergency revascularisation
with either PTCA or CABG. Primary endpoint was survival at 30 days.
RESULTS and CONCLUSIONS: In this small study, 32 patients had emergency
revascularisation (27 had PTCA, successful in 23) and had a 30-day mortality
of 69%. 23 were randomised to medical management and had a 30-day
mortality of 78%, this result was not statistically significant. The study stopped
early because of low recruitment.
Europ Heart 1997;18:586.

STARS: Stent Anti-Thrombotic Regimen Study

1650 patients undergoing PTCA with stent deployment were randomised to
receive aspirin alone, aspirin + warfarin, or aspirin + ticlopidine. In all patients
less than three stents were required in vessels of 3.0–5.0 mm diameter and
there was optimal deployment with no evidence of coronary dissection and
< 10% residual stenosis post-procedure. Patients were reassessed at 30 days
with particular emphasis on rate of subacute stent thrombosis.

RESULTS	Aspirin alone (n = 557)	Aspirin + coumadin (n = 550)	Aspirin + ticlopidine (n = 546)	p value
Subacute thrombosis*	3.6%	2.7%	0.5%	0.001
Death	0.2%	0.0%	0.0%	–
TLR	3.4%	2.5%	0.5%	0.002
Thrombosis on angiography	2.9%	2.7%	0.5%	0.005

*i.e. death, target lesion revascularisation, MI, thrombus on angiography.

CONCLUSIONS: Aspirin in addition to ticlopidine was superior to either
aspirin alone, or in combination with coumadin in preventing subacute in-
stent thrombosis after successful stent deployment.
NEJM 1998;339:1665–71.

START: STent versus directional coronary Atherectomy Randomised Trial

122 lesions suitable for both Palmaz–Schatz stenting and directional
atherectomy (DCA) were randomised to one of the procedures. IVUS was used
to aggressively debulk in the DCA patients and to quantify lumen diameter.

RESULTS:	Stent (n = 62)	DCA (n = 60)	p value
Post-procedural lumen diameter (mm)	2.79	2.90	
6 month lumen diameter (mm)	1.89	2.18	0.023
Intimal proliferation (mm)	3.1	1.1	< 0.0001
Restenosis of > 50% (%)	32.8	15.8	0.032
Target vessel failure at 6 months (%)	33.9	18.3	0.056

Appendix A

CONCLUSIONS: Aggressive DCA may provide better angiographic results than stenting.
JACC 34(4):1057–7, 1999 Oct.

START: STents And Radiation Therapy

476 patients with in-stent restenosis (> 50%) in a single vessel of 2.7–4.0 mm diameter underwent balloon angioplasty and were randomised to vascular brachytherapy with strontium^{90}/yttrium^{90} source or placebo. All received either ticlopidine or clopidogrel. They were followed-up over 8 months with a primary endpoint of target vessel revascularisation (TVR).

RESULTS:	Sr^{90}	Placebo	Reduction	p value
TVR	16.0%	24.1%	34%	0.026
Major adverse cardiac event*	18.0%	25.9%	31%	0.039

*No significant difference in risk of death

CONCLUSIONS: Use of brachytherapy with beta radiation significantly improved clinical and angiographic outcomes at 8 months with no evidence of an increased risk of late subacute stent thrombosis.
Results presented at ACC meeting 2000.

STRATUS: Study To Determine Rotablator And Transluminal Angioplasty Strategy

500 patients with coronary stenosis of < 20 mm in length in a vessel < 3.25 mm suitable for rotablator therapy. They were randomised to an aggressive approach with burr:artery ratio 0.7–0.9 with no or low pressure (1 atmosphere) adjunctive balloon inflation or, a more conservative approach with burr:artery ratio 0.6–0.8 and routine adjunctive balloon inflation with Bar 1.1–1.3 and balloon pressure of 3 atmospheres. Primary endpoints were clinical adverse cardiac events and angiographic restenosis at 6 months.

RESULTS:	Aggressive strategy (n = 250)	Conservative strategy (n = 250)	p value
MLD at 6 months (mm)	1.22 ± 0.72	1.31 ± 0.69	
Death	6 (2.5%)	12 (5.1%)	NS
MI	6 (2.5%)	2 (1%)	NS
Target lesion revascularisation	85 (34.5%)	65 (27.4%)	0.08

CONCLUSIONS: An aggressive approach to rotablation does not reduce adverse events or restenosis at 6 months.
JACC 1998;31:455A.

Appendix A

STRESS: The Stent REStenosis Study

410 patients with symptomatic coronary stenoses > 70% diameter were randomised to have angioplasty with or without Palmaz–Schatz stent deployment. Lesions were <15 mm in length and vessel diameter >3.0 mm. All patients were reassessed at 6 months with repeat angiography to look for evidence of restenosis.

RESULTS:	Stent (n = 205)	PTCA (n = 202)	p value
MLD pre (mm)	0.77 ± 0.27	0.75 ± 0.25	0.48
MLD post (mm)	2.49 ± 0.43	1.99 ± 0.47	< 0.001
Diameter stenosis post (%)	19 ± 11	35 ± 14	< 0.001
MLD follow-up (mm)	1.74 ± 0.6	1.56 ± 0.65	0.007
Diameter stenosis follow-up (%)	42 ± 18	49 ± 19	0.001
Restenosis (%)	31.6	42.1	0.046
Death (%)	1.5	1.5	1
MI (%)	6.3	6.9	0.81
CABG (%)	4.9	8.4	0.15
Any major adverse cardiac event i.e. death, MI, CABG, re-PTCA (%)	19.5	23.8	0.16

CONCLUSIONS: Stenting results in a larger luminal diameter on angiography compared with angioplasty alone, and reduces the rate of restenosis at 6 months. NEJM 1994;331:496–501.

STRESS I and II (Small Vessel Substudy): The STent REStenosis Study Group

331 patients with symptomatic coronary disease were randomised to angioplasty with or without a Palmaz–Schatz stent. Inclusion criteria were as for STRESS except the vessel diameter < 3.0 mm.

RESULTS:		Stent (n = 163)	PTCA (n = 168)	p value
Reference diameter (mm)		2.69 (2.05–2.99)	2.64 (1.93–2.99)	NS
MLD post-procedure (mm)		2.26 ± 0.36	1.80 ± 0.36	< 0.001
Diameter stenosis post (%)		17 ± 11	34 ± 15	< 0.001
At 6 months	MLD (mm)	1.54 ± 0.54	1.27 ± 0.53	< 0.001
	DS (%)	44 ± 19	54 ± 20	< 0.001
	Restenosis (%)	34	55	< 0.001
1 year free of death, MI, CABG, or PTCA (%)		78	67	0.019

CONCLUSIONS: Stenting in small vessels is superior to angioplasty alone and reduces rate of restenosis.

JACC 1998;31:307–11.

Appendix A

TOSCA: Total Occlusion Study of CAnada

410 patients with native coronary artery lesion (TIMI 0 or 1 flow) in a vessel >3.0 mm diameter within 72 hours onset of ST-elevation in whom the lesion could be crossed with a guidewire, were randomised to balloon angioplasty alone or a heparin-coated stent. Primary endpoint was death, MI, or target vessel revascularisation and TIMI grade 3 flow on angiography at 6 months.

RESULTS:		PTCA (n = 208)	Stent (n = 202)	p value
In-hospital	Max. balloon pressure (bar)	10.0 ± 3.3	15.4 ± 3.3	NS
	Complete procedural success*	143 (68.8%)	169 (83.7%)	NS
At 6 months	Target vessel revascularisation	32 (15.4%)	17* (8.4%)	0.03
	Any MI	8 (3.8%)	24 (11.9%)	0.01
	Any major event[†]	48 (23.1%)	32 (15.8%)	0.08
	Failed patency (TIMI flow < 3)	39 (19.5%)	21 (10.9%)	0.024

*< 50% residual stenosis and TIMI 3 flow without crossover, target vessel revascularisation. MI or death pre-discharge from hospital.
[†]Excluding peri-procedural MI with CK-MB elevation <5 times.

CONCLUSIONS: In this situation, use of a stent improves patency and reduces restenosis at 6 months though there was no significant difference in adverse cardiac events.
Circulation 1999;100:236–42.

VANOWISH: Veterans Affairs Non-Q-Wave Infarction Strategies In-Hospital

920 patients with ECG and CK confirmation of non-Q wave MI were randomised to standard conservative therapy versus intervention with PTCA. All were followed-up over a 1-year period to assess risk of death or MI.

RESULTS	Invasive group (n = 462)	Conservative group (n = 458)	p value
In-hospital death or MI	36 (7.8%)	15 (3.3%)	0.0004
1-month death or MI	48 (10.4%)	26 (5.7%)	0.012
1-month death	23 (4.9%)	9 (2.0%)	0.0004
1-year death or MI	111 (24.0%)	85 (18.6%)	0.05
1-year death	58 (12.6%)	36 (7.9%)	NS

CONCLUSIONS: Those who had intervention had a significantly higher in-hospital death / MI rate compared to a conservative strategy. At 1 year the difference was not significant but with a trend still in favour of the conservative approach.
NEJM 1998;338:1785–92.

WRIST: Washington Radiation for In-Stent Restenosis Trial

100 patients undergoing angioplasty for in-stent restenosis in a native coronary vessel and 30 patients with in-stent restenosis in a saphenous vein

Appendix A

graft were randomised as to whether or not they received adjunctive gamma radiation with Iridium[192]. Lesions had to be <47 mm in length in a vessel 3.0–5.0 mm diameter and all had left ventricular ejection fractions >30%.

RESULTS:	Iridium-192 (n = 65)	Placebo (n = 65)	p value
6-month adverse cardiac event (%)	29.2	67.7	0.001
6-month restenosis on angiography (%)	23.7	60.7	0.001

CONCLUSIONS: Vascular brachytherapy with gamma radiation using Iridium-192 reduces restenosis and adverse cardiac events when used for in-stent restenosis.
Lancet 1972; 354:49–56.
Circulation 1998;98 Suppl. 17:1–651.

A comparison of immediate coronary angioplasty with intravenous streptokinase in acute myocardial infarction (Zwolle data)

142 patients aged <76 years with pain and ECG criteria of acute myocardial infarction were randomised to 1.5 MU streptokinase or primary angioplasty. All received 300 mg aspirin, IV nitroglycerin to maintain bp of 110 mmHg, and IV heparin to keep APTT 2–3× normal. Study endpoints were recurrent ischaemia during admission, LV ejection fraction pre-discharge on radionuclide scanning, and vessel patency assessed on angiography at a later stage.

RESULTS:	Streptokinase (n = 72)	Angioplasty (n = 70)*	p value
Reccurence of infarct	9	0	0.003
Unstable angina	14	4	0.02
LV ejection fraction	45 ± 12%	51 ± 11%	0.004
Infarct-related artery patency	68%	91%	0.001
% stenosis on QCA	76 ± 19%	36 ± 20%	< 0.001

*Technically successful procedure in 64 out of 65 patients

CONCLUSIONS: Immediate angioplasty was associated with less ischaemia, less LV impairment, and a higher rate of artery patency compared with streptokinase.
NEJM 1993;328:680–4.

Immediate angioplasty compared with the administration of a thrombolytic agent followed by conservative treatment for myocardial infarction (Mayo Clinic)

108 patients with acute myocardial infarction were randomised to thrombolysis with t-PA or immediate angioplasty, all received heparin. Patients were < 80 years and within 12 hours of onset of chest pain and had ECG

Appendix A

criteria of acute MI. Cardiogenic shock was a contraindication. Primary endpoint was a change in size of perfusion defect on technetium^{99m} sestamibi scans carried out on admission and discharge.

RESULTS:		t-PA (n = 56)	PTCA (n = 47)
Mean time from onset of pain to intervention (i.e. start of infusion or first balloon inflation)		232 ± 174 minutes	277 ± 144 minutes
Myocardial salvage	Anterior infarct	27 ± 21%	31 ± 21%
	Inferior infarct	7 ± 13%	5 ± 10%
In-hospital death		2	2
Revascularisation procedure within 6 months		12	4*

*p = 0.075

CONCLUSIONS: There was no significant difference between the two groups of ejection fraction at discharge and at 6 weeks, no difference in recurrent infarction or death at 6 months. Primary angioplasty therefore does not appear to result in greater myocardial salvage compared to standard lytic therapy. NEJM 328(10):685–91.

Appendix B

Contact details for societies, manufacturers' details, key websites

British Cardiovascular Intervention Society
Dr Mike Norell (Hon. Secretary)
Hull Royal Infirmary
Hull
HU3 2JZ
Tel: 01482 674 224
Fax: 01482 321 128
Email: secretary@bcis.org.uk
Website: www.bcis.org.uk

The European Society of Cardiology
The European Heart House
2035 Route des Colles
B.P. 179, Les Templiers,
FR 06903 Sophia Antipolis
France
Tel: 33 4 92 94 76 00
Fax: 33 4 92 94 7601
Email: webmaster@escardio.org
Website: www.esc.be

Central Cardiac Audit Database
Royal Postgraduate Medical School
Hammersmith
London
Tel: 0208 383 1902
Fax: 0208 383 1902
Email: ccad@compuserve.com
Website: www.ccad3.biomed.gla.ac.uk

British Society of Echocardiography
9 Fitzroy Square
London
W1P 5AH
Tel/Fax: 0208 981 0397
Website: www.cardiac.org.uk

European Society for Cardio-thoracic Surgery
EACTS Executive Secretariat
4 Cavendish Square
London
W1M 0BX
Tel: 0207 870 8923
Fax: 0207 629 3233

Cardiovascular and Interventional Society of Europe
Läubli Brigit, Executive Director
Bellerivestrasse 42
CH-8008 Zurich
Switzerland
Tel: 41 1 384 9330
Fax: 41 1 384 9339
Email: office@cirse.org
Website: www.cirse.org

British Institute of Radiology
36 Portland Place
London
W1N 4A1
Tel: 0207 307 1400
Fax: 0207 307 1414
Website: www.bir.org.uk

Medical Devices Agency
Hannibal House
Elephant and Castle
London
SE1 6TQ
Tel: 0207 972 8000
Email: mail@medical-devices.gov.uk
Website: www.medical-devices.gov.uk

British Medical Association
BMA House
Tavistock Square
London
WC1H 9JP
Tel: 0207 387 4499
Fax: 0207 383 6400
Email: membership@bma.org.uk
Website: www.bma.org.uk

Appendix B

British Cardiac Society
9 Fitzroy Square
London, W1P 5AH
Tel: 0207 383 3887
Fax: 0207 388 0903
Email: enquiries@bcs.com
Website: www.cardiac.org.uk

American College of Cardiology
Heart House
911 Old Georgetown Road
Bethesda MD 20814 1699, USA
Tel: 1 800 253 4636/301 897 5400
Fax: 1 301 897 9745
Website: www.acc.org

American Medical Association
515 North State Street
Chicago, IL 60610, USA
Tel: 001 312 464 5000
Website: www.ama-assn.org

American Heart Association
National Center
7272 Greenville Avenue
Dallas, TX 75231
Website: www.americanheart.org

World Health Organization
Avenue Appia 20
1211 Geneva 27, Switzerland
Tel: 41 22 791 21 11
Fax: 41 22 7 91 07 46
Email: info@who.nt
Website: www.who.org

The Society of Thoracic Surgeons
401 North Michigan Avenue
Chicago, IL 60611–4267, USA
Tel: 1 312 644 6610
Fax: 1 312 527 6635
Email: sts@sba.com
Website: www.sts.org

British Pacing and Electrophysiology
Group
9 Fitzroy Square
London, W1P 5AH

Tel: 0208 980 0654
Fax: 0208 980 0725
Website: www.heart.org.uk

European Univon of Medical
Specialists
Hans L. Liebbrandt
5683 Liebbrandt
Kievietlaann 4
5683 RC Best
The Netherlands
Tel/fax: 31 499 39 82 60
Email: libbran@iaehv.nl
Website: www.iae.nl

Society for Cardiovascular and
Interventional Radiology
10201 Lee Highway
Suite 500
Fairfax, VA 22030, USA
Tel: 1 800 488 7284/1 703 691 1805
Fax: 1 703 691 1855
Email: info@scvir.org
Website: www.scvir.org

American Society for
Echocardiography
4101 Lake Boone Trail
Suite 201
Raleigh, NC 27607, USA
Tel: 1 919 787 5181
Fax: 1 919 787 4916
Website: www.asecho.org

The American Association of
Cardiovascular and Pulmonary
Rehabilitation
AACVPR
7611 Elmwood Avenue Ste 201
Middleton, WI 53562, USA
Tel: 1 608 831 6989
Fax: 1 608 831 5122
Email: aacvpr@tmahq.com
Website: www.aacvpr.org

International Society for Heart
Research
Dr Roberto Bolli, Secretary General
(ISHR)

Department of Medicine,
ACB Third Floor
550 South Jackson Street
University of Louisville
Louisville, KY 40292, USA
Tel: 1 502 852 1837
Fax: 1 502 852 6474

**American Society of Nuclear
Cardiology**
9111 Old Georgetown Road
Bethesda, MD 20814–1699, USA
Tel: 1 301 493 2360
Fax: 1 301 493 2376
Email: admin@asnc.org
Website: www.asnc.org

**The American Society of
Hypertension**
515 Madison Avenue
New York, NY 10022, USA
Tel: 1 212 644 0650
Fax: 1 212 644 0658
Email: ash@ash-us.org
Website: www.ash-us.org

Useful Websites

www.medica-devices.gov.uk:
Medical Devices Agency: The website
of the Agency which is to safeguard
public health by working with users,
manufacturers and legislators to
ensure that medical devices meet
appropriate standards of safety,
quality and performance.

www.acc.org/clinical/guidelines:
ACC/AHA Practice Guidelines.

www.2.umdnj.edu/~shindler/trials:
Acronyms for Clinical Trials.

www-east.elsevier.com/jac/2705/
jac1313fla: Clinical Trials in
Cardiology.

www.bcis.org.uk
British Cardiovascular Intervention
Society

www.centrewatch.com: Center
Watch Clinical Trials Listing: Allows
you to find a variety of information
related to clinical trials. Designed to
be a resource both for patients and
research professionals.

www.ncbi.nlm.nih.gov/PubMed/
medline: Search Medline.

www.isinct.com: Institute for
Scientific Information.

www.adref.com: Info-Med Uk Ltd.:
This Contains links to medical
websites and a reference resource for
health care professionals.

Electronic Journals

European Heart Journal:
www.hbuk.co.uk/wbs/ehj

American Heart Journal:
http://www.medscape.com/mosby/
AmHeartJ/public/journal.AmHeartJ.
html

Arteriosclerosis, Thrombosis and
Vascular Biology:
http://atvb.ahajournals.org/

British Medical Journal:
http://www.bmj.com/

Cardiovascular Research:
http://www.elsevier.nl:80/homepage/
sab/cardio/

Chest: http://w3.edoc.com/chest/

Clinical Cardiology:
http://www.clinical-cardiology.org/

Appendix B

Heart:
http://heartjul.com

Heart (British Heart Journal):
http://www.bmjpg.com/data/hea.htm

HeartWeb:http://www.heartweb.org/

Journal of Thoracic and
Cardiovascular Surgery:
http://www.mosby.com/jtcvs/

Journal Watch – Cardiology:
http://www.jwatch.org/card/

Lancet: http://www.thelancet.com/

Nature: http://www.nature.com/

Nature Medicine:
http://medicine.nature.com/

Science Magazine:
http://www.sciencemag.org/

Contact Details For Industry

AVE Inc
Castle Yard House
2 Castle Yard
Richmond
Surrey TW10 6TF
Tel: 0800 001033
Fax: 0208 848 8988

Bard Limited
Forest House
Brighton Road
Crawley
West Sussex, RH11 9BP

Biocompatibles
Frensham House
Frensham Business Park
Heydon Lane
Farnham
Surrey, GU9 8QL

Tel: 01252 732 732
Fax: 01252 732 777

Biotronik Limited
Biotronik House
Weston Business Park
Weston on the Green
Oxfordshire
OX6 8SY
Tel: 01869 343 777
Fax: 01869 343 888

Boston Scientific Corporation
New England House
Sandridge Park
Porters Wood
St Albans
Hertfordshire, AL3 6PH
Tel: 01727 831 666
Fax: 01727 865 862

Cardiocare Limited
(Eclipse Surgical Technologies)
Seos Building
Marchants Way
Burgess Hill
West Sussex, RH15 8QY
Tel: 01444 892 377
Fax: 01444 892 377

Cardiovision Ltd.
66 Harley Street
London
W1N 1AE
Email: general@cardiovision.co.uk
Web address: www.cardiovision.co.uk
Tel: 0207 580 6649
Fax: 0207 323 1939

Cook (UK) Limited
Monroe House
Letchworth
Hertfordshire, SG6 1LN
Tel: 01462 482 884
Fax: 01462 480 944

Cordis (Johnson and Johnson Co)
Coronation Road

408

Appendix B

South Ascot
Berkshire
SL5 9EY
Tel: 01344 871000
Fax: 01344 872599

Eli Lilly
Dextra Court
Chapel Hill
Basingstoke,
Hampshire
RG21 6SY
Tel: 01256 473 241
Fax: 01256 485 858

Guidant Limited
Hants International Business Park
Crockford Lane
Chineham
Basingstoke
RG24 5WJ
Tel: 01256 374 000
Fax: 01256 347 001

Interventional Technologies
Mrs Cheryl Shanks
Lisnenan
Letterkenny
County Donegal
Republic of Ireland
Email: shanks.derby@brinternet.com
Tel: 0800 801 042
Fax: 00 353 74 27456

JoMed
Orchard Villa
Porters Park Drive Shenley
Radlet
Hertfordshire
Tel: 01923 855 663
Fax: 01923 855 770

Mallinckrodt Medical (UK) Limited
Imaging Division
10/11 North Portway Close
Round Spinney

Northampton,
NN3 8RQ
Tel: 01604 498 307
Fax: 01604 646 884

Medtronic Limited
Suite One, Sherbourne House
Croxley Business Centre
Watford
DW1 8YE
Tel: 01923 212 213
Fax: 01923 241 004

Nycomed (UK) Limited
2111 Coventry Road
Sheldon
Birmingham
Tel: 0121 7422 444
Fax: 0121 7222 130

Schneider UK
Ash House
Fairfield Avenue
Staines
Middlesex
TW18 4AN
Tel: 01784 453 232
Fax: 01784 440 048

Sherwood Davis and Geck
Cynamid House
Farehman Road
Gosport
Hampshire,
PO13 OAS
Tel: 01329 224 000
Fax: 01329 220 213

Vascular Therapies
2 Kings Ride Park
Kings Ride
Ascot
Berkshire
SL5 8BP
Tel: 01344 746666
Fax: 01344 874 911

Index

Page numbers in *italic* refer to figures and tables. *a* denotes appendix.

411

Index

Index

Index

Index

415

Index

Index

Index

Index